Neuro-oncology

Primary malignant brain tumours

Neuro-oncology
Primary malignant brain tumours

Edited by
David G T Thomas FRCP (Glas) FRCS (Ed)

*Senior Lecturer in Neurological Surgery,
The Institute of Neurology; Consultant Neurosurgeon,
The National Hospitals for Nervous Diseases Queen Square
and Maida Vale and Northwick Park Hospital, Harrow.*

Edward Arnold
A division of Hodder & Stoughton
LONDON MELBOURNE AUCKLAND

© 1990 David GT Thomas

First published in Great Britain 1990

British Library Cataloguing in Publication Data
Neuro-oncology.
  1. Man. Brain. Tumours
  I. Thomas, David G. T. (David Glyndor Trehane)
  616.99'281

  ISBN 0-7131-4586-2

All rights reserved. No part of this publication may be reproduced or transmitted in any form or by any means, electronically or mechanically, including photocopying, recording or any information storage or retrieval system, without either prior permission in writing from the publisher or a licence permitting restricted copying. In the United Kingdom such licences are issued by the Copyright Licensing Agency: 33-34 Alfred Place, London WC1E 7DP.

Whilst the advice and information in this book is believed to be true and accurate at the date of going to press, neither the author nor the publisher can accept any legal responsibility or liability for any errors or omissions that may be made.

Typeset in 10/11pt Plantin by Colset Pte Ltd, Singapore
Printed and bound in Great Britain for Edward Arnold, a division of Hodder and Stoughton Limited, Mill Road, Dunton Green, Sevenoaks, Kent TN13 2YA, by Butler & Tanner Ltd, Frome, Somerset

Preface

The outlook for patients with primary malignant brain tumours remains gloomy. These lethal tumours make a particular impact not only in neurological medicine and surgery but also in society in general. This is because they are not uncommon and they have peaks of incidence in the first and fifth decades of life. Thus, children or adults in the prime of life are frequently and rapidly rendered disabled by paralysis, dysphasia, loss of vision or epilepsy. Many soon die, despite prodigious efforts at therapy. Such tragic events can lead to, and often have done in the past, an attitude of nihilism towards investigation and therapy of these neoplasms. More recently many workers in the neurosciences, both clinical and non-clinical, have been spurred to make advances in neuro-oncology. Although these steps forward largely parallel, and sometimes borrow from, developments in the understanding and management of patients with cancers at other sites, it is because the nervous system is so different from the rest of the body that neuro-oncology has both specific problems and achievements when compared with oncology in general. This book attempts to review such areas, as well as the practical matters involved in the management of patients with brain tumours, like clinical presentation and terminal care. The audience addressed consists both of postgraduate clinicians in the relevant fields of neurology, neurosurgery and oncology, and basic neuroscientists interested in the field. The contributors have expert scientific knowledge or extensive clinical experience. The intention of the editor, and the purpose of the text, is to present an up to date and authoritative view of the neuro-oncology of primary malignant brain tumours.

For over 50 years it has been recognized that human cerebral malignant gliomas are easy to grow in tissue culture in the laboratory, and it has been found that this native ability to grow *in vitro*, as well as the absence of fibroblast or bacterial contamination in surgical biopsy material from the brain, makes them uniquely suitable amongst human solid tumours for cell biological studies.

There has also in the last 40 years been an explosive expansion in technical methods for cellular neurobiology, and, most recently, molecular biological methods in the neurosciences. Application of such methods, and the application of molecular biological methods taken from cancer research in general, has produced new data leading to new hypotheses about the nature of neuroepithelial tumours, particularly cerebral gliomas. The first four chapters in this book outline many approaches made with cellular and molecular neurobiological approaches to primary brain tumours. It is hoped that this will be not only of academic interest to the reader, but that a better understanding of the basic biology of these tumours and of the factors which influence their growth will in the foreseeable future lead to new and better methods of diagnosis and treatment. Classification, grading and staging of brain tumours involve problems which are largely different from those found in other human solid tumours. Thus, the most malignant and most common single type of cerebral glioma, that is the grade IV malignant glioma or glioblastoma multiforme, does not metastasize but in spite of this causes death usually within six months. Even the classification of this common and lethal tumour has presented difficulties and caused controversy within neuropathology. A critical review of neuropathological concepts and methods as applied to the classification of brain tumours is provided in Chapter 5. Methods of imaging the brain have rapidly improved and have been applied to diagnosis, accurate control of surgery and to follow up. The relatively non-invasive-methods of positron emission tomography and magnetic resonance spectroscopy can now reveal the physiological condition of a brain tumour in the intact patient. Neuro-radiological imaging and *in vivo* metabolic studies are described in Chapters 6 and 7. The epidemiology, incidence, and common patterns of clinical manifestation of primary malignant brain tumours are set out in Chapter 8. New approaches to surgery for these tumours, often employing image guidance from scan data, are outlined in Chapter 10. Some aspects of clinical management are well known and are described in a didactic fashion in the text. However, other aspects are more controversial, for example the relative utility and risk of a high rate of histological verification of diagnosis by stereotactic biopsy, or the value of maximal image directed tumour resection. These topics receive fuller treatment and discussion in the text. Paediatric brain tumours have special biological and clinical features and their management requires separate treatment. This is given in Chapter 11. Here a neurosurgeon and radiotherapist/oncologist, both of whom have an extensive specialist paediatric practice, review modern management of this important age group of patients. Adjuvant therapy for many kinds of malignant brain tumour may be beneficial. The technical aspects of such therapy and its results are critically reviewed in three chapters on radiotherapy, chemotherapy and therapy by biological response modifiers. Radiotherapy of brain tumours both by conventional external beam techniques and by newer methods, like interstitial radiation, are reviewed in detail. The results of empirical chemotherapy trials are examined closely and the utility of chemotherapy in conventional neurological practice is described and carefully assessed. The biological basis of biological response modifier therapy and very many pilot clinical studies are examined in detail. An indication of the relative established values in the management of brain tumours of these three modalities is in the length of text devoted to them, which is found to be inversely proportional to current practical utility of the therapy. Thus more space is required for a critical evaluation of chemotherapy than for radiotherapy, which is a modality with a better established efficiency. Biological response modifiers require even more space because it is necessary to outline both the biological rationale of the methods and to evaluate critically the evidence from limited clinical trials in order to present a state of the art review. At present all treatment of primary malignant brain tumours is palliative only, therefore the final chapter on terminal care of such patients is an especially important contribution to a postgraduate textbook on this subject. It is not only an essential chapter on this account, but it also serves to reinforce the will to maximize the beneficial effects for the patient which may be obtained from the optimum employment of current management methods and is a spur to pursuing lines of research aimed at achieving better results in the future.

DGT Thomas
1989

Contents

Preface	v
List of Contributors	xiii

1) *The in vitro biology of human brain tumours* John L Darling   **1**
   Introduction   1
   Cell culture as an experimental tool in neuro-oncology   1
   Application of *in vitro* techniques to clinical neuro-oncology   15
   References   19

2) *Oncogene expression and control of growth in malignant brain tumours*
   Bengt Westermark, Monica Nistér, Nils-Erik Heldin and Carl-Henrik Heldin   **26**
   Introduction   26
   Functional aspects of oncogenes   27
   Antioncogenes   30
   Interplay between oncogenes and antioncogenes in neoplastic development   30
   Oncogenes in glioma   30
   Concluding remarks   36
   References   37

3) *Growth factors and glial cell markers in human malignant brain tumours* Bryn Watkins, Karen Bevan, Deon Venter and Mark Noble   **40**
   Introduction   40
   Glial cell development in the rat optic nerve   40
   Glial and neuronal development in the retina and the cortex   42
   Ramifications of current developmental studies for neuropathology   44
   A serological analysis of gliomas   45
   Conclusions   48
   References   48

x *Contents*

4) *Pathology of experimental brain tumours* Geoffrey J Pikington and Peter L Lantos	**51**
Tumours induced by oncogenic agents	51
Transplantable tumours	60
References	70
5) *The classification of intracranial tumours* RO Barnard	**77**
Tumours of neuroepithelial tissue	77
Tumours of nerve sheath cells	83
Meningiomas	84
References	92
6) *Neuroradiological imaging of brain tumours* D Kingsley	**94**
Computed tomography	94
Magnetic resonance	96
Cerebral angiography	101
Imaging in tumour assessment	102
References	116
7) In vivo *metabolism of human cerebral tumours* David J Brooks	**122**
Introduction	122
Positron emission tomography	122
Surface-coil nuclear magnetic resonance spectroscopy	123
The oxygen and glucose metabolism of cerebral tumours	124
The pH of cerebral tumours	128
Amino acid metabolism of human cerebral tumours	128
Blood-brain barrier function in human cerebral tumours	129
Uptake of cytotoxic agents by human cerebral tumours	130
Conclusions	131
References	131
8) *The Epidemiology of brain tumours* Ronald O McKeran, Edward S Williams and Helen Thornton Jones	**135**
Introduction	135
The general background	135
Genetic and environmental factors in causation	138
Conclusion	139
References	140
9) *Clinical manifestations of brain tumours* David GT Thomas and Ronald O McKeran	**141**
Introduction	141
Symptoms of focal neurological deficit and raised intracranial pressure	142
Brain tumour syndromes	143
Epilepsy in relation to malignant brain tumours	146
Differential diagnosis	146
Conclusions	146
References	147

10) *Advances in surgery for malignant brain tumours* R Bradford and DGT Thomas	**148**
Introduction	148
Pathological diagnosis of malignant glioma	149
CT-directed stereotactic biopsy	149
MRI-directed stereotactic biopsy	154
Stereotactic biopsy of brain-stem lesions	156
Computer-interactive stereotactic tumour excision	157
Conclusions	161
References	161
11) *Brain and spinal cord tumours in children* Jeffrey S Tobias and Richard D Hayward	**164**
Introduction	164
Pathological classification of childhood brain tumours	165
Tumours of the posterior fossa	167
Tumours of the pituitary region	178
Tumours of the pineal region	182
Cerebral hemisphere tumours	184
Tumours of the spinal cord	189
References	190
12) *Radiotherapy in the treatment of cerebral astrocytomas* Steven A Leibel and Glenn E Sheline	**193**
Introduction	193
Tolerance of the brain to therapeutic irradiation	193
Classification of astrocytic gliomas	198
Astrocytoma	199
Anaplastic astrocytomas and glioblastoma multiforme	204
New directions	210
Summary	213
References	214
13) *Chemotherapy for malignant gliomas in adults* Edward J Dropcho and M Stephen Mahaley	**222**
Introduction	222
Single-agent therapy	223
Combination therapy	227
Intra-arterial therapy	227
Blood-brain barrier disruption	233
References	234
14) *Biological response modifier therapies for patients with malignant gliomas* G Yancey Gillespie and M Stephen Mahaley	**242**
Introduction	242
Classifications	242
Coda	271
References	271

15) *The terminal care of brain tumour patients* Margaret H Wheildon and
Ronald O McKeran **283**
    Introduction 283
    The place of death 283
    Support structures 284
    The management of specific clinical problems arising from
        neurological dysfunction in patients with brain tumours 285
    Symptom control 288
    The role of the hospice movement 290
    Conclusion 291
    References 292
    Suggested further reading 292

Index   **293**

List of Contributors

RO Barnard MD, Consultant Neuropathologist, The National Hospital, Maida Vale, London W9

R Bradford MBBS, BSc, MD, FRCS, Consultant Neurosurgeon and Senior Lecturer, The Royal Free Hospital, Pond Street, London NW3

DJ Brooks BA, MD, MRCP, Senior Lecturer in Neurology, Royal Postgraduate Medical School, Du Cane Road, London W12 and Institute of Neurology, Queen Square, London WC1N 3BG

John L Darling MSc, PhD, Lecturer in Neuro-oncology, Gough-Cooper Department of Neurological Surgery, Institute of Neurology, Queen Square, London WC1N 3BG and The Radiotherapy Research Unit, Institute of Cancer Research, Clifton Avenue, Belmont, Sutton, Surrey SM2 5PX

Edward J Dropcho MD, Department of Neurology and Brain Tumour Research and Treatment Program, University of Alabama at Birmingham, Alabama 35294, USA

G Yancey Gillespie PhD, Division of Neurological Surgery, University of Alabama at Birmingham, Alabama 35294, USA

Richard D Hayward FRCS, Consultant Neurosurgeon, Hospital for Sick Children, Great Ormond Street, St Mary's Hospital and The National Hospital for Nervous Diseases, Queen Square, London WC1N 3BG

Carl-Hennik Heldin PhD, Professor, Ludwig Institute for Cancer Research Biomedical Center, Box 593, S-751 93 Uppsala Sweden

Nils-Erik Heldin PhD, Department of Pathology, University Hospital, S-751 85 Uppsala, Sweden

Helen Thornton Jones BSC, Director, The Thames Cancer Registry, Belmont, Surrey

DPE Kingsley FRCS, FRCR, DMRD, Consultant Neuroradiologist, The Hospital for Sick Children, Great Ormond Street, and The National Hospital for Nervous Diseases, London

Peter L Lantos MD, PhD, FRCPath, Professor of Neuropathology, Department of Neuropathology, Institute of Psychiatry, London SE5 8AF

Steven A Leibel MD, Department of Radiation Oncology, University of California, San Francisco School of Medicine, San Francisco, California, USA

Ronald O McKeran BSc, MD, FRCP, Consultant Neurologist Atkinson Morley's Hospital, Wimbledon, St George's Hospital, Tooting and St Helier's Hospital, Carshalton

M Stephen Mahaley MD, PhD, Division of Neurological Surgery, Brain Tumour Research and Treatment Program, University of Alabama at Birmingham, Birmingham, Alabama 35294 USA

Monica Nistér MD, PhD, Senior Resident, Department of Pathology, University Hospital, S-751 85 Uppsala, Sweden

Mark Noble PhD, The Ludwig Institute of Cancer Research, The Middlesex Hospital Medical School, 91 Riding House Street, London W1P 8BT

Geoffrey J Pilkington PhD, Senior Lecturer, Department of Neuropathology, Institute of Psychiatry, London SE5 8AF

Glenn E Sheline MD, Formerly, Department of Radiation Oncology, University of California San Francisco School of Medicine, San Francisco, California, USA

DGT Thomas MA, FRCP, FRCS, Consultant Neurosurgeon, The National Hospitals, Queen Square and Maida Vale, and Northwick Park Hospital, Harrow, Senior Lecturer in Neurological Surgery, Institute of Neurology, The National Hospital, Queen Square, London WC1N 3BG

Jeffrey S Tobias MD, MCCP, FRCR, Consultant in Radiotherapy and Oncology, University College Hospital, Gower Street, London WC1

Bryn Watkins PhD, The Gough-Cooper Department of Neurological Surgery, The Institute of Neurology, Queen Square, London WC1N 3BG and The Ludwig Institute for Cancer Research, The Middlesex Hospital Medical School, 91 Riding House Street, London W1P 8BT

Bengt Westermark PhD, Professor of Tumour Biology, Department of Pathology, University Hospital, S-751 85 Uppsala, Sweden

Margaret H Wheildon FFARCS, Director, St Raphael's Hospice, Cheam and Consultant Anaesthetist, Merton and Sutton Health Authority

Edward S Williams PhD, MD, FRCP, FRCR, Chief Medical Officer to Croydon Health Authority

1 The *in vitro* biology of human brain tumours

John L Darling

Introduction

It is doubtful whether major improvements can be made through the pragmatic clinical study of brain tumours alone. Although there is some potential for fine tuning of treatment, without significant biological input changes in the currently grim outlook for patients with malignant glioma will change little. Surgery is limited by the infiltrative nature of the tumour, radiotherapy by the intrinsic radioresistance of glioma cells and poor normal tissue tolerance, and chemotherapy by the availability of largely ineffective drugs coupled with unfavourable pharmakokinetics. These fundamental hindrances to treatment may well be capable of resolution if there is a basic understanding of the biological processes responsible for them. This review will attempt to summarize some aspects of the biology of human malignant gliomas, particularly those which can be elucidated by *in vitro* experiments and where there is likely to be a direct and obvious clinical benefit.

Cell culture as an experimental tool in neuro-oncology

The isolation of cell cultures from human tumours has been a major area of research in the last 20 years. However, the ability to produce cultures which retain the characteristics of a tumour have not been realized in most cases. The overgrowth of stromal fibroblasts or other adventitious elements is an important problem, as is bacterial and fungal contamination. Perhaps most importantly it is apparent that there is a basic deficiency in our understanding of the *in vitro* growth requirements of most tumour cell types.

One tumour type which appears to be abnormal in these respects is the malignant glioma. It was realized quite early that such tumours usually yielded vigorous short-term cultures which were apparently derived from the tumour cells and not the stroma. In an unprecedented proportion of cases, perhaps 30 to 40 per cent, these short-term lines gave rise to established permanent cell lines.[1-3]

The dynamic nature of cell culture is one of its major advantages. The ability to examine and manipulate cells under defined environmental conditions is unique and impossible using either experimental animal models or human pathological material. The physicochemical environment (pH, gas phase composition, temperature, growth substratum) can be controlled precisely, and the medium, if supplemented with fetal calf serum from the same batch, is at least consistent between experiments although not completely defined. Variation between serum batches is likely to become less of a problem with the development of serum extenders or defined chemical media. However, it could be argued that the behaviour of cells in culture differ from their behaviour *in situ*. Not only is there the difficult question of cell selection at the time of initial plating and later during serial passage, but also the problem of a lack of cell-to-cell contact and cell–extracellular matrix interaction, both factors which are poorly understood, but affect cell behaviour *in situ*.

A major advantage of using human glioma *in vitro* is that a comparison is possible between tumour cells and their normal counterparts. Cell cultures have been prepared from both operative samples[4] and post-mortem samples of normal human brain.[5] These glioma-derived cells appear to retain aspects of astroglial function *in vitro*. They express glutamine synthetase, but at a lower specific activity than cells derived from gliomas. They exhibit the high-affinity uptake of gamma-aminobutyric acid (GABA) and have low levels of nucleotide phosphohydrolase activity.

Methods for producing short-term cultures

Collagenase digestion

Normal, good-quality tissue culture-treated plasticware without specific surface coating can be used successfully to grow cells from many types of intracranial tumour. A method which uses crude collagenase to disaggregate tumour biopsies has been used extensively by the author and co-workers.[6, 7] As the incubation is carried out in the presence of serum, tumour biopsies can be exposed to enzyme for relatively long periods of time.

1. Tumour biopsies are collected in Ham's F-10 or F-12 medium, buffered with 20 mM HEPES and supplemented with 200 units/ml of penicillin, 200 μg/ml streptomycin, 100 μg/ml kanamycin or gentamycin and 2.5 μg/ml amphotericin B. Samples are generally transported to the laboratory within 1 h of removal, although cultures can be successfully produced from biopsies taken several days previously if these have been kept at 4°C in a large excess of culture medium to ensure adequate oxygenation.
2. The biopsies are placed in a petri dish, together with some fresh biopsy collection medium, and dissected free of obvious non-tumour material. The tissue fragments are then transferred to a fresh dish with medium and chopped into 1–2 mm pieces using crossed scalpels. The blades are changed between biopsies to ensure that sharpness is maintained and the biopsy is cleanly cut.
3. The fragments are transferred to a 30 ml universal container and biopsy collection medium is added, the larger pieces are allowed to settle under gravity and the supernatant discarded. The tissue is washed on two further occasions and the supernatants discarded after each wash. This removes necrotic material and some non-cellular material.

4. Most of the last wash is removed and the tissue fragments are re-suspended in complete culture medium (Ham's F-10 or F-12, buffered with 20 mM HEPES and supplemented with 10 per cent v/v selected fetal calf serum and 100 units/ml penicillin and 100 μg/ml streptomycin).
5. A sufficient volume of a × 10 concentration of crude collagenase solution is added to give a final working concentration of 200 units/ml. Suitable preparations include Sigma, grade I or Worthington CLS grade.
6. The tissue is then incubated for a period of 4–18 h at 37°C and examined periodically for signs of disaggregation. Once this has occurred and the tissue is reduced to small cell aggregates (rather than a single cell suspension) the preparation is pipetted several times to further reduce the preparation and transferred to a sterile centrifuge tube. The tissue suspension is then centrifuged (gently, at approx 250 G) and the supernatant discarded.
7. The cells are then re-suspended in fresh complete growth medium and plated into a 25 cm^2 flask. This is incubated at 37°C overnight and the medium and non-adherent material discarded. The culture is re-fed with fresh medium and examined twice a week and re-fed as required.
8. There is considerable heterogeneity in the time taken for a primary culture to become confluent although a majority will be capable of being passaged within 2–4 weeks. It is the author's practice to passage the total contents of the primary cultures (using 1 in 300 trypsin) from 25 cm^2 flasks into a 75 cm^2 flask (in effect, a 1 to 3 split).
9. Cultures are routinely frozen down between passage level 2 and 3. At this stage it is usually possible to freeze at least 3 million cells (in 10 per cent DMSO in complete culture medium and frozen at a rate of 1°C per minute) and store these in the liquid phase of a liquid nitrogen refrigerator. The overall success rate of this procedure for intracranial tumours, in terms of producing a culture capable of being frozen down, is about 75 to 80 per cent.

Other methodologies

Although the method detailed above is capable of producing short-term cultures from glioma with great ease, other methods have found favour with other workers. In soft tumours like malignant glioma vigorous pipetting or passage through hypodermic needles produces a crude cell suspension which has been reported to develop into satisfactory cultures.[1, 8] Mechanical disaggregation can produce considerable cell damage and is ineffective against tough tumour tissue like meningiomas. The use of trypsin as a disaggregating agent has been advocated[2, 9] and if only applied for short periods of time (5–20 min) yields a good cell suspension, but at the risk of producing some damage to the cells through both the action of the enzyme and the need to carry out the disaggregation in the absence of serum. The use of enzyme cocktails has been advocated using aggressive regimens including pronase, collagenase and DNAase.[10]

The need for enzymatic or mechanical disaggregation is obviated by the use of explant cultures where small pieces of tumour (commonly 1 × 1 × 1 mm) are allowed to adhere to the plastic surface of a cell culture flask either in the absence of medium or in the presence of very small quantities of medium. After 15–45 min incubation at 37°C, in a humidified incubator to allow attachment, medium is gently added to the flasks to avoid dislodging the explants and gradually over a period of days built up to 5–10 ml per 25 cm² flask.[11, 9, 8] A simple explant method has been developed in the author's laboratory, primarily for the culture of small biopsies taken during stereotactic neurosurgical procedures, which yields cultures in the same proportion of cases as collagenase digestion.[12]

There have been no comparative studies between the different methods for producing brain tumour cultures although this may well influence the cellular subpopulations which grow from a biopsy. Aggressive mechanical or enzyme treatment may kill delicate cells and favour the growth of tissue culture-adapted cell types. Conversely, gentle enzymatic treatment or explantation may favour the growth of more representative cells. The question may be of particular importance in tumours like medulloblastoma and ependymoma which are difficult to grow and where cell death at an early stage of culture preparation may be an important factor.

Characteristics of glioma cells in culture

Cell attachment and spreading

Studies with established cell lines from human glioma and cultures derived from normal brain indicate that glioma cells attach and detach to the substratum more readily than normal cells[13] indicating the relative anchorage independence of these cells. There were, however, considerable differences between lines and between subpopulations of cells within a single line, in their ability to detach from and re-attach to the substratum. A comparison of the spreading of normal human and malignant glia[14] indicated that normal cells tended to retain their shape in suspension whilst glioma cells tended to adopt a spherical shape. Glioma cells also spread less quickly and more thinly than normal glia when placed on the substratum.

Cell motility

Cells derived from malignant glioma are more motile than cells derived from other intracranial tumours. Cells from explant cultures of human glioma are highly motile and irreversibly inhibited by cytochalasin B.[15] Cells cultured from normal brain are motile in sparse culture but have a tendency to form adhesions along areas of mutual contact and, as a monolayer forms, cells become essentially immobile.[16] There is also a relationship between the motility of tumour astrocytes and expression of GFAP. Stellate-shaped cells containing high levels of GFAP are relatively immobile and possess rigid cell processes.[17] Using an automatic Visicon autotracking system, Koga[18] has been able to examine the motility of brain tumour cells continuously. Cell motility was higher in cultures derived from malignant astrocytomas (mean motility 0.8 μm/min) than in cultures derived from low-grade astrocytomas (mean motility 0.24 μm/min).

Cytogenetics of human glioma cells in vitro

In human glioma there does not appear to be a consistent rearrangement of chromosomes, although there are certain, non-random patterns of chromosomal abnormalities. The most common of these include the loss of a single sex chromosome (the X in the female and the Y in males) and the loss of chromosomes 10 and 22. Chromosomes most frequently gained include 7 and 20. There may also be double minutes present and structural abnormalities of 9 p.[19(a, b)]

Establishment of cell lines from specific types of brain tumour

Although short-term cultures are sufficient for many biological studies, they rarely provide enough cells for long-term studies or for biochemical examination. It is therefore of considerable importance to be able to produce established cell lines from tumours of different histological types.

Malignant astrocytomas

A recent report has been published which has extensively reviewed the *in vitro* characteristics of cell lines established from high-grade malignant gliomas.[3] Table 1.1 summarizes the *in vitro* data on 12 lines of which the characterization has been reported subsequent to the above publication. All the lines have been established from malignant glioma (Kernohan grades III and IV). It is apparent the GFAP (glial fibrillary acidic protein) expression is a rare event in established cell lines, and the only group to report measurable levels in their lines used immunoblot analysis which is capable of detecting low levels of GFAP. Only two of these lines, 992 and 215 had significant levels of the antigen. There have been a number of reports which indicate that although many primary cultures derived from glioma have significant numbers of GFAP-positive cells, these are lost from most cultures during subsequent passage.[21-25] Most lines were positive for fibronectin, but all had abnormal karyotypes. As discussed above, common abnormalities include chromosomes 1, 7, 9, 10 and 22 and the presence of double minutes. Saturation densities are higher than those reported for normal glia-like cells and range between 7.5×10^4 and 8.5×10^5 cells/cm^2. The doubling time for some lines, even those which have gross chromosomal changes, can be quite long and short doubling times (<24 h) are not an invariable consequence of establishment in culture. There was no correlation between colony-forming efficiency in either suspension or in monolayer and the ability of these cells to form tumours in immune-deficient mice. Establishment *in vitro* is not always associated with the ability to produce tumours in athymic mice. Jacobsen and colleagues[11] have reported that three of their glioma cell lines expressed desmin and myoglobin. This could indicate that some glioma cells are capable of expressing some features of striated muscle cells, or that stromal elements capable of expressing these antigens can be stably incorporated into established cell lines. Rutka and colleagues[10] have shown that one of their glioma-derived cell lines produces collagen suggesting that vascular mesenchymal elements can be present in these lines.

Gliosarcomas

Two reports have been produced which describe cell lines from gliosarcomas (Table 1.2). One of these lines expresses type IV collagen and type III procollagen, laminin and fibronectin[20], and in nude mice this cell line produces a spindle cell sarcoma rather than a glioma.

Table 1.1 Cell lines derived from malignant gliomas

Cell line and passage level studied	Derived from	Growth in nude mice	Chromosomes	Marker antigens FN	Marker antigens GFAP	Marker antigens S-100	Marker antigens GS	Culture characteristics — Colony formation Suspension (%)	Culture characteristics — Colony formation Monolayer (%)	Doubling time (h)	Saturation density (cells/cm²)	Reference no.
LN308 (p26)	IV astrocytoma (60 ♂)	+	81, xxy 2 markers	ND	+[1]	±	ND	0.47	ND	>96	$7.5 \times 10^{4[2]}$	Studer et al. (1985) 8
LN992 (p42–45)	IV astrocytoma (67 ♂)	ND	84, xxyy 5 markers	ND	+[1]	+	ND	0.28	ND	$132^{[2]}$	$7.5 \times 10^{4[2]}$	
LN215 (p83–90)	IV astrocytoma (60 ♀)	ND	66, xx 3 markers	ND	+[1]	−	ND	0.58	ND	$36^{[2]}$	$2.5 \times 10^{5[2]}$	
LN235 (p62–63)	IV astrocytoma (38 ♂)	ND	116 xxxxyyyy	ND	+[1]	−	ND	0.46	ND	$72^{[2]}$	$1.9 \times 10^{5[2]}$	
2607 (p52)	III astrocytoma (41 ♂)	+	80–98	+	−	−	ND	4.6	2.6	32	2.5×10^5	Jacobsen et al. (1987) 11
2981 (p46)	III astrocytoma (37 ♂)	+	79–111	+	−	−	ND	8.1	3.7	26	1.5×10^5	
5737 (p51)	IV giant cell glioblastoma (60 ♀)	+	74–98	+	−	−	ND	13.0	7.3	29	8.5×10^5	

Table 1.1 Cont'd

Cell line and passage level studied	Derived from	Growth in nude mice	Chromosomes	Marker antigens				Culture characteristics					Reference no.
				FN	GFAP	S-100	GS	Colony formation		Monolayer (%)	Doubling time (h)	Saturation density (cells/cm^2)	
								Suspension (%)					
SF-126 (p54)	IV astrocytoma (50♀)	–	Hypertriploid + double minutes	+	–	ND	–	2.9	42		29	2.4×10^5	Rutka et al., (1987) 10
SF-188 (p70)	IV astrocytoma (8♂)	–	Hypertriploid + double minutes	+	–	ND	–	10	40		28	2.8×10^5	
SF-210 (p45)	IV astrocytoma (72♀)	–	Hyperdiploid	+	–	ND	–	0.65	34		28	2.0×10^5	
SF-268 (p51)	III/IV astrocytoma (24♀)	–	Hyperdiploid	–	–	ND	–	0.85	43		32	2.0×10^5	
SF-295 (p42)	IV astrocytoma (67♀)	–	Hypertriploid + double minutes	–	–	ND	–	4.43	30		34	2.4×10^5	

+ = Present or positive, – = absent or negative; ND = not determined or negative; (1) confirmed by immunoblot analysis; (2) determined from published graph. FN = fibronectin; GFAP = glial fibrillary acidic protein; GS = glutamine synthetase.

Table 1.2 Cell lines derived from gliosarcomas

Cell line and passage level studied	Derived from	Growth in nude mice	Chromosomes	Marker antigens					Culture characteristics				Reference no.
				FN	GFAP	LAM	COLLIV	PROIII	Colony formation		Doubling time (h)	Saturation density (cells/cm^2)	
									Suspension (%)	Monolayer (%)			
SF539BT (p42–45)	Recurrent IV astrocytoma with spindle cell sarcoma (gliosarcoma) (34♀)	+	64 (40–184)	+	–	+	+	+	0.2	22	32	5.2×10^4	Rutka et al., 1986; 26
Nu74 (p103)	Gliosarcoma (64♂)	+	77–114	+	–	ND	ND	ND	9.0	41	24	2.0×10^5	Jacobsen et al., 1987; 11

+ = Present or positive, – = absent or negative; ND = not determined or implicitly stated in paper. FN = fibronectin, GFAP = glial fibrillary acidic protein, LAM = laminin, COLLIV = type IV collagen, PROIII = type III procollagen.

Oligodendrogliomas

Transformed oligodendrocytes can be produced in cultures of brains from rats transplacentally treated with ethylnitrosourea[27] which express the specific oligodendrocyte marker 2'3'-cyclic nucleotide 3'-pyrophosphohydrolase. Although in explant cultures from both normal and neoplastic human oligodendrocytes, cells with refractive haloes, pulsation and tug-of-war movements have been noted[28], there few reports in the literature about the establishment of cell lines from oligodendrogliomas. Miyake established a line from a mixed glioma from a 13-year-old girl (KG-1).[29] After eight months in culture, cells with strong perinuclear haloes were observed growing on a layer of epithelial and fibroblastic cells. The glial cells were isolated by pipetting and subcultured. They were globose or bi- or multipolar and expressed S-100 protein but not GFAP. By passage 23, the culture had a long doubling time (41 h) and did not reach high saturation densities. The cells reacted following treatment with dibutryl cyclic AMP, by retracting their cytoplasm. The karyotype was aneuploid, with a modal number of 102.

Medulloblastoma

Complete excision of medulloblastoma is rarely possible and radiation therapy remains the most effective treatment modality. When prophylactic craniospinal irradiation is given about 40 to 60 per cent of patients who complete a full course survive five years.[30, 31] The ability to investigate the experimental biology of these tumours *in vitro* would be of immense value in improving radiotherapy and investigating the role of chemotherapy.

Medulloblastoma appears to grow relatively well in short-term cultures, and cells at least persist *in vitro* for many months although such cultures tend to degenerate or become overgrown with adventitious agents.[32-35] The identity of cells which grow from medulloblastoma has not been examined in any detail, although Waghe *et al.*[36] were able to demonstrate the presence of proliferating cells in these cultures using tritiated thymidine. Establishment of these cells in culture is a rare event and Table 1.3 summarizes some of the biological data on four lines which have been reported in the literature. The cell line, D283 Med is not anchorage-dependent and grows as floating aggregates.[37] It is possible that many medulloblastomas may prefer growing in suspension and this explains the paucity of adherent cell lines. In general, culture doubling times are longer than those seen in malignant astrocytoma cell lines and some have apparently diploid or near-diploid karyotypes although they are capable of forming tumours in immune-deficient mice. Some established medulloblastoma cell lines exhibit glial as well as neuronal markers. GFAP is not expressed by any of the lines although two, D283 Med and TE671 express glutamine synthestase.[38] The presence of neuron-specific enolase has been detected in TE671[39, 40] and D283 Med.[37] Neurofilament proteins and MAP-2 have both been demonstrated in TE671 cells[40] and D283 Med expresses all the three neurofilament protein subunits.[41]

Cell kinetics of malignant gliomas

The cell kinetics of human brain tumours are poorly understood, although such information is likely to lead to the rational design and development of improved

Table 1.3 Cell lines derived from medulloblastomas

Cell line and passage level studied	Derived from	Growth in nude mice	Chromosomes	Marker antigens GFAP	VM	NF	NSE	S100	Colony formation Suspension (%)	Monolayer (%)	Doubling time (h)	Saturation density (cells/cm^2)	Reference no.
TE671 (p22–27)	L Cerebellum cerebellar medulloblastoma (6♀)	+	93 near tetraploid 4 markers	−	ND	+	+	−	16	26	27	2×10^6	McAllister et al., 1977 126 Friedman et al., 1983 127 Mork et al., 1986 40 Friedman et al., 1985 37
D283Med (p20–25)	Peritoneal metastasis of cerebellar medulloblastoma (60♂)	+	47 3 markers	−	ND	+	+	−	1.8	N/A	53	N/A	Friedman et al., 1985 37 Trojanowski et al., 1987 41
DAOY (p48)	Desmoplastic cerebellar medulloblastoma (4♀)	+	93 14 markers	−	ND	ND	−	−	41	13	34	1.2×10^6	Jacobsen et al., 1985 128
PE161 (p7)	Classic cerebellar medulloblastoma with no desmoplastic aspects	ND	Bimodal peaks, at 46 and 92	−	+	+	−	ND	ND	0.8	ND	5.4×10^4	Gerosa et al., 1986 129

+ = Present or positive, − = absent or negative, ND = not determined or implicitly stated in the paper. GFAP = glial fibrillary acidic protein, VM = vimentin, NF = neurofilament protein, NSE = neurone-specific enolase.

therapy protocols. Cells within tumours which have short cell cycle times or high labelling indices are inadequately controlled because cell production exceeds cell killing *in situ*. By accelerating the radiotherapy or chemotherapy regimens it should be possible to shift the balance the favour of greater cell kill. The application of cell kinetic studies to benign tumours is also of importance because if these cannot be removed completely by surgery or tend to progress to a more aggressive form, and the likelihood of recurrence could be predicted, then radio- or chemotherapy could be considered at an early stage.

Cell labelling with tritiated thymidine

Much of the early work which used thymidine labelling to determine the labelling index (LI) of intracranial tumours has been reviewed by Steel.[42] The results produced by Hoshino and colleagues,[43] summarized in Table 1.4 are typical of the data presented by other workers. It is apparent that high-grade gliomas have higher labelling indices, as a group, than low-grade gliomas or benign tumours.

Table 1.4 A comparison of S-phase labelling index data as determined by ^{3}H-thymidine or bromodeoxyuridine uptake *in situ*

	As measured by ^{3}H-thymidine uptake* (%)		As measured by BUdR labelling† (%)	
Glioblastoma multiforme (‡)	(n = 13)	9.3	(n = 6)	10
Highly anaplastic astrocytoma	(n = 7)	4.0§		8.9
Moderately anaplastic astrocytoma	ND			2.0
Fibrillary astrocytoma	(n = 3)	0.8		ND
Ependymoma	(n = 1)	1.9	(n = 2)	<1
Medulloblastoma	(n = 4)	12	(n = 3)	15.2

* Data from ref. 43.
† Data from ref. 45.
‡ Histological groupings as defined in ref. 45.
§ May include some tumours now classified as moderately anaplastic astrocytoma.
ND = no data presented.

Cell labelling with bromodeoxyuridine

The administration of tritiated thymidine is not without hazard and consequently there have been moves to use non-toxic ligand which can detect S-phase cells *in situ*. Bromodeoxy-uridine (BUdR), an analogue of thymidine, which is incorporated into DNA and can be detected by anti-BUdR monoclonal antibody[42] has been used. The agent is administered, like thymidine, during operation but is not myelotoxic at the doses used. The BUdR LI or S-phase fraction is determined by counting the number of labelled cells in tissue sections or by producing single cell suspensions from biopsies, denaturating the DNA, staining with an FITC-conjugated anti-BUdR monoclonal antibody and counting the number of fluorescent cells by flow cytometry. Using either of these methods, the results of which are comparable,[45, 46] a result can be produced within 2 to 3 h of the operation instead of the 5 to 10 weeks needed for autoradiography. The method correlates well with conventional methods (Table 1.4). Because of the relative lack of toxicity, the BUdR technique can be applied to benign tumours. A recent study with histologically benign meningiomas indicated that the mean LI was only 0.45 per cent but in those where there was histological evidence of malignancy the LI was 3.9 per cent. Recurrent meningiomas had higher mean LI than primary meningiomas, and meningiomas with LIs greater than 1 per cent grew faster and tended to recur more frequently than those with LIs less than 1 per cent.[41, 48]

Some data have been presented on small groups of patients which indicate that there is a correlation between labelling index and mean survival time, but these studies do not take into account any effect of treatment or possible confounding effects of clinical prognostic variables. Although it seems unlikely that data using tritiated thymidine will be available in sufficient numbers of patients to prove the relationship between these two parameters, with the advent of BUdR and Ki-67 labelling techniques such results may be attained in the future.

Labelling with Ki-67 monoclonal antibody

Ki-67 recognises an antigen expressed on the nuclear surface of proliferating cells. This antigen is expressed during G_1, G_2, S and M phases of the cell cycle but not by G_0 cells.[49] It has proved possible to determine the growth fraction of cells from a variety of neoplasms, including brain tumours, from frozen sectioned material stained with the monoclonal antibody that recognizes this antigen.[50, 51] The antibody can also be used on smear preparations from gliomas and will be of use in stereotactic neurosurgical procedures as an adjunct to histology in these small tumour samples. The LIs determined from Ki-67 labelling studies are very similar to those produced by both BUdR and thymidine labelling[52] although it might be expected that as Ki-67 is present in all proliferating cells irrespective of cell cycle phase the LIs produced using this method should be higher than those produced by the other methods.

Relevance of cell kinetics to treatment

Using thymidine labelling and autoradiography it has been possible to determine cytokinetic parameters for glioma. Steel indicated that the potential doubling time of malignant gliomas was of the order of 10 days.[42] Clearly, this rapid rate of growth is unlikely and it has been suggested that this indicates that there is a high cell loss factor – estimates for this have been as high as 85 per cent.[53] It is unlikely that removal of cells from the brain can match this and therefore it may be that the growth fraction is smaller than experimental determinations indicate. Like most solid tumours malignant glioma has a relatively slow growth fraction. This indicates that drugs which are most effective against resting cells will have more antitumour effect than those which are only active against cells during specific parts of the cell cycle. Animal experiments suggest that non-specific agents can only achieve a 1 log cell kill even if present throughout the entire cell generation time.[54] The growth fraction is also likely to alter during chemotherapy. If a cycle non-specific drug such as CCNU or procarbazine is administered a proportion of tumour cells will be killed and, in order to repopulate the tumour, quiescent cells will begin to divide. One approach to this would be to administer a cycle-specific agent sequentially to act against this pool of newly proliferating cells. Repopulation of the 9L gliosarcoma, growing intracranially, begins 2 to 4 days after BCNU treatment and exponential cell proliferation is observed 4 to 12 days after BCNU treatment.[55] Administration of the cell-cycle specific drug 5-FU during this period produces significant increases in the number of long-term survivors.[56] There is also evidence from experimental observations with the 9L gliosarcoma that vincristine, if administered after an appropriate period following treatment with a cell cycle non-specific agent also improves survival.[57]

Heterogeneity of malignant glioma

Human glioma, like most other human tumours are not composed of a biologically homogeneous population of cells.[58] The question of tumour cell heterogeneity has considerable clinical as well as biological importance.[59] Most pathologists agree that morphological heterogeneity is a characteristic of malignant glioma[28] and it is now apparent that heterogeneity covers a wide range of phenotypic and genotypic characteristics which are demonstrable *in vitro* and *in vivo*.

Heterogeneity in DNA content and karyotype

Using flow cytometry, Hoshino *et al.*[60] examined a series of well-differentiated gliomas, meningiomas, medulloblastomas and metastatic brain tumours, and found a fairly homogeneous diploid cellular population. However, in malignant gliomas the DNA composition was extremely varied ranging from diploid to hypertetraploid between tumours and between different areas of the same tumour. Supporting evidence for multiploid chromosomal variation within human glioma has come from karyotypic studies.[61,62] In the largest of these studies, Mark[63] found that 47 out of 50 gliomas had aberrant chromosomal numbers, and that 40 per cent of the tumours studied had multiple karyotypic patterns.

Antigenic heterogeneity of glioma

There are large differences in GFAP levels between tumours of the same histological type.[64,65] In an extensive study of established glioma cell lines, only two out of 15 expressed this antigen.[66] In one line, U251MG, about 80 per cent of cells expressed GFAP, whilst in a spindle cell derivative of this line, U251MGsp, all cells expressed the antigen. Immunoperoxidase staining of surgical biopsies from malignant astrocytomas often reveals a heterogeneous pattern with single GFAP-positive cells or small islands of positive cells standing out against a GFAP-negative background.[67] A similar pattern can be observed in biopsy specimens stained for glutamine synthetase (GS).[68] In a panel of primary cultures from glioma, West *et al.*[5] found that GS activity ranged from 10 to 45 nmol of product/min/mg of protein.

The advent of monoclonal antibodies (MCA) has been instrumental in confirming the cell-surface heterogeneity of gliomas. Monoclonal antibodies with some specificity for gliomas, have been extensively screened against a large panel of cell lines.[69] These antibodies, although preferentially binding to glioma cell lines, showed quantitative differences in binding capacity between them. Using MCAs raised against glioma cell lines or human fetal brain, McComb *et al.*[70] were able to show that there was considerable heterogeneity in binding capacity between different lines.

Heterogeneity in growth potential in vivo

Bradley et al.[71] found that only 44 per cent of malignant glioma biopsies could be successfully grown subcutaneously in immune-deficient mice. Although other authors, using multiple implantations, have reported higher take rates[72, 73] it is apparent that there was considerable heterogeneity in the growth rate between different tumours and the take rate and subsequent growth of different portions taken from the same tumour. Differences in growth rate could be observed even after a considerable period of *in vivo* growth.[74] When 15 established glioma cell lines were implanted subcutaneously into athymic nude mice only four proved tumorigenic.[75]

Biochemical heterogeneity of malignant glioma

2′3′-Cyclic nucleotide 3′-phosphohydrolase (CNPase) is present in Schwann cells and neoplastic astrocytes[76] at levels which exceed those typically found in non-glial cells. In 13 biopsy samples of malignant astrocytomas the levels of CNPase ranged 230-fold from 0.02 to 4.6 μmol/min/mg soluble protein[77] and between 0 and 0.213 μmol/min/mg soluble protein in a panel of glioma cell lines.[66] Similar figures have been reported for short-term cultures of human glioma.[5] The levels of adenylate cyclase in these cells also varied widely between 0.11 and 14.71 pmol cAMP produced/min/mg protein.[5]

Cell-surface mucopolysaccharides have been investigated both on normal glial and astrocytoma cells. While the production, composition, distribution and turnover of these mucopolysaccharides are remarkably uniform on normal glial cells they are more heterogeneous on glioma cells.[78] Changes in cell surface molecules may well affect changes in surface activity and, certainly the ability of glioma cells to be agglutinated by plant lectins appears to be much more heterogeneous than normal glia.[79] The ganglioside composition of plasma membranes from glioma cell cultures also exhibits considerable heterogeneity.[80]

Heterogeneity in cell biological characteristics

Cells derived by enzymatic disaggregation from 10 malignant glioma biopsies had an 85-fold range of CFE, from 0.006 to 0.513 per cent[81] and the morphology of colonies derived from the same tumour biopsy varied, as did the expression of GFAP.[82] Yung et al.[83] have produced cloned cell lines with different morphologies and levels of GFAP expression from the same tumour biopsy. The growth rates and saturation densities of glioma cell cultures reported by Bigner et al.[66] however, showed relatively small ranges of variation (2.25-fold and 4.4-fold, respectively).

Many authors have documented the morphological and biochemical alterations which take place in glioma cultures treated with dbcAMP.[84] It is clear that not all the cells in a culture respond to stimulation by exogenous dbcAMP, and Bullard et al.[85] and Maunoury[2] have shown that anywhere between 5 and 100 per cent of cells are capable of responding.

Application of *in vitro* techniques to clinical neuro-oncology

In vitro chemosensitivity testing

Microtitration assays for brain tumours

As short-term cultures can be prepared with relative ease from most biopsy samples of malignant glioma, there is the distinct advantage of being able to use intermediate duration microtitration assays to measure chemosensitivity.[86] These can be automated and are capable of producing results in most clinical samples sent for assay. Clinical correlations using cell counting assays have been reported in small groups of patients with glioma.[87] An assay based on ^{35}S-methionine uptake to measure protein synthetic activity has been developed by the author and others and used for a correlative study between drug sensitivity *in vitro* and clinical progress in patients with malignant glioma.[6,7] In the initial study, 40 patients had chemosensitivity assays performed *in vitro* and had undergone adjuvant chemotherapy with procarbazine (PCB), CCNU and vincristine (VCR) with sufficient follow-up to render them evaluable.[88] To date, a total of 157 patients (63 with grade III and 94 with grade IV tumours, age range 18–76) have been treated with adjuvant radiotherapy and chemotherapy with PCB (100 mg/m^2, p.o., days 1–10), CCNU (80 mg/m^2, p.o., day 1) and VCR (1.5 mg/m^2, i.v. day 1). Samples were available from 62 patients and chemosensitivity to each drug was determined. By comparing the ID$_{50}$ obtained for each drug to a large training set of cultures derived from malignant gliomas it was possible to classify each patient's culture as either sensitive or insensitive to each of the drugs used clinically. It was found that those patients with cultures that were sensitive to PCB and/or CCNU *in vitro* had a more favourable prognosis than those whose cultures were not (Lee-Desu Statistic = 19.2; d.f. = 1; $p < 0.0001$). Further examination of the relationship between known prognostic variables and chemosensitivity *in vitro* indicates that chemosensitivity acts as a independent prognostic variable. Further work is needed to define the exact role this has in developing new chemotherapeutic strategies for glioma.

An assay like the ^{35}S-methionine uptake assay clearly has potential for rapid screening of new drugs with potential activity against human gliomas using large panels of short-term cultures.

Clonogenic assays for brain tumours

There has been considerable interest in developing clonogenic assays for brain tumours that will predict the stem cell response to chemotherapy. Monolayer cloning assays have been developed for animal[89] and human[90] brain tumours. In these assays, tumour biopsies are disaggregated with proteolytic enzymes, treated with drugs and plated together with heavily irradiated 9L gliosarcoma feeder cells. The resultant colonies have glial- and malignancy-related characteristics[82] but colony-forming efficiencies rarely exceed 0.1 per cent. Initial studies indicate that there is a relationship between *in vitro* resistance and clinical resistance.[91] In a series of six patients, only one tumour showed a cell kill greater than 50 per cent against BCNU and this patient responded clinically to the drug. The remaining five patients had maximum cell kills in the range 0–42 per cent and none responded clinically.[91] In larger series it is apparent that the clonogenic assay tends to over-predict clinical sensitivity[82] but has good predictive power for clinical resistance. Another interesting feature of this assay is the apparent relationship between patient age and *in vitro* cell kill[92] with younger glioma patients tending to have tumour cells more sensitive to BCNU *in vitro*.

Organ culture

Organ culture systems, where explants of tumours are grown on Gelfoam matrices, or rafts in liquid medium, have a number of theoretical advantages over monolayer cell cultures. Cellular interactions are maintained and the function of the tissue is to some extent intact, with repair mechanisms and metabolic co-operation between cells still operating. Brain tumour fragments grown on Gelfoam rafts[93] will infiltrate the matrix in a similar manner to their *in situ* infiltration of normal brain.[94] Saez, Campbell and Laws[95] have used Gelfoam matrix as a substrate for the growth of malignant astrocytomas and have been able to make microfluorimetric estimates of NADH as a quantitative index of the chemosensitivity although no clinical correlations were reported. It has been possible to quantitate the effects of PCB, CCNU VCR and 5-FU on organ cultures of malignant gliomas using ^{125}IUdR uptake and demonstrate a good correlation between this method and both inhibition of protein synthesis and growth delay of flank tumours in immune-deprived mice.[96]

Multicellular tumour spheroids (MTS)

These are tumour cells growing in a three-dimensional structure, simulating the growth and microenvironmental conditions of tumours *in situ*. Their preparation was first described by Sutherland *et al.*[97], who noted that V79 Chinese hamster lung carcinoma cells removed from monolayer culture and inoculated into spinner flasks initially underwent a rapid phase of aggregation to form clumps of cells. These clumps then continued to grow, by cell proliferation, and increase in size.

Multicellular tumour spheroids provide several advantages over monolayer or suspension cell cultures. Not only are the oxygenation characteristics of human tumours modelled, but also the intimate contacts between cells and cell-cycle heterogeneity (e.g. within some areas of a single spheroid, cells divide at rates comparable to cells in monolayer culture and in other areas they become arrested in Go phase).

Extensive screening of animal and human cell lines has revealed that most cell lines derived from tumours will form MTS *in vitro* while normal cell lines will not. Established human glioma cell lines have also been grown as MTS,[98] but the general histological and ultrastructural pattern of a thin rim encompassing a large volume of non-proliferating cells was not observed. In addition, these spheroids did not show central degeneration, although readily reaching diameters in excess of 600 μm.[99] Conversely, MTS produced from early passage cultures of human gliomas, by plating cells on to agarose-coated petri dishes[100, 82], did have a thin outer rim and a large area of central necrosis. The 9L rat gliosarcoma cell line undergoes MTS formation[101, 102] when grown in suspension culture and the cell-cycle characteristics and growth fraction of cells within the spheroid closely resembled those of the intracranial tumour.

It is possible to produce MTS from single cell suspensions obtained from a variety of human brain tumour biopsies samples by collagenase digestion.[103, 104] Such spheroids have been used to test the antiproliferative effects of interferons[105] and cyclic nucleotides.[106]

Invasion of human glioma and its measurement *in vitro*

A major obstacle in the surgical treatment of malignant glioma has been the property of these tumours to invade normal brain making complete surgical extirpation impossible. Little is known about the cellular and molecular biology of this process, and there have been considerable difficulties in developing adequate test systems for investigating this property *in vitro*.[107] Studies using organ cultures of neonatal mouse cerebrum or cerebellum attached to cellulose polyacetate strips to investigate metastatic cell attachment and invasion have been reported.[108] One model system which has been reported in detail is the embryonic chick heart fragment confrontation assay.[109] In this system, disaggregated cells or fragments of tumour tissue are cultured in gyratory shakers forming spherical aggregates. Fragments of 9-day-old embryonic chick heart ventricles are also cultured in the same way. The normal heart aggregates consist of a central core of myoblasts and fibroblasts surrounded by some extracellular material and some fibroblastoid cells on the periphery. To assay invasiveness, single tumour spheroids are confronted with single heart fragments in dishes which have been based-coated with agar to reduce adhesion. After a period of time to allow two spheroids to attach to each other, the confronting pairs are transferred to flasks and incubated on a shaker. After 7 to 10 days incubation, aggregates are taken and examined histologically, using either conventional histology or immunocytochemistry with antibody against chick heart cells. The degree of invasion is determined visually. With this method it has been possible to demonstrate that there was some correlation between the degree of invasion *in vitro* and the take rate and latency of tumour development *in vivo* with established cell lines.[110] When the glioma cells replaced more than 50 per cent of the heart fragment, these lines formed tumours with short latencies while apparently better differentiated cell lines, which expressed GFAP, which did not invade chick heart fragments to the same degree, were less tumorigenic *in vivo*.

Similar studies have been described which use the interaction between rat glioma cell lines and co-cultured normal rat brain fragments.[111, 112] All these studies suffer from the disadvantage that either non-neural cells are confronted with glioma cells or that the invasion is monitored by subjective histological examination. It is imperative to develop an objective quantitative system to measure human brain tumour invasion *in vitro*. Studies have been reported which use the penetration of cells through millipore membranes. With the suitable construction of chambers and perhaps labelling of cells ^{125}IUdR it should be possible to quantitate such systems. However, it is not a true measure of tumour cell invasion, which is a multifactorial process involving extracellular proteinase activity and other uncharacterized factors, which cannot be measured in a system using an essentially inert barrier like a filter.

The ability of cells from a short-term culture of a medulloblastoma to degrade extracellular matrix labelled with tritiated proline, produced by rat smooth muscle cells, has been described[113] and quantitative model systems like this deserve further study.

Phenotypic modification and induction of differentiation *in vitro*

Defined *in vitro* culture conditions allow an examination of the way in which particular chemicals or environmental conditions can effect the phenotype of human glioma. There are a number of well-characterized astrocytic- and malignancy-related marker changes which can be assayed *in vitro*. The ultimate clinical aim of such studies is to be able to modify the malignant character of glioma *in situ*.

A variety of so-called biological response modifiers are capable of suppressing the growth of glioma cells *in vitro* including glucocorticoids,[114] interferons,[105, 115] glial maturation factor,[116] gangliosides,[115] and lectins[117] which are apparently related to differentiation in cells. For example, dexamethasone and pig brain extract increase the level of GFAP,[118] induce glutamine synthetase activity, GABA uptake, and decrease plasminogen activator levels[114] in glioma cell lines. However, treatment with simple agents like ethanol can also increase the levels of glutamine synthetase and GFAP in such cells[119] and whether this can be termed a differentiation event is debatable. In any event, such changes in glial differentiation markers occur in the absence of changes in cell morphology, cell numbers, total protein concentration or protein synthesis, all of which might be regarded as gross indications of cell damage. The question of cell–cell interaction and cell–extracellular matrix interaction in inducing differentiation and modulating response to chemotherapy and radiotherapy has not been investigated. The relationship between cell proliferation and differentiation is well documented. When C6 rat glioma cells become overcrowded in culture and cease to proliferate the proportion of GFAP-positive cells increases.[120] Malignant glioma cells will proliferate on confluent monolayers of normal glia, whilst cells derived from normal brain will not.[121, 122] Malignant glioma cells will also proliferate on preformed monolayers of human fetal intestinal epithelieum and human fetal skin fibroblasts.[122] Cells from glioma cultures which exhibit more differentiated characteristics, like GFAP expression and high glutamine synthetase activity, are inhibited by growing them on cell feeder layers.

An interaction between glioma cells and extracellular matrix material (ECM), which induces apparent phenotypic differentiation has been observed.[123, 124] A cell line (SF514P) derived from normal human leptomeninges[125] produces a ECM which remains attached to the plastic substratum after removal of the cells with alkali and detergent. This material appears to be capable of inhibiting the growth, altering the morphological appearance and inducing GFAP in cells of the U343MG-A glioma cell line when plated on to the matrix material. The component of the matrix responsible for these changes is unknown as no single ECM component was capable of producing these effects to the same degree as the complete matrix, although type I and type IV collagen did have some effect. The secretion of a 65 000 kDa metalloprotinase by U343MG-A was also inhibited by growth on the matrix. It has been suggested that the mechanism of growth inhibition may be due to the reduced secretion of the enzyme, protecting the matrix, which prevents migration and proliferation, from degradation. It does seem however that this is quite a specific interaction and it is by no means certain that all ECM material is capable of inhibiting the growth and producing phenotypic changes in all glioma cell lines. It may well be that only certain lines like U343MG-A are capable of phenotypic modification by interaction with ECM material. Why this is so and to what extent it may be therapeutically important are interesting questions for the future.

Acknowledgements

Much of the work by the author described here has been supported by grants from the Brain Research Trust and The Cancer Research Campaign. It is a pleasure to acknowledge the technical assistance of Karen Armitage, Grazyna Lewandowicz and Suzanne Clark. The continual interest and support of David GT Thomas is acknowledged. Miss C Jones assisted with the preparation of the manuscript.

References

1. Westermark B, Ponten J, Hugosson R. Determinants for the establishment of permanent tissue culture lines from human gliomas. *Acta Pathologica et Microbiologica Scandinavica* (Section A). 1973; **81**, 791-805.
2. Maunoury R. Establishment and characterisation of 5 human cell lines derived from a series of 50 primary intracranial tumours. *Acta Neuropathologica* (Berlin). 1977; **39**, 33-41.
3. Collins VP. Cultured human glial and glioma cells. *International Reviews of Experimental Pathology*. 1983; **24**, 135-202.
4. Ponten J, Macintyre EH. Long-term culture of normal and neoplastic human glia. *Acta Pathologica et Microbiologica Scandinavica*. 1968; **74**, 465-6.
5. West GM, Vaughan PFT, Freshney RI, McNamee HB, Graham DI. Isolation of primary cultures from post-mortem samples of human brain. *Biochemical Society Transactions*. 1982; **10**, 53-4.
6. Thomas DGT, Darling JL, Freshney RI, Morgan D. *In vitro* chemosensitivity assay of human glioma by scintillation autofluorography. In: Paoletti P, Walker MD, Butti G, Knerich R, eds. *Multidisciplinary Aspects of Brain Tumor Therapy*. Amsterdam: North Holland, 1979: 19-35.
7. Morgan D, Freshney RI, Darling JL, Thomas DGT, Celik F. Assay of anticancer drugs in tissue culture: Cell cultures from biopsies of human astrocytoma. *British Journal of Cancer*. 1983; **47**, 205-14.
8. Studer A, de Tribolet N, Diserens AC, Guide AC, Matthieu JM, Carrel S, Stavrun D. Characterisation of four human malignant glioma cell lines. *Acta Neuropathologica* (Berlin). 1985; **66**, 208-17.
9. Cravioto H. Human and experimental gliomas in tissue culture. *Progress in Neuropathology*. 1986; **6**, 165-88.
10. Rutka JT, Giblin JR, Dougherty DV, Liu HC, McCulloch JR, Bell CW, Stern RS, Wilson CB, Rosenblum ML. Establishment and characterisation of five cell lines derived from human malignant gliomas. *Acta Neuropathologica* (Berlin). 1987; **75**, 92-103.
11. Jacobsen PF, Jenkyn DJ, Papadimitriou JM. Four permanent cell lines established from human malignant gliomas: Three exhibiting striated muscle differentiation. *Journal of Neuropathology and Experimental Neurology*. 1987; **46**, 431-50.
12. Thomas DGT, Darling JL, Watkins BA, Hine MC. A simple method for the growth of cell cultures from small biopsies of brain tumours taken during CT-directed stereotactic procedures. *Acta Neurochirurgica Supplementum*. 1984; **33**, 243-45.
13. Benediktsson G, Carlsson J, Nilsson S, Jakobsson PA, Ponten J. The detachment, attachment and growth capacity of human glioma and glia cells in culture. *Acta Pathologica et Microbiologica et Immunologica Scandinavica* (Sect. A). 1983; **91**, 291-6.
14. Forsby N, Collins VP, Westermark B. The spreading of human normal glial and malignant glioma cells in culture. *Acta Pathologica et Microbiologica et Immunologica Scandinavica* (Sect. A). 1985; **93**, 235-49.

15. Haynes LW, Weller RO. The effects of cytochalasin B and colchicine on cell motility and ultrastructure in primary cultures of malignant gliomas. *Acta Neuropathologica* (Berlin). 1978; **44**, 21–30.
16. Ponten J, Westermark B, Hugosson R. Regulation of proliferation and movement of human glia-like cells in culture. *Experimental Cell Research*. 1969; **58**, 393–400.
17. Duffy PE, Huang Y-Y, Rapport MM. The relationship of glial fibrillary acidic protein to the shape, motility, and differentiation of human astrocytoma cells. *Experimental Cell Research*. 1982; **139**, 145–57.
18. Koga H. Study of the motility and contractibility of cultured brain tumor cells. *Journal of Neurosurgery*. 1985; **62**, 906–11.
19. Bigner SH, Mark J, Mahaley MS, Bigner DD. Patterns of the early, gross chromosomal changes in malignant gliomas. *Hereditas*. 1984; **101**, 103–13.
20. Bigner SH, Bjerkvig R, Laerum OD. DNA content and chromosomal composition of malignant gliomas. *Neurologic Clinics*. 1985; **35**, 769–84.
21. Lolait SJ, Harmer JH, Anteri G, Pedersen JS, Toh BH. Expression of glial fibrillary acidic protein, actin, fibronectin and factor VIII antigen in human astrocytomas. *Pathology*. 1983; **15**, 373–78.
22. Franks AJ, Burrow HM. *In vitro* heterogeneity in human gliomas. Are all transformed cells of glial origin? *Anticancer Research*. 1986; **6**, 625–30.
23. Kennedy PGE, Watkins BA, Thomas DGT, Noble MD. Antigenic expression by cells derived from human gliomas does not correlate with morphological classification. *Neuropathology and Applied Neurobiology*. 1987; **13**, 327–47.
24. Lipsky RH, Silverman SJ. Effects of mycophenolic acid on detection of glial filaments in human and rat astrocytoma cultures. *Cancer Research*. 1987; **47**, 4900–04.
25. Kennedy PGE, Watkins BA, La Thangue NB, Clemens GB, Thomas DGT. A cultured human oligodendroglioma cell line and herpes simplex virus-infected cells share antigenic determinants. *Journal of Neuro-oncology*. 1987; **4**, 389–96.
26. Rutka JT, Giblin JR, Hoitodt HK, Dougherty DV, Bell CW, McCulloch JR, Davis RL, Wilson CB, Roseblum ML. Establishment and characterisation of a cell line from a human gliosarcoma. *Cancer Research*. 1986; **46**, 5893–902.
27. Bressler JP, Cole R, deVellis J. Neoplastic transformation of newborn rat oligodendrocytes in culture. *Cancer Research*. 1983; **43**, 709–15.
28. Russell DS, Rubinstein LJ. *Pathology of Tumours of the Nervous System*. 5th edn. London: Edward Arnold, 1989.
29. Miyake E. Establishment of a human obligodendroglial cell line. *Acta Neuropathologica* (Berlin). 1979; **46**, 51–5.
30. Bloom HJG. Medulloblastoma in children: Increasing survival rates and further prospects. *International Journal of Radiation Oncology, Biology, Physics*. 8, 2023–7.
31. Jacobi G, Kornhuber B. Malignant brain tumors in children. In: Jellinger K, ed. *Therapy of malignant brain tumors* Wien: Springer-Verlag, 1987: 396–493.
32. Wilson CB, Barker M, Slagel DE. Tumors of the central nervous system in monolayer tissue culture. *Archives of Neurology*. 1966; **15**, 275–282.
33. Barker M, Wilson B, Hoshino T. Tissue culture of brain tumours. In: Kirsch WM, Grossi-Paoletti E, Paolettis P, eds. *The Experimental Biology of Brain Tumors*. Springfield, Illinois: Charles C. Thomas, 1972: 57.
34. Manuelidies EE. Long term lines of tissue cultures of intracranial tumors. *Journal of Neurosurgery*. 1965; **22**, 368–73.
35. Lumsden CE. The study by tissue culture of tumours of the nervous system. In: Russell DS, Rubinstein LJ, eds. *Pathology of Tumours of the Nervous System*. 3rd edn. London: Edward Arnold, 1971; 334–420.
36. Waghe M, Kumar S, Steward JK. Tissue culture studies of children's tumours. *Journal of Pathology*. 1973; **111**, 117–24.

37. Friedman HS, Burger PC, Bigner SH, Trojanowski JO, Wikstrand CJ, Haplerin EC, Bigner DD. Establishment and characterisation of the human medulloblastoma cell line and transplantable xenograft. D283 Med. *Journal of Neuropathology and Experimental Neurology*. 1985; **44**, 592-605.
38. Friedman HS, Schold SC. Rational approaches to the chemotherapy of medulloblastoma. *Neurology Clinics*, 1985; **3**, 843-53.
39. Zelter PM, Schneider SL, Von Hoff DD. Morphologic, cytochemical and neurochemical characterisation of the human medulloblastoma cell line, TE671. *Journal of Neuro-oncology*. 1984; **2**, 35-45.
40. Mork SJ, May EE, Papasozomenos CH, Vinores SA. Characteristics of human medulloblastoma cell line TE-671 under different growth conditions *in vitro*: A morphological and immunohistochemical study. *Neuropathology and Applied Neurobiology*. 1986; **12**, 277-89.
41. Trojanowski JQ, Friedman HS, Burger PC, Bigner DD. A rapidly dividing human medulloblastoma cell line (D283MED) expresses all three neurofilament subunits. *American Journal of Pathology*. 1987; **126**, 358-63.
42. Steel GG. Growth kinetics of brain tumours. In: *Brain Tumours: Scientific Basis, Clinical Investigations and Current Therapy*. London: Butterworths, 1980: 10-20.
43. Hoshino T. A commentary on the biology and growth kinetics low-grade and high-grade gliomas. *Journal of Neurosurgery*. 1984; **61**, 895-900.
44. Gratzner HG. Monoclonal antibody to 5-bromo and 5-iododeoxyuridine: A new reagent for detection of DNA replication. *Science* 1982; **218**, 474-6.
45. Hoshino T, Nagashima T, Murovic JA, Wilson CB, Edwards SB, Gulin PH, Davis RL, DeArmond SJ. *In situ* cell kinetic studies of human neuroectodermal tumours with bromodeoxyuridine labelling. *Journal of Neurosurgery*. 1986; **64**, 453-9.
46. Nagashima T, DeArmond SJ, Murovic J, Hoshino T. Immunocytochemical demonstration of S-phase cells by antibromodeoxyuridine monoclonal antibody in human brain tumour tissues. *Acta Neuropathologica* (Berlin). 1985; **67**, 155-9.
47. Hoshino T, Nagashima T, Murovic, JA, Wilson CB, Davis RL. Proliferative potential of human meningiomas of the brain: A cell kinetic study with bromodeoxyuridine. *Cancer* 58: 1466-72.
48. Hoshino T. Bromodeoxyuridine (BUdR) labelling indices in human tumour biopsies. *Journal of Neuro-oncology*. 1987; **5**, 173.
49. Gerdes J, Lemke H, Baisch H, Wacker HH, Schwals O, Stein H. Cell cycle analysis of a cell proliferation associated human nuclear antigen defined by the monoclonal antibody Ki-67. *Journal of Immunology*. 1984; **133**, 1710-15.
50. Gerdes J. An immunohistological method for estimating cell growth fractions in rapid histopathological diagnosis during surgery. *International Journal of Cancer*. 1985; **35**, 169-71.
51. Burger PC, Shibata T, Kleihues P. The use of the monoclonal antibody Ki-67 in the identification of proliferating cells: Application to surgical neuropathology. *American Journal of Surgery Pathology*. 1986; **10**, 611-17.
52. Kleihues P, Shibata T, Landolt AM, Ostertag C, Burger PC. Assessment of the growth fraction in human brain tumors as defined by the monoclonal antibody Ki-67. *Journal of Neuro-oncology*. 1986; **5**, 175.
53. Hoshino T, Barker M, Wilson CB, Boldrey EB, Fewer D. Cell kinetics of human gliomas. *Journal of Neurosurgery*. 1972; **49**, 13-21.
54. Rosenblum ML, Knebel KD, Vasquez DA, Wilson CB. Brain tumor therapy: quantitative analysis using a model system. *Journal of Neurosurgery*. 1977; **46**, 145-54.
55. Rosenblum ML, Knebel KD, Vasquez DA, Wilson CB. *In vivo* clonogenic tumor cell kinetics following 1,3,-bis(2-chroroethyl)-1-nitrosourea brain tumour therapy. *Cancer Research*. 1976; **36**, 3718-25.

56. Levin VA, Hoffman WF, Pischer TL, Seager ML, Boldrey EB, Wilson CB. BCNU-5-fluorouracil combination therapy for recurrent malignant brain tumors. *Cancer Treatment Reports.* 1978; **62**, 2071–76.
57. Levin VA, Wilson CB. Correlations between experimental chemotherapy in the murine glioma and effectiveness of clinical therapy regimens. *Cancer Chemotherapy and Pharmacology.* 1978; **1**, 41–8.
58. Bigner DD, Pedersen HB, Bigner SH, McComb R. A proposed basis for the therapeutic resistance of gliomas. *Seminars in Neurology.* 1981; **1**, 169–79.
59. Schnipper LE. Clinical implications of tumor-cell heterogeneity. *New England Journal of Medicine.* 1986; **314**, 1423–31.
60. Hoshino T, Nomura K, Wilson CB, Knebel KD, Gray JW. The distribution of nuclear DNA from human brain tumour cells: Flow cytometric studies. *Journal of Neurosurgery.* 1978; **49**, 13–21.
61. Guner M, Freshney RI, Morgan D, Freshney MG, Thomas DGT, Graham DI. Effects of dexamethasone and betamethasone on *in vitro* cultures from human astrocytoma. *British Journal of Cancer* 1977; **35**, 439–47.
62. Shapiro JR, Yung W-KA, Shapiro WR. Isolation, karyotype and clonal growth of heterogeneous subpopulations of human malignant gliomas. *Cancer Research.* 1981; **41**, 2349–59.
63. Mark J. Chromosomal characteristics of neurogenic tumours in adults. *Hereditas.* 1971; **68**, 61–100.
64. Palfreyman JW, Thomas DGT, Ratcliffe JG, Graham DI. Glial fibrillary acidic protein (GFAP) purification from human fibrillary astrocytoma, development and validation of a radio-immuno assay for GFAP-like immunoactivity. *Journal of the Neurological Sciences.* 1979; **41**, 101–13.
65. Rasmussen S, Bock E, Warecka K, Althage G. Quantitation of glial fibrillary acidic protein in human brain tumours. *British Journal of Cancer.* 1980; **41**, 113–16.
66. Bigner DD, Bigner SH, Ponten J, Westermark B, Mahaley MS, Jr, Ruoslahti E, Herschman H, Eng LF, Wikstrand CJ. Heterogeneity of genotypic and phenotypic characteristics of fifteen permanent cell lines derived from human gliomas. *Journal of Neuropathology and Experimental Neurology.* 1981; **40**, 201–29.
67. van der Meulen JDM, Houthoff HJ, Ebels EJ. Glial fibrillary acidic protein in human gliomas. *Neuropathology and Applied Neurobiology.* 1978; **4**, 177–90.
68. Pilkington GJ, Lantos PL. The role of glutamine synthetase in the diagnosis of cerebral tumours. *Neuropathology and Applied Neurobiology.* 1982; **8**, 227–36.
69. deMuralt B, de Tribolet N, Diserens AC, Carrel S, Mach J-P. Reactivity of antiglioma monoclonal antibodies for a large panel of cultured gliomas and other neuroectodermially derived tumours. *Anticancer Research.* 1983; **3**, 1–6.
70. McComb RD, Wikstrand CJ, Bourdon MA, Bigner SH, Bigner DD. Antigenic heterogeneity of human malignant gliomas (MGs) demonstrated by reactivity with 10 monoclonal antibodies (MCAs). *Journal of Neuropathology and Experimental Neurology.* 1983; **42**, 308.
71. Bradley NJ, Bloom HJG, Davies AJS, Swift SM. Growth of human gliomas in immune deficient mice: A possible model for pre-clinical therapy studies. *British Journal of Cancer.* 1978; **38**, 263–72.
72. Shapiro WR, Basler GA, Chernik NL, Posner JB. Human brain tumor transplantation into nude mice. *Journal of the National Cancer Institute.* 1979; **62**, 447–53.
73. Schold SC, Jr, Bullard DE, Bigner SH, Jones TR, Bigner DD. Growth, morphology and serial transplantation of anaplastic human gliomas in athymic mice. *Journal of Neuro-oncology.* 1983; **1**, 5–14.
74. Basler GA, Shapiro WR. Brain tumor research with nude mice. In: Fogh J, Giovanella BC, eds. *The Nude Mouse in Experimental and Clinical Research.* Vol 2. New York: Academic Press 1982; 475–90.

75. Bullard DE, Schold SC, Bigner SH, Bigner DD. Growth and chemotherapeutic response in athymic mice of tumours arising from human glioma-derived cell lines. *Journal of Neuropathology and Experimental Neurology.* 1981; **40**, 410–27.
76. Pfeiffer SE, Wechsler W. Biochemically differentiated neoplastic clone of Schwann cells. *Proceedings of the National Academy of Science* (USA). 1972 **69**, 2885–89.
77. Dohan FC, Jr, Kornblith PL, Wellum GR, Pfeiffer SE, Levine L. S-100 protein and 2',3'-cyclic nucleotide-3'-phosphohydrolase in human brain tumours. *Acta Neuropathologica* (Berlin). 1977; **40**, 123–28.
78. Glimelius B, Norling B, Westermark B, Wasterson A. A comparative study of glycosaminoglycans in cultures of human normal and malignant glial cells. *Journal of Cell Physiology.* 1979; **98**, 527–737.
79. Glimelius B, Westermark B, Ponten J. Agglutination of normal and neoplastic human cells: Concanavalin A and Ricinus communis agglutinin. *International Journal of Cancer.* 1974; **14**, 314–25.
80. Manuelidis L, Yu RK, Manuelides EE. Ganglioside content and pattern in human gliomas in culture: Correlation of morphological changes with altered gangliosides. *Acta Neuropathologica* (Berlin). 1977; **38**, 129–35.
81. Rosenblum ML, Dougherty DV, Deen DF, Wilson CB. Potentials and limitations of a clonogenic cell assay for human brain tumors. *Cancer Treatment Reports.* 1981; **65**, (Suppl. 2) 61–6.
82. Rosenblum ML, Gerosa MA, Wilson CB, Barger GR, Pertuiset BF, de Tribolet N, Dougherty DV. Stem cell studies of human malignant brain tumours. Part 1. Development of the stem cell assay and its potential. *Journal of Neurosurgery.* 1983; **58**, 170–76.
83. Yung WKA, Shapiro JR, Shapiro WR. Heterogeneous chemosensitivities of subpopulations of human glioma cells in culture. *Cancer Research.* 1982; **42**, 992–8.
84. Haynes LW, Weller RO. Induction of some features of glial differentiation in primary cultures of human gliomas by treatment with cyclic AMP. *British Journal of Experimental Pathology.* 1978; **59**, 259–76.
85. Bullard DE, Bigner SH, Bigner DD. The morphologic response to cell lines derived from human gliomas to butyryl adenosine 3'5'-cyclic monophosphate. *Journal of Neuropathology and Experimental Neurology.* 1981; **40**, 231–46.
86. Darling JL, Thomas DGT. Results obtained using assays of intermediate duration and clinical correlations. In: Dendy PP, Hill BT, eds. *Human Tumour Drug Sensitivity Testing in vitro: Techniques and Clinical Applications.* London: Academic Press, 1983: 269–80.
87. Kornblith PL, Smith BH, Leonard LA. Response of cultured human brain tumors to nitrosoureas correlation with clinical data. *Cancer.* 1981; **47**, 255–65.
88. Thomas DGT, Darling JL, Paul EA, Mott TJ, Godlee JN, Tobias JS, Capra L, Collins CD, Mooney C, Bozek T, Finn GP, Arigbabu SO, Bullard DE, Shannon N, Freshney RI. Assay of anticancer drugs in tissue culture: Prediction of relapse free interval in patients with malignant cerebral glioma using an *in vitro* chemosensitivity assay. *British Journal of Cancer.* 1985; **51**, 525–32.
89. Rosenblum ML, Knebel KD, Wheeler KT, Barker M, Wilson CB. Development of an *in vitro* colony formation assay for the evaluation of *in vivo* chemotherapy of a rat brain tumour. 1956; **44**, 264–73.
90. Rosenblum ML, Vasquez DA, Hoshino T, Wilson CB. Development of a clonogenic cell assay for human brain tumours. *Cancer.* 1978; **41**, 2305–14.
91. Rosenblum ML, Dougherty DV, Deen DF, Hoshino T, Wilson CB. Analysis of clonogenic human brain tumor cells: preliminary results of tumor sensitivity testing with BCNU. *Cancer.* 1980; **41**, Suppl. IV, 181–85.
92. Rosenblum ML, Gerosa M, Dougherty DV, Reese C, Barger GR, Davis RL, Levin VA, Wilson CB. Age-related chemosensitivity of stem cells from human malignant brain tumors. *Lancet.* 1982; **i**, 885–7.

93. Raafat M, El-Bolkainy N, Rifaat M, Sorour O. A new technique for growing intracranial tumours *in vitro*. *Medical Journal of Cairo University*. 1972; **11**, 1-13.
94. Sorour O, Raafat M, El-Bolkainy N, Rifaat M. Infiltratative potentiality of brain tumors in organ culture. *Journal of Neurosurgery*. 1975; **43**, 742-48.
95. Saez RJ, Campbell RJ, Laws ER. Chemotherapeutic trials of human malignant astrocytomas in organ culture. *Journal of Neurosurgery*. 1977; **46**, 320-27.
96. Darling JL, Masters JRW, Bradley NJ. Comparison of chemosensitivities of human glioma in experimental systems. *Journal of Neuro-oncology*. 1984; **2**, 291.
97. Sutherland RM, McCreadie JA, Inch WR. Growth of multicell spheroids in tissue culture as a model for nodular carcinomas. *Journal of the National Cancer Institute*. 1971; **46**, 113-20.
98. Haji-Karim M, Carlsson J. Proliferation and viability in cellular spheroids of human origin. *Cancer Research*. 1978; **83**, 1457-64.
99. Carlsson J, Brunk U. The fine structure of three-dimensional colonies of human glioma cells in agarose culture. *Acta Pathologica et Microbiologica Scandinavica* (Sect. A). 1977; **85**, 183-92.
100. Pertuiset BF, Rosenblum ML, Poisson M, Haum JJ, Deen DF, Buge A. Cinétique de spheroides multicelulares developpés à partir d'un glioblastome humain et action de la 1,3,-bis-(2-chloroethyl)-1-nitrosouree. *Semaine des Hôpitaux de Paris*. 1983; **59**, 468-72.
101. Deen DF, Hoshino T, Williams ME, Muraoko I, Knebel KD, Barker M. Development of a 9L rat brain tumour cell multicellular spheroid system and its response to 1,3-bis(2-chloroethyl)-1-nitrosourea and radiation. *Journal of the National Cancer Institute*. 1980; **64**, 1373-81.
102. Sano Y, Deen DF, Hoshino T. Factors that influence initiation and growth of 94L rat brain gliosarcoma multicellular spheroids. *Cancer Research*. 1982; **42**, 1223-26.
103. Darling JL, Oktar N, Thomas DGT. Multicellular tumour spheroids derived from human brain tumours. *Cell Biology International Reports*. 1983; **7**, 23-30.
104. Darling JL, Oktar N, Thomas DGT. *In vitro* chemosensitivity testing of human brain tumours using muticellular spheroids. *Advances in the Biosciences*. 1986; **58**, 121-34.
105. Bradley NJ, Darling JL, Oktar N, Bloom HJG, Thomas DGT, Davies AJS. The failure of human lymphocyte interferon to influence the growth of human glioma cell populations: *in vitro* and *in vivo* studies. *British Journal of Cancer*. 1983; **48**, 819-25.
106. Oktar N, Darling JL, Thomas DGT. An experimental trial of cyclic nucleotides on multicellular spheroids for human brain tumour. *Journal of Neuro-oncology*. 1987; **5**, 83-9.
107. Laerum OD, Bjerkvig R, Steinsvag SK, deRidder L. Invasiveness of primary brain tumours. *Cancer Metastasis Reviews*. 1984; **3**, 223-36.
108. Wang T-Y, Nicolson GL. Metastatic tumour cell invasion of brain tissue cultured on cellulose polyacetate strips. *Clinical Experimental Metastasis*. 1983; **1**, 327-39.
109. Mareel M, Klint J, Meyvisch C. Methods of study of the invasion of malignant C_3H mouse fibroblasts into embryonic chick heart *in vitro*. *Virchows Archw* (Zellpathologie). 1979; **30**, 95-111.
110. deRidder LI, Laerum OD, Mark SJ, Bigner DD. Invasiveness of human glioma cell lines *in vitro*: relation to tumorigenicity in athymic mice. *Acta Neuropathologica* (Berlin). 1987; **72**, 207-13.
111. Steinsvag SK. Interaction between glioma cells and normal brain tissue in organ culture studied by scanning electron microscopy. *Invasion Metastasis*. 1985; **5**, 255-69.
112. Steinsvag SK, Laerum OD. Invasion of glioma cells into brain tissue in organ culture. *Journal of the National Cancer Institute*. 1985; **74**, 24-32.
113. Bogenmann E, Mark C, Isaacs H, Neustein HB, DeClerk YA, Lang WE, Jones PA. Invasiveness properties of primary pediatric neoplasmas *in vitro*. *Cancer Research*. 1983; **43**, 1176-86.

114. McLean JS, Frame MC, Freshney RI, Vaughan PFT, Mackie AE, Singer I. Phenotypic modification of human glioma and non-small cell lung carcinoma by glucocorticoids and other agents. *Anticancer Research*. 1986; **6**, 1101-06.
115. Yates AJ, Stephens RE, Elder PJ, Markowitz DL, Rice JM. Effects of interferon and gangliosides on growth of cultured human glioma and fetal brain cells. *Cancer Research*. 1985; **45**, 1033-39.
116. Lim R, Hicklin DJ, Ryken TC, Han X-M, Lin K-N, Miller JF, Baggenstoss BA. Suppression of glioma growth *in vitro* and *in vitro* by glial maturation factor. *Cancer Research*. 1980; **46**, 5241-47.
117. Liwnicz BH. Mitogenic lectin receptors of nervous system tumors: Study of gliomas, neural crest tumours and meningiomas *in vitro* using phylohemagglutinin and concanavalin A. *Journal of Neuropathology and Experimental Neurology*. 1982; **41**, 281-297.
118. Frame MC, Freshney RI, Vaughan PFT, Graham DI, Shaw R. Interrelationship between differentiation and malignancy associated properties in glioma. *British Journal of Cancer*. 1984; **49**, 269-80.
119. Patel AJ, Weir MD, Darling JL, Thomas DGT, Hunt A. Biochemical studies of primary cultures from human astrocytomas: observations on cell growth and regulation of glutamine synthetase. In: Walker MD, Thomas DGT, eds. *Biology of Brain Tumour*. Boston: Martines Nijhoff, 1986: 15-25.
120. Freshney RI, Morgan D, Hassanzadah M, Shaw R, Frame M. Glucocorticoids, proliferation and the cell surface. In: Richards RJ, Rajan KT, eds. *Tissue Culture in Medical Research*. Oxford: Pergamon Press, 1981: 125-32.
121. Westermark B. Growth control of normal and neoplastic human glia-like cells in culture. *Acta Universitatis Upsalensis*. 1973; **164**.
122. MacDonald CM, Freshney RI, Hart E, Graham DI. Selective control of human glioma cell proliferation by specific cell interaction. *Experimental Cell Biology*. 1985; **53**, 130-7.
123. Rutka JT. Effects of extracellular matrix proteins on the growth and differentiation of an anaplastic glioma cell line. *Canadian Journal of Neurological Science*. 1986; **13**, 301-6.
124. Rutka JT, Giblin JR, Apoclaca G, DeArmond SJ, Stern R, Rosenblum ML. Inhibition of growth and induction of differentiation in a malignant human glioma cell lines by normal leptomeningeal extracellular matrix proteins. *Cancer Research*. 1987; **47**, 3515-22.
125. Rutka JT, Giblin JR, Dougherty DV, McCulloch JR, DeArmond SJ, Rosenblum ML. Ultrastructural and immunocytocyhemical analysis of leptomeningeal and meningioma cultures. *Journal of Neuropathology and Experimental Neurology*. 1986; **45**, 285-303.
126. McAllister RM, Isaacs H, Rongey R, Peer M, Au W, Soukup SW, Gardner MB. Establishment of a human medulloblastoma cell line. *International Journal of Cancer*. 1977; **20**, 206-12.
127. Friedman HS, Bigner SH, McComb RD, Schold SC, Pasternak JF, Groothuis DR, Bigner DD. A model for human medulloblastoma: growth, morphology and chromosomal analysis *in vitro* and in athymic mice. *Journal of Neuropathology and Experimental Neurology*. 1983; **42**, 485-503.
128. Jacobsen PF, Jenkyn DJ, Papadimitriou JM. Establishment of a human medulloblastoma cell line and its heterotransplantation into nude mice. *Journal of Neuropathology and Experimental Neurology*. 1985; **44**, 472-85.
129. Gerosa MA, Rosenblum ML, Stevanomi G, Tommasi M, Raimondi E, Nicolato A, Bricolo A, Tridente G. Toward medulloblastoma cell lines: Preliminary report. *Advances in the Biosciences*. 1986; **58**, 105-16.

2 Oncogene expression and control of growth in malignant brain tumours

Bengt Westermark, Monica Nistér, Nils-Erik Heldin and Carl-Henrik Heldin

Introduction

The phenotypic properties of a cancer cell deviate from normal in several respects, the most important characteristics being uncontrolled growth, invasiveness and immortality. Development of the fully malignant phenotype is generally thought to be a stepwise process involving several genetic lesions. One might thus envisage a situation whereby a cell is afflicted by mutations which lead to the escape of growth control; the neoplastic progenitor cell then gives rise to an offspring that undergoes progressive genetic changes leading to the emergence of even more malignant variants. As pointed out by Klein and Klein,[1] three classes of genes may be distinguished which are involved in the expression of the malignant phenotype. The first class includes the oncogenes, which are defined by their ability to transform cells in tissue culture and render them tumorigenic *in vivo*. The second class of genes is defined as antioncogenes or tumour suppressor genes which are thought to have a normal function in growth regulation and differentiation and to be deleted or incapacitated in malignant cells[2,3] (see also Fig. 2.1). The last group contains so-called modulator genes which have no inherent transforming potential but influence the neoplastic behaviour of the cell, e.g. by encoding proteolytic enzymes or factors that allow the cell to escape immunosurveillance.

Glioblastoma multiforme is the most common primary tumour of the central nervous system. As suggested by the term 'multiforme', the tumour is characterized by a pleomorphic cellular picture with the occurrence of a plethora of tumour cell types. Despite the advanced phenotypic heterogeneity, detailed karyotypic analyses using chromosome banding techniques[4,5] have given no indication of a true polyclonality but rather suggest that the tumour may have evolved from a single malignant progenitor cell and that the phenotypic as well as the genotypic heterogeneity is the result of secondary, progressive events in the dividing population.

The complex biology and resistance to therapy make glioblastoma multiforme a great challenge for investigation. In this review we will discuss the impact that the current knowledge of the structure and function of oncogenes has had on our

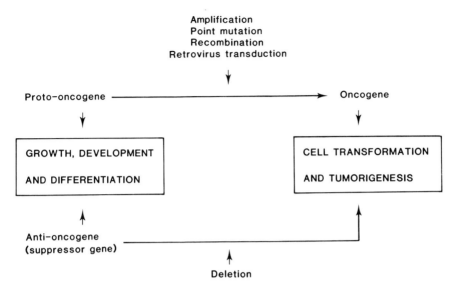

Fig. 2.1 Oncogenes and antioncogenes in transformation and tumorigenesis. Proto-oncogenes are normal cellular genes involved in the regulation of normal growth and development. A proto-oncogene can be converted to a transforming oncogene by mechanisms that affect the level of expression and/or structure of the coding sequences. Antioncogenes (or tumour suppressor genes) are normally involved in differentiation and growth control processes. Deletion of such genes leads to the loss of a regulatory, growth restraining function. Tumour growth may thus result from the generation of an aberrant growth stimulus in combination with the loss of growth restraint.

understanding of the biology of human glioma (for general reviews on oncogenes, see refs. 1, 6–10).

Functional aspects of oncogenes

Oncogenes represent altered versions of normal cellular genes (proto-oncogenes or c-*onc*). Most of the known oncogenes have been identified as parts of the genomes of acutely transforming retroviruses (v-*onc*); these viruses evolve through genetic recombination such that a mutated version of a proto-oncogene is integrated into a usually partially deleted retroviral genome.[6] This converts the virus from a principally innocent particle to a transforming and oncogenic variant. The generation of acutely transforming retroviruses is an extremely rare event in nature and has never been found to occur in man. However, genetic mechanisms other than transduction by retroviruses operate in the activation of oncogenes in human neoplasms, such as chromosomal rearrangement, point mutation and gene amplification.[1] These events lead to the expression of qualitatively and/or quantitatively aberrant protein products.

Recent studies on the structure and function of polypeptide growth factors in relation to oncogenes and their protein products have yielded a unifying concept of neoplastic transformation and normal mitogenesis. The basic finding is that a number of proto-oncogene products have been identified as proteins with defined roles in mitogenicity, e.g. growth factors, growth factor receptors, coupling factors or other cell cycle-related proteins. The consensus of opinion is that oncogenes encode qualitatively and/or quantitatively aberrant proteins which cause transformation by subverting the mitogenic pathway.[8, 10] The generation of an endogenous growth signal may thus be one of the essential steps in malignant conversion. This concept is briefly outlined below (see also Fig. 2.1 and Fig. 2.2).

One of the most striking examples of the close relationship between transformation and growth stimulation is the finding that the oncogene v-*sis* of simian sarcoma virus (SSV) is homologous to the cellular gene encoding the B subunit of platelet-derived growth factor (PDGF).[10–13] This finding implies that SSV transformation is mediated by a PDGF-like growth factor that stimulates the infected cell by an autocrine pathway. Recent information of the structure and function of the v-*sis* protein product provides strong support of this idea (reviewed by Westermark et al.[14, 15]). An important finding is that the phenotype of SSV-transformed cells can be reverted by specific and nonspecific PDGF antagonists.[16, 17]

The PDGF B-chain gene is so far the only growth factor gene found to be transduced by an acutely transforming retrovirus. However, there is experimental evidence that other growth factors may also have transforming potential. Thus, transfection of susceptible cells with transforming growth factor alpha (TGF-α)[18] or epidermal growth factor (EGF)[19] DNA expression vectors confers growth factor independence in culture and renders the cells tumorigenic *in vivo*. As both EGF and TGF-α exert their cellular function via the EGF receptor, these findings show that an autocrine activation of the EGF receptor pathway may generate a transforming signal.

Direct evidence for a transforming potential of a growth factor receptor has been provided by the finding that the oncogene v-*erb* B of avian erythroblastosis virus encodes a truncated version of the EGF receptor.[20] Deletion of amino- and carboxy-terminal protein sequences are thought to render the intrinsic receptor tyrosine protein kinase constitutively active, i.e. the cell cannot and need not bind EGF in order to fire mitogenic signals. Another example is the retroviral oncogene v-*fms* which encodes a mutated form of the receptor for the hematopoietic growth factor CSF-1 (colony-stimulating factor 1).[21]

The finding of these two retroviral oncogenes which represent transduced cellular growth factor receptor genes provides strong support for the idea that growth factor receptors have oncogenic potential when properly activated by structural alterations. Further support for this view is derived from the finding that the normal homologues of several other oncogenes have the general structure of growth factor receptors, although the corresponding ligands have not yet been identified (Fig. 2.2). One example is the *neu* gene which was identified in the DNA of an intracerebral tumour of a rat exposed to a carcinogen (ethylnitrosourea, ENU) *in utero*.[22] As the product of the *neu* gene is similar to the EGF receptor (EGF-R),[23] it is generally thought to be the receptor for an as yet unidentified growth factor. A single point mutation in the transmembrane domain converts the normal *neu* gene to a transforming variant.[24] This change could possibly lead to a conformation change of the

Functional aspects of oncogenes 29

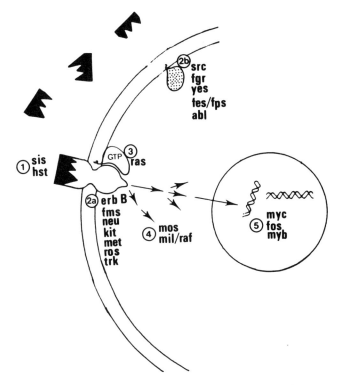

Fig. 2.2 The molecular mechanism of mitogenesis and its relation to transformation. Normal growth stimulation occurs through the binding of a growth factor to its receptor. The signal is transduced through the activated receptor and specific coupling factors. The mitogenic signal is then transmitted to the nucleus and cell cycle related genes are being expressed. Proto-oncogenes encode regulatory factors along the mitogenic pathway. The corresponding oncogenes cause transformation by subverting the mitogenic pathway: (1) *sis* and probably also *hst* encode growth factors; (2) *erb* B and *fms* encode known growth factor receptors and *neu, kit, yes, fes/fps* and *abl* encode tyrosine kinases which are functionally related to the cytoplasmic domain of growth factor receptors; (3) the *ras* gene family encodes putative coupling factors; (4) *mos* and *mil/raf* encode cytoplasmic serine/threonine protein kinases; and (5) *myc, fos* and *myb* encode nuclear proteins. For details and references, see text and refs. 10 and 15. (Adapted from ref. 55.)

receptor, mimicking the effect of ligand binding and thus render the catalytic domain of the receptor constitutively activated.

In several hormone-regulated systems, the transduction of an extracellular signal is mediated by GTP-binding proteins (G proteins).[25] Three members of the *ras* gene family (Ha-*ras*, Ki-*ras*, N-*ras*) encode similar 21 kDa proteins which are attached to the inner leaflet of the plasma membrane and which share amino acid sequences with G proteins.[26] This finding has led to the assumption that the *ras* proteins may function as coupling factors associated with, e.g., growth factor receptors. The *ras* genes are converted to transforming variants by single amino acid substitutions in two regions of the molecule (reviewed by Gibbs et al.[27]). This small change in the primary structure generally leads to a loss of GTPase activity, possibly leading to a constitutively active coupling factor.

Studies on early gene expression in growth-stimulated cells have shown increased levels of the mRNA of certain proto-oncogenes, such as c-*fos* and c-*myc* (reviewed by Heldin et al.[10]). Both genes encode nuclear proteins. Their function is still largely unknown but they are thought to control gene transcription and modify the expression of genes related to the the cell cycle. The involvement of the c-*myc* gene in tumorigenesis has been the focus of much attention in recent years. The conversion of the *myc* proto-oncogene to a transforming variant is in general related to changes in the level of expression with no alteration of the protein structure. A number of studies have thus shown that overexpression of c-*myc* caused by chromosomal rearrangement or gene amplification may be a contributory event in the genesis of "spontaneous" human tumours, particularly of haematopoietic or lymphoid origin.[1]

Two other members of the *myc* family have been identified so far, viz, N-*myc* and L-*myc*. N-*myc* gene amplification has been found in advanced stages of neuroblastoma[28] and in small-cell lung carcinoma.[29] In the latter cell type, L-*myc* amplification has also been detected.[30]

Antioncogenes

Non-random deletion of chromosomes or chromosome segments may be indicative of the loss of antioncogenes or tumour suppressor genes. The best studied example is the familial form of retinoblastoma in which deletion of segments of the long arm of chromosome 13 led to the discovery of a putative antioncogene (rb¹) (reviewed by Knudson[2]). Moreover, the familial form of Wilms' tumour is typically associated with deletion of chromosome 11p13. Direct proof for the existence of genetic information on chromosome 11 that can suppress malignancy of Wilms' tumour cells has been obtained from studies on single chromosome transfer.[31]

Interplay between oncogenes and antioncogenes in neoplastic development

A simplified model for the basic mechanisms of neoplastic development is depicted in Fig. 2.1. An aberrant growth stimulus is generated by the protein products of activated oncogenes as described above. The effect of the activated oncogenes is synergized by the deletion of antioncogenes, and results in the loss of negative growth signals normally involved in growth control and differentiation.

Oncogenes in glioma

In the molecular analysis of primary tumours or cultured cell lines, the distinction between proto-oncogenes and oncogenes is not always simple to make.

Proto-oncogenes have an essential role in the control of growth and differentiation. The mere expression of a particular proto-oncogene in a tumour, such as a glioma, may thus only be a marker of cell type, stage of development or growth rate without any direct and causative role in the pathogenesis of the tumour. Since to date we have but a rudimentary knowledge of the pattern of proto-oncogene expression in normal glia at different stages of development, it is difficult and sometimes impossible to interpret findings on the pattern of oncogene expression in glioma properly. It is only when the expression at the mRNA or protein level can be matched by corresponding abnormalities at the genomic level that we can argue for a pathogenetic role of the particular gene with any degree of certainty.

Human glioma cells are particularly easy to grow in tissue culture, thus in unselected material we were able to grow about 20 per cent of glioblastoma multiforme cells as continuous cell lines.[32] The relative ease with which such cell lines can be established has made them widely used as model systems for studies on the biology of glioma. When we interpret findings on established cell lines, however, we should be aware of the fact that they may not be true representatives in all respects of glioma cells *in vivo*. The cell lines are highly selected and may have undergone extensive genotypic and phenotypic changes during their long-term growth in culture. Studies on permanent glioma cell lines should therefore be regarded only as a first screen; potentially important findings on, e.g., oncogene expression, must be corroborated by studies on biopsy material from primary tumours.

In the following sections we will give an update on the state of the art of oncogenes in glioma. In doing so, we will try to take the above considerations into account.

Expression of the c-*sis* gene and production of PDGF-like factors in human glioma cells

An involvement of the c-*sis*/PDGF B-chain gene in the pathogenesis of glioma can be inferred from the pioneering studies by Deinhardt and collaborators.[33] They found that an intracerebral injection of SSV together with its helper virus resulted in the induction of gliomas in newborn marmoset monkeys at a relatively high frequency. Some of these tumours were found to have the classical hallmarks of glioblastoma, i.e. cellular pleomorphism, increased vascularity, endothelial cell proliferation and vast necrosis. In previous communications we have discussed these findings in relation to the molecular biology of SSV transformation in culture and proposed the idea that SSV *in vivo* induces a polyclonal glial cell expansion through an autocrine stimulation of the PDGF receptor.[14, 15] However, we consider it unlikely that an autocrine stimulation of growth alone can explain the development of a complex malignancy such as glioblastoma. We have therefore suggested that the proliferating SSV-transformed cells *in vivo* form a fertile ground for the occurrence of secondary genetic changes which lead to the emergence of the truly malignant population. Expression of an integrated v-*sis* gene and autocrine growth stimulation is then only the initial event in a multistep process. Renewed studies on SSV-induced gliomas using the modern techniques of molecular biology will hopefully reveal the true nature of these tumours.

Because of the oncogenic effect of SSV in the central nervous system it is relevant to ask the question whether the cellular homolog of v-*sis*, i.e. the c-*sis*/PDGF B-chain gene, is involved in the pathogenesis of human glioma. This question relates to studies performed in our laboratory in recent years in which we have analysed our panel of human glioblastoma lines with regard to the production of PDGF-like growth factors and the expression of PDGF receptors. Our initial observation was that the clonal cell line U-343 MGa Cl 2 produces relatively large quantity of a factor that is structurally, immunologically and functionally related to PDGF.[34] Northern blot hybridization analysis of PDGF A-chain and B-chain transcripts showed that glioblastoma cell lines express both genes at high frequency.[35] The level of expression varies independently, even between clones derived from a single glioma line (U-343 MGa).[36] Southern blot analysis did not reveal any gross amplification or rearrangement of the PDGF A- or B-chain genes.

Analysis of PDGF receptor mRNA and ^{125}I-PDGF binding in the glioma lines provided evidence for the biosynthesis and expression of PDGF receptors on a number of lines that concomitantly express PDGF A- and B-chain genes. This finding raises the question whether such glioma cells are stimulated by an autocrine mechanism in analogy to SSV transformed cells. However, attempts to block the autocrine pathway by PDGF antibodies, which are known to block the growth of SSV transformed cells[16] have so far failed to retard the growth of glioma cells. Obviously, this finding does not immediately invalidate the autocrine hypothesis in spontaneous glioma. If autocrine growth stimulation is an early event in a multihit process, one might envisage that the successive changes during the evolution of the tumour lead to a state of absolute growth factor independence, including the endogenously produced factor. Examples from other cell systems illustrate this phenomenon.[10] Moreover, several autocrine pathways may be activated in glioma cells as these have been found to express mRNA of both TGF-α[35] and acidic FGF,[37] in addition to PDGF A- and B-chain. Perhaps all existing autocrine pathways have to be blocked until growth is retarded.

Hopefully, studies on the involvement of PDGF-like growth factors in experimental tumours will be helpful in our attempts to evaluate the role of autocrine stimulation of the PDGF receptor pathway in glioma. However, one should also regard the possibility that the synthesis of PDGF-like growth factors, as well as other growth factors, by glioma cells only reflects an activity of the normal progenitor cell which persists in the malignant offspring. Critical analyses of the growth factor synthesis in the intact brain at various stages of development are thus warranted.

Amplification and expression of the c-*erb* B/EGF receptor gene in glioma

A number of studies have shown that normal glia-derived cells in culture respond to EGF with an increased rate of proliferation.[38-40] Schlessinger and collaborators addressed the question as to the expression and function of the EGF receptor in human glioma cells. In their initial studies they made the observation that the EGF receptor kinase activity was higher in membranes prepared from malignant glioma tissue than in those prepared from normal brain tissue.[41] This finding was substantiated by analyses at the gene level; using human c-*erb* B/EGF receptor cDNA probes, a six- to 60-fold amplification of the EGF receptor gene was found in four out of 10 malignant gliomas.[42] No amplification was found in low-grade astrocytoma or in meningioma. The occurrence of abnormal restriction fragments was taken as an indication of possible rearrangement of the gene; this possibility has, however, not

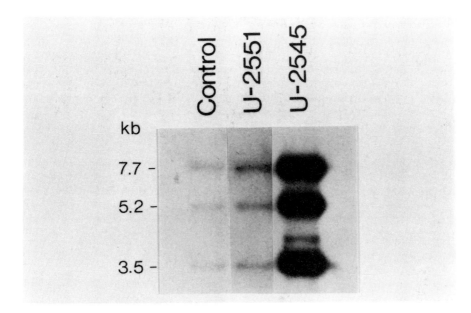

Fig. 2.3 Amplification of the c-erb B/EGF receptor gene in human glioma. DNA from two gliomas was digested with Eco R1 and subjected to Southern blot hybridization analysis using a ^{32}P-labelled c-erb B cDNA probe corresponding to the cytoplasmic portion of the EGF receptor (kindly provided by Dr J Schlessinger). Note the amplification of the EGF receptor gene in the U-2545 glioma compared to normal human DNA or to the U-2551 glioma.

been analysed in detail. In a recent publication Bigner *et al.* have confirmed the findings of Schlessinger and collaborators.[43] In a series of 33 malignant human glioma biopsies, 15 showed amplification of the EGF receptor gene. A similar frequency was observed in a series of glioma biopsies in our laboratory. Figure 2.3 shows a Southern blot analysis of two glioma biopsies one of which shows EGF receptor gene amplification. In our experience, amplification of the EGF receptor gene is invariably accompanied by an increased cell surface EGF receptor expression. Figure 2.4 shows the occurrence of EGF receptors on glioma cells in primary cultures of the two biopsies. EGF receptors were visualized by indirect immunofluorescence using a mouse anti-human EGF receptor monoclonal antibody (kindly provided by Dr Hilary Koprowski, The Wistar Institute, Philadelphia, PA). Note the very strong, patchy fluorescence on glioma cells carrying an amplified receptor gene. Similar results are obtained by immunohistochemical analysis of frozen sections of primary glioma tissue (not shown).

In experimental studies, gene amplification and overproduction of the corresponding protein has been shown to be induced by applying a selection pressure on a cell population. One of the best known examples is the amplification of the dehydrofolate reductase gene in cells that are selected for resistance to methotrexate.[44] Amplification of an oncogene, such as *erb* B, and overproduction of the corresponding protein are likely to confer growth advantages by an analogous dominant mechanism and allow the cell to grow under conditions where growth is normally inhibited. It is not

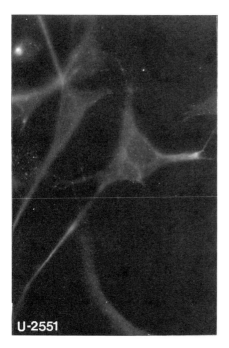 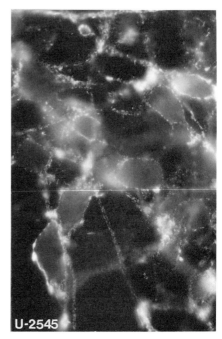

Fig. 2.4 Expression of EGF receptors on human glioma cells in primary culture. EGF receptors were visualized by indirect immunofluorescence using monoclonal antibodies directed against the external portion of the receptor (kindly provided by Dr H Koprowski). Note the high level of expression in the U-2545 glioma (with EGF receptor gene amplification) compared to U-2551 (without gene amplification).

clear, however, in what way overexpression of the EGF receptor may confer growth advantage. One possibility is that there is a suboptimal concentration of EGF (or TGF-α) in the extracellular fluid; cells with an overexpressed receptor will then at a given moment have an increased number of occupied (= activated) receptors compared to cells with a normal receptor number. Alternatively, the tumour cells may produce a low amount of TGF-α, the autocrine response to which is augmented by an increased receptor number. Recent studies by Nistér et al. have shown expression of TGF-α mRNA in human glioma cell lines suggesting that the second alternative may hold true.[35] Another possibility is that the EGF receptor may even in the absence of a bound ligand have a low, constitutive activity; if the receptor number is increased, the activity may reach a level high enough to trigger growth. Lastly, the overexpressed receptor may be structurally abnormal (as is the v-*erb* B product) and be constitutively active. Overexpression of such a receptor would then generate a strong mitogenic signal.

The findings of changes at the genomic level strongly suggest a pathogenetic role for the EGF receptor in malignant glioma. The finding of an amplified EGF receptor gene only in high-grade glioma in conjunction with the apparent requirement for repeated cell cycling for amplification to occur,[44] makes it likely that it is a progressive event in glioma development. This view is supported by circumstantial evidence from other tumours showing gene amplification, e.g. neuroblastoma, in which N-*myc* amplification occurs only in advanced stages of the disease.[28] High-grade gliomas are considered by many investigators to evolve from more highly differentiated tumours. It is possible that a progressive increase in EGF receptor level, brought about by an increased gene copy number, confers a selective growth advantage on a clonal or subclonal population that will constitute the glioblastoma proper.

As mentioned above, a transforming, point mutated *neu*/HER2 gene was isolated from the DNA of an experimental brain tumour in the rat. This finding obviously raises the question whether the *neu* gene is involved in human spontaneous brain tumours. To our knowledge, this subject has not been thoroughly investigated and to date there has been no report on mutation, rearrangement, or amplification of *neu*/HER2 in glioma although *neu* amplification has been reported in other human malignancies such as mammary carcinoma.[45, 46] In a survey of established glioma cell lines, Libermann found only low levels of *neu* mRNA (personal communication).

Amplification of c-*myc* and N-*myc*

Amplification of c-*myc* and N-*myc* has been found to occur in primary human glioma, albeit at a low frequency. Southern blot analysis of DNA from low passage cultures of one particular glioblastoma cell line demonstrated a several-fold amplification of c-*myc* where hybridization with 17 other oncogene probes only showed a normal gene copy number.[47] Since the result was not confirmed by an analysis of primary tissue, one cannot entirely rule out the possibility that c-*myc* amplification in this case occurred as a result of cell multiplication in culture although the use of low passage cultures argues against this notion.

In their analysis of glioma biopsies, Bigner et al. found one case of N-*myc* amplification, whereas none had amplified c-*myc*.[43] Since this series included as many as 33 specimens, one may draw the conclusion that amplification of *myc* genes is not a frequent event in glioma.

Oncogenes and antioncogenes in glioma: what can we learn from cytogenetical analyses?

The pioneering work on karyotype analysis of human primary glioma was performed by Mark.[48] More recently, Bigner and Mark have addressed the problem in a collaborative effort and found that the primary gross deviations could be categorized into three groups, i.e. (1) loss of a gonosome, (2) gains of No. 7 and at the same time often losses of No. 10 and (3) loss of No. 22.[4, 5] The most frequent structural aberration was the presence of double minute chromosomes (DMs) which could be demonstrated in about 50 per cent of the cases.

The high incidence of DMs in human glioma is interesting since DMs are known to harbor amplified gene sequences.[44] Bigner and collaborators addressed the question as to whether the majority of DMs in glioma represent the chromosomal manifestation of EGF receptor gene amplification and found that the majority of gliomas with DMs indeed showed amplification of the EGF receptor gene. The single glioma with N-*myc* amplification also had DMs.

In an elegant study by Kinzler et al. the occurrence of DMs in a particular glioma allowed the identification and molecular cloning of a novel putative oncogene.[49] Knowing that DMs are indicators of gene amplification, the investigators analysed DNA from the tumour with a large number of known oncogene probes. As they could not identify the amplified sequences by this strategy, they made an effort to clone the amplified DNA and found a sequence that probably constitutes the amplified gene. It was given the name *gli* from its occurrence in glioma. The *gli* gene has recently been found to encode a putative transcription factor.[56]

As the EGF receptor gene is located on the short arm of chromosome 7 (7p12–13),[50] the occurrence of extra copies of No. 7 should indicate a corresponding increase in EGF-receptor gene dosage. It is at present unclear if this increase in gene copy number confers any significant increase in EGF receptor expression in primary tumours. In our study on primary human glioma cultures, high numbers of cell-surface EGF receptors were invariably found to coincide with such a degree of gene amplification that could not be explained only by an increased chromosome number. A high level of EGF-receptor mRNA has been reported in glioma cell lines with multiple copies of chromosome 7.[51,52] In a study on a large number of human glioma cell lines we found a broad range in ^{125}I-EGF-binding with a 50-fold difference between the extremes despite the fact that all cell lines analysed, even those with overexpression of EGF receptors, have a normal or near-normal EGF-receptor gene dosage.[35,36] Thus, whereas gene amplification may be the main cause of EGF receptor overexpression *in vivo*, other mechanisms seem to operate in cultured cell lines, in which, for an unknown reason to DMs, are not commonly present.

The possible role of antioncogene deletion in the pathogenesis of glioma has not been elucidated. However, the finding of non-random loss of chromosomes is highly suggestive. The loss of one copy of chromosome 22 is particularly intriguing since this is typical also of other, albeit distantly related, intracranial tumours, viz. meningioma[53] and acoustic neurinoma.[54] It is interesting to speculate on the possibility that chromosome 22 carries the locus for a gene that is involved in the control of growth and differentiation of, e.g. glial cells, Schwann cells and meningocytes (*cf.* Fig. 2.1), the loss of which results in abnormal growth.

Concluding remarks

The reports on oncogene expression in human glioma cells described in this review form the beginning of a new research avenue which will lead us to a better understanding of the molecular biology of human gliomas. We can certainly foresee an interesting future, since traditional investigators in brain tumour research are starting to exploit the recent advances in molecular genetics, while molecular biologists are beginning to appreciate glioma as a challenging tumour. We anticipate that an insight into the basic molecular mechanisms involved in the pathogenesis of glioma may lead to the development of better therapeutic modalities, that will be more specific in their action than those available at present. In this respect, growth factors and their receptors are potential targets for intervention, since they are expressed at the cell surface and therefore are more accessible to interference than cytoplasmic or nuclear oncogene products. It is hoped that further studies on glioma suppressor genes will also unravel novel features of the abnormal growth behaviour of glioma cells and give clues to its reversal.

References

1. Klein G, Klein E. Evolution of tumours and the impact of molecular oncology. *Nature.* 1985; **315,** 190–5.
2. Knudson AG, Jr. Hereditary cancer, oncogenes and antioncogenes. *Cancer Research.* 1985; **45,** 1437–43.
3. Stanbridge EJ. A case for human tumour-suppressor genes. *BioEssays.* 1985; **3,** 252–5.
4. Bigner SH, Mark J, Mahaley MS, Bigner DD. Patterns of the early gross chromosomal changes in malignant human gliomas. *Hereditas.* 1984; **101,** 103–13.
5. Bigner SH, Mark J, Bullard DE, Mahaley MS, Jr, Bigner DD. Chromosomal evolution in malignant human gliomas starts with specific and usually numerical deviations. *Cancer Genetics and Cytogenetics.* 1986; **22,** 121–35.
6. Bishop JM. Cellular oncogenes and retroviruses. *Annual Review of Biochemistry.* 1983; **52,** 301–54.
7. Bishop JM. Viral oncogenes. *Cell.* 1985; **42,** 23–38.
8. Heldin CH, Westermark B. Growth factors: Mechanism of action and relation to oncogenes. *Cell.* 1984; **37,** 9–20.
9. Weinberg RA. The action of oncogenes in the cytoplasm and nucleus. *Science.* 1985; **230,** 770–6.
10. Heldin C-H, Betsholtz C, Claesson-Welsh L, Westermark B. Subversion of growth regulatory pathways in malignant transformation. *Biochemica et Biophysica Acta.* Cancer Reviews 1987; **907(3),** 219–44.
11. Devare SG, Reddy EP, Law JD, Robbins KC, Aaronson SA. Nucleotide sequence of the simian sarcoma virus genome. Demonstration that its acquired cellular sequences encode the transforming gene product p28^{sis}. *Proceedings of the National Academy of Sciences of the United States of America.* 1983; **80,** 731–5.
12. Doolittle RF, Hunkapiller MW, Hood LE, Devare SG, Robbins KC, Aaronson SA, Antoniades HN. Simian sarcoma virus oncogene, v-sis, is derived from the gene (or genes) encoding a platelet-derived growth factor. *Science.* 1983; **221,** 275–7.
13. Waterfield MD, Scrace GT, Whittle N, Stroobant P, Johnsson A, Wasteson A, Westermark B, Heldin C-H, Huang JS, Deuel TF. Platelet-derived growth factor is structurally related to the putative transforming protein p28^{sis} of simian sarcoma virus. *Nature.* 1983; **304,** 35–9.
14. Westermark B, Johnsson A, Betsholtz C, Heldin C-H. Biological properties of simian sarcoma virus and its oncogene product. In: Retroviruses, oncogenes and growth factors. *Contributions to Oncology.* 1986; **24,** 51–61.
15. Westermark B, Betsholtz C, Johnsson A, Heldin C-H. Acute transformation by simian sarcoma virus is mediated by an externalized PDGF-like growth factor. In: Kjeldgaard NO, Forchhammer J, eds. *Viral Carcinogenesis.* Copenhagen: Munksgaard, 1987: 445–7.
16. Johnsson A, Betsholtz C, Heldin C-H, Westermark B. Antibodies against platelet-derived growth factor inhibit acute transformation by simian sarcoma virus. *Nature.* 1985; **317,** 438–40.
17. Betsholtz C, Johnsson A, Heldin C-H, Westermark B. Efficient reversion of SSV-transformation and inhibition of growth factor-induced mitogenesis by suramin. *Proceedings of the National Academy of Sciences of the United States of America.* 1986; **83,** 6440–4.
18. Rosenthal A, Lindquist PB, Bringman TS, Goeddel DV, Derynck R. Expression in rat fibroblasts of a human transforming growth factor-α cDNA results in transformation. *Cell.* 1986; **46,** 301–9.
19. Stern DF, Hare DL, Cecchini MA, Weinberg RA. Construction of a novel oncogene based on synthetic sequences encoding epidermal growth factor. *Science.* 1987; **235,** 321–5.

20. Downward J, Yarden Y, Mayes E, Scrace G, Totty N, Stockwell P, Ullrich A, Schlessinger J, Waterfield MD. Close similarity of epidermal growth factor receptor and v-erb-B oncogene protein sequences. *Nature*. 1984; **307**, 521–7.
21. Sherr CJ, Rettenmier CW, Sacca R, Roussel MF, Look AT, Stanley ER. The c-fms proto-oncogene product is related to the receptor for the mononuclear phagocyte growth factor, CSF-1. *Cell*. 1985; **41**, 665–76.
22. Schechter AL, Stern DF, Vaidyanathan L, Decker SJ, Drebin JA, Greene MI, Weinberg RA. The neu oncogene: an erbB-related gene encoding a 185, 000 Mr tumour antigen. *Nature*. 1984; **312**, 513–6.
23. Bargmann CI, Hung M-C, Weinberg RA. The neu oncogene encodes an epidermal growth factor-related protein. *Nature*. 1986; **319**, 226–30.
24. Bargmann CI, Hung M-C, Weinberg RA. Multiple independent activations of the neu oncogene by a point mutation altering the transmembrane domain of p185. *Cell*. 1986; **45**, 649–57.
25. Gillman AG. G proteins and dual control of adenylate cyclase. *Cell*. 1984; **36**, 577–9.
26. Hurley JB, Simon MI, Teplow DB, Robishaw JD, Gilman AD. Homologies between signal transducing G proteins and ras gene products. *Science*. 1984; **226**, 860–2.
27. Gibbs JB, Sigal IS, Scolnick EM. Biochemical properties of normal and oncogenic ras p21. *Trends in Biological Science*. 1985; **9**, 350–3.
28. Brodeur GM, Seeger RC, Schwab M, Varmus HE, Bishop JM. Amplification of N-myc in untreated human neuroblastomas correlates with advanced disease stage. *Science*. 1984; **224**, 1121–4.
29. Nau MM, Brooks BJ, Jr, Carney DN, Gadzar AF, Battey JF, Sausville EA, Minna JD. Human small-cell lung cancers show amplification and expression of the N-myc gene. *Proceedings of the National Academy of Sciences of the United States of America*. 1986; **83**, 1092–6.
30. Nau MM, Brooks BJ, Battey J, Sausville E, Gazdar AF, Kirsch IR, McBride OW, Bertness V, Hollis GF, Minna JD. L-myc, a new myc-related gene amplified and expressed in human small cell lung cancer. *Nature*. 1985; **318**, 69–73.
31. Weissman BE, Saxon PJ, Pasquale SR, Jones GR, Geiser AG, Stanbridge EJ. Introduction of a normal human chromosome 11 into a Wilms' tumour cell line controls its tumorigenic expression. *Science*. 1987; **236**, 175–80.
32. Westermark B, Pontén J, Hugosson R. Determinants for the establishment of permanent tissue culture lines from human gliomas. *Acta Pathologica et Microbiologica Scandinavica*, Sect. A. 1973; **81**, 791–805.
33. Deinhardt F. The biology of primate retrovirus. In: Klein G, ed. *Viral Oncology*. New York: Raven Press, 1980: 359–98.
34. Nistér M, Heldin C-H, Wasteson Å, Westermark B. A glioma-derived analog to platelet-derived growth factor: demonstration of receptor competing activity and immunological cross-reactivity. *Proceedings of the National Academy of Sciences of the United States of America*. 1984; **81**, 926–30.
35. Nistér M, Libermann TA, Betsholtz C, Pettersson M, Claesson-Welsh L, Heldin C-H, Schlessinger J, Westermark B. Expression of messenger RNAs for platelet-derived growth factor and transforming growth factor- and their receptors in human malignant glioma cell lines. *Cancer Research*. 1988; **48**, 3910–18.
36. Nistér M, Wedell B, Betsholtz C, Bywater M, Pettersson M, Westermark B, Mark J. Evidence for progressional changes in the human malignant glioma line U-343 MGa: Analysis of karyotype and expression of genes encoding the subunit chains of platelet-derived growth factor. *Cancer Research*. 1987; in press. 47, 4935–60.
37. Libermann TA, Friesel R, Jaye M, Lyall RM, Westermark B, Drohan W, Schmidt A, Maciag T, Schlessinger J. An angiogenic factor is expressed in human glioma cells. *EMBO J*. 1987; **6**, 1627–32.

38. Westermark B. Density dependent proliferation of human glia cells stimulated by epidermal growth factor. An angiogenic growth factor is expressed in human glioma cells. *Biochemistry and Biophysics Research Communications.* 1976; **69**, 304–10.
39. Leutz A, Schachner M. Epidermal growth factor stimulates DNA-synthesis of astrocytes in primary cerebellar cultures. *Cell Tissue Research.* 1981; **220**, 393–404.
40. Simpson DL, Morrison R, de Villis J, Herschmann HR. Epidermal growth factor binding and mitogenic activity on purified populations of cells from the central nervous system. *J. Neuroscience Research.* 1982; **8**, 453–62.
41. Libermann TA, Razon N, Bartal AD, Schlessinger J. Expression of epidermal growth factor receptors in human brain tumours. *Cancer Research.* 1984; **44**, 753–60.
42. Libermann TA, Nusbaum HR, Razon N, Kris R, Lax I, Soreq H, Whittle N, Waterfield MD, Ullrich A, Schlessinger J. Amplification, enhanced expression and possible rearrangement of EGF receptor gene in primary human brain tumours of glial origin. *Nature.* 1985; **313**, 144–7.
43. Bigner SH, Wong AJ, Mark J, Kinzler KW, Vogelstein B, Bigner DD. Relationships between gene amplification and chromosomal deviations in malignant human gliomas. *cancer Genetics and Cytogenetics.* 1987; 29(1), 165–70.
44. Schimke RT. Gene amplification in cultured animal cells. *Cell.* 1984; **37**, 705–13.
45. King CR, Kraus MH, Aaronson SA. Amplification of a novel v-erbB-related gene in a human mammary carcinoma. *Science.* 1985; **229**, 974–6.
46. Slamon DJ, Clark GM, Wong SG, Levin WJ, Ullrich A, McGuire WL. Human breast cancer: correlation of relapse and survival with amplification of the HER-2/neu oncogene. *Science.* 1987; **235**, 177–82.
47. Trent J, Meltzer P, Rosenblum M, Harsh G, Kinzler K, Mashal R, Feinberg A, Vogelstein B. Evidence for rearrangement, amplification, and expression of c-myc in a human glioblastoma. *Proceedings of the National Academy of Sciences of the United States of America.* 1986; **83**, 470–3.
48. Mark J. Chromosomal characteristics of neurogenic tumours in adults. *Hereditas.* 1971; **68**, 61–100.
49. Kinzler KW, Bigner SH, Bigner DD, Trent JM, Law ML, O'Brien SJ, Wong AJ, Vogelstein B. Identification of an amplified, highly expressed gene in human glioma. *Science.* 1987; **236**, 70–3.
50. Shimizu N, Hunts J, Merlino G, Wang-Peng J, Xu Y-H, Yamamoto T, Toyoshima K, Pastan I. Regional mapping of the EGF receptor (EGFR)/c-erbB proto-oncogene. *Cytogenetics and Cell Genetics.* 1985; **40**, 743–4.
51. Henn W, Blin N, Zang KD. Polysomy of chromosome 7 is correlated with overexpression of the erbB oncogene in human glioblastoma cell lines. *Human Genetics.* 1986; **74**, 104–6.
52. Bell C, Harsh G, IV, Rosenblum M, Meltzer P, Trent J. Numeric and structural alterations of chromosome 7 in human brain tumours: Correlation with expression of epidermal growth factor receptor (EGFR). *Proceedings of the American Association for Cancer Research.* 1986; **27**, 37.
53. Mark J. Chromosomal abnormalities and their specificity in human neoplasms: An assessment of recent observations by banding techniques. *Advances in Cancer Research.* 1977; **124**, 165–222.
54. Seizinger BR, Martuza RL, Gusella JF. Loss of genes on chromosome 22 in tumorigenesis of human acoustic neurinoma. *Nature.* 1986; **322**, 644–7.
55. Westermark B, Nistér M, Heldin C-H. Growth factors and oncogenes in human malignant glioma. *Neurologic Clinics.* 1985; **3**, 785–99.
56. Kinzler KW, Ruppert JM, Bigner SH, Vogelstein B. The GLI gene is a member of the *Kruppel* family of zinc finger proteins. *Nature.* 1988; **332**, 371–74.

3 Glial cell markers in the study of CNS development and human gliomas

Bryn Watkins, Karen Bevan, Deon Venter and Mark Noble

Introduction

What happens when the paradigms of morphological analysis are tested with the tools of cellular biology? This question is central to a consideration of the classification of different neoplasias. For example, the development, by Bailey and Cushing,[1] of a systematic approach to glioma classification was based upon the particular understanding of CNS development which prevailed in the first quarter of the twentieth century. The major investigative tools of this era were the light microscope and cytochemical stains, which together allowed the recognition that cells of the CNS could be divided into various morphological categories. On the basis of a hypothesis that the relationship between different cell-types could be elucidated through a careful study of cellular morphology, cells were grouped not only into distinct morphological classes but also into "transitional forms" thought to recognize intermediate stages involved in the differentiation of one cell-type (generally a precursor cell) into another cell-type (generally a fully differentiated end-stage cell). The outcome of this approach to glioma classification is shown in Figure 3.1. Although subsequent simplification of this initial classification system has been steadily pursued,[2,3] the simplifications have been generally based on the assumptions (i) that morphological analysis is a sufficient tool for classification of different cell-types, and (ii) that the lineage relationships between different CNS cell-types proposed by early investigators of this subject were generally correct.

Although still in their early stages, contemporary studies have already set the foundation for a substantial reappraisal of earlier hypotheses on CNS development. These studies have used the tools of cellular and molecular biology to investigate three particular areas of the CNS: the optic nerve, the retina and the cortex. We will first review studies on normal development, and then go on to review our current studies on glioma classification.

Glial cell development in the rat optic nerve

The starting point for a cellular biological analysis of glial development was the optic nerve, the simplest part of the CNS. This tissue has been particularly useful for

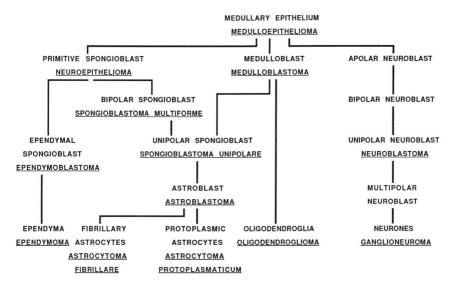

Figure 3.1 Lineage relationships, cell-types and classification of neuronal and glial tumours, as proposed by Bailey and Cushing.[1]

developmental studies because of the limited number of cell-types it contains. All of the neurones which send their axons through the optic nerve have their cell bodies located elsewhere, either in the retina or in the brain. Thus, the only neuroectodermally derived cells in this tissue are the astrocytes and oligodendrocytes, and their progenitor cells. Until 1983 the major question related to development of these optic nerve glia was whether they came from a single progenitor cell, or whether astroblasts and oligodendroblasts represented two distinct glial lineages. However, since this time, it has become clear that the optic nerve is a substantially more complex tissue that was previously appreciated.

The first glial cell type to appear in the optic nerve during embryonic development is the *type-1 astrocyte*. This population of astrocytes appears to be specifically derived from the optic stalk,[4] the outpouching of the neural tube which represents the embryonic anlage of the optic nerve. Type-1 astrocytes, and their precursors, seem to contribute to the morphogenetic development of the optic nerve by offering a preferred substrate for growing axons.[5, 6] These cells also apparently interact with endothelial cells to induce formation of the blood-brain barrier,[7] and (as discussed below) are a source of mitogen for other cells in the nerve.[8-10]

The next two glial cell types to appear during development of the rat optic nerve are both derived from a single progenitor cell, the *oligodendrocyte-type-2 astrocyte (O-2A) progenitor cell*,[11] which migrates into the optic nerve from the optic chiasm during embryogenesis.[4] *In vitro* studies suggest strongly that division of the O-2A progenitor cells is promoted by the type-1 astrocytes derived from the optic stalk, through the secretion of platelet-derived growth factor.[8-10] Beginning at the time of birth,[12] dividing O-2A progenitors begin to generate *oligodendrocytes*, and these cells go on to enwrap large axons of the CNS with myelin sheaths. After another 7–10 days, the first *type-2 astrocytes* appear in the optic nerve;[12] these cells are thought to extend processes which are associated with axons at the nodes of Ranvier,[13, 14] the regions between consecutive myelin sheaths where ion fluxes occur during transmission of impulses along the myelinated axon. Thus, the O-2A lineage appears to be specialized to create the anatomical specializations which characterize the myelinated tracts of the CNS.[13]

A further member of the O-2A lineage is the O-2A^{adult} progenitor cell, which differs from its perinatal counterpart in antigen expression, morphology, cell-cycle length, motility, time-course of differentiation, in the manner in which it generates oligodendrocytes and seemingly also in its capacity for extended self-renewal.[15-17] Two properties of O-2A^{adult} progenitors are particularly noteworthy. First, they express several properties which suggest they are specialized to be more in keeping with the physiological requirements of the adult nervous system than O-2A^{perinatal} progenitors.[15, 16] Second, they appear to be derived from a subpopulation of O-2A^{perinatal} progenitors.[16, 17] This generation of O-2A^{adult} progenitors from O-2A^{perinatal} progenitors suggests that progenitor populations are developmentally nested, such that cells with properties appropriate for early development give rise not only to terminally-committed end-stage cells but also to a new group of precursor cells with properties more appropriate for later developmental periods. The relationship between all of the presently known cell-types of the rat optic nerve is summarized in Figure 3.2.

Glial and neuronal development in the retina and the cortex

The analysis of cellular relationships in the retina and the cortex has been pursued rather differently than in the optic nerve. Although cellular biological studies have played some role in these studies, the most critical contributions have come from the use of retroviruses (i.e., RNA viruses) to label clones of related cells (for review, see ref. 18). In these studies, the first step is to genetically engineer the genome of a retrovirus to encode bacterial β-galactosidase, an enzyme which can be visualized histochemically. A small number of retroviral particles are then injected into a region of the developing nervous system, where occasional retroviruses will successfully infect single cells and have their viral genome incorporated into the cellular DNA. Following a productive integration of viral genes, all progeny resulting from an infected cell with express the β-galactosidase gene, and can subsequently be recognized. By initially injecting small numbers of viral particles, the frequency of successful infection is brought low enough to allow the subsequent identification of groups of clonally related cells.

The lineage relationships between the cells of the retina, as revealed by retroviral labelling, have been surprising. All possible relationships between the different cell-types of the retina have thus far been demonstrated, and clones have been visualized which consist only of neurones, only of retinal Müller cells (the retinal macroglial cell), and of both Müller cells and neurones.[19] Although these results are consistent with the view that the earliest retinal progenitors are all plutipotent cells, capable of giving rise to all retinal populations, it is also possible that even the earliest retinal progenitor cells will turn out to be heterogeneous in their developmental potential.

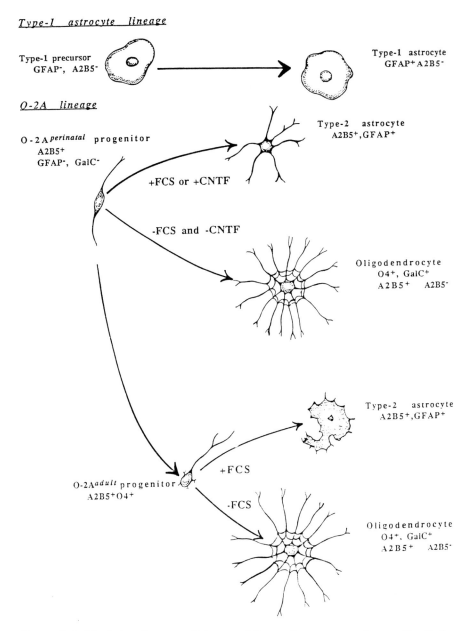

Figure 3.2 All of the diverse cell-types of the optic nerve can be readily distinguished from each other *in vitro* on the basis of antigen expression and morphology. Some of the defining antibodies are mentioned in this figure. As also shown, O-2A progenitors grown in the presence of appropriate inducing factors (e.g., fetal calf serum or ciliary neurotrophic factor) differentiate into type-2 astrocytes, while growth in the absence of inducing agents is associated with differentiation of O-2A progenitors into oligodendrocytes (refs 11, 28, 40, 41). For comprehensive reviews on differentiation in the optic nerve, see refs 17, 42, 43.

An additional surprising insight into retinal development has come with the observations that the astrocytes which are found in the retinas of many species are not even derived from the retinal progenitor cells. These astrocytes instead appear to be derived from astrocyte precursors of the optic nerve, and migrate into the retina during embryonic development.[20] Thus, although the cells which form the retina begin development as just a further portion of the same neural tube outpouching which forms the embryonic optic stalk, the retina develops into a tissue remarkably different from the optic nerve. The retinal progenitors develop into many different kinds of neurones and into retinal Müller cells, while the progenitor cells of the embryonic optic nerve give rise only to one population of astrocytes.

Developmental studies on the cortex have been as surprising as studies on the retina. Injection of β-galactosidase expressing retroviruses into the cortex of embryonic day 16 rats has led to the identification of several different kinds of clones.[21] Some clones appear to consist only of astrocytes, while other clones appear to consist only of neurones. However, the neuronal clones are not confined to one type of neuron. Even in clones with two identifiable members, these two β-galactosidase expressing neurones may be very different types of cells (e.g., pyramidal and non-pyramidal neurones). In addition, some clones consist of both obvious neurones and cells which are organized horizontally in the white matter tracts. As the only cells thus far known to be horizontally organized in the white matter are cells of the O-2A lineage, it may well be that at least some progenitor cells give rise to neurones, oligodendrocytes and type-2 astrocytes.

Ramifications of current developmental studies for neuropathology

Three concepts emerge from contemporary developmental neurobiological studies: (1) The lineage relationships between the cell types of the CNS are different from those predicted by earlier investigators; (2) the range of cell-types present in the CNS is different from that envisaged by earlier investigators; and, (3) the rules which govern development in one region of the CNS may not necessarily be valid in other regions.

Two additional important concepts have also specifically emerged from studies on the O-2A lineage. First, our studies on this lineage indicate that the very critieria used in assessing cells morphologically is not supported when tested against cellular biological analysis. Specifically, morphologists have used the presence of 10 nm (intermediate) filaments as a significant identifying element for "astroblasts" and the absence of such filaments as an identifying element for "oligoblasts". Yet, the O-2A^{perinatal} progenitor cell is rich in vimentin intermediate filaments[22] while the O-2A^{adult} progenitor cell has no detectable intermediate filaments.[15] Thus, these cells would have been classified by ultrastructural criteria as "astroblasts" or "oligoblasts" respectively, even though both of the progenitors can develop into either oligodendrocytes or type-2 astrocytes. Second, the demonstration that division of O-2A progenitors is promoted by cells of a different glial lineage (i.e., type-1 astrocytes) demonstrates that control of cell division in the CNS can be mediated by mitogens secreted by normal glial cells.

A serological analysis of gliomas

The first technique we applied to glioma analysis was immunostaining, and we examined the antigenic phenotype of glioma cells *in vitro* and *in situ* with antibodies which have been useful in studying normal glial populations in rodents and in humans (see ref. 23 for details). The antibodies used in these studies, and their cellular distribution, are summarized in Table 3.1. Of these antibodies, four were particularly useful: anti-fibronectin, anti-glial fibrillary acidic proten (GFAP) and the A4 and A2B5 monoclonal antibodies. Fibronectin is a glycoprotein of the extracellular matrix and is associated with many cell types, such as fibroblasts and endothelial cells, but is usually not found on normal CNS cells except during early embryonic development.[24, 25] GFAP, an intermediate filament protein, is specifically expressed by astrocytes within the CNS.[26-28] Monoclonal antibody A2B5[29] has been used in studies of the rat optic nerve to distinguish between type-1 astrocytes (and their precursors) and cells of the O-2A lineage. Type-1 astrocytes are large flat cells which are A2B5$^-$, while type-2 astrocytes are A2B5$^+$ process-bearing cells with small cell bodies.[11, 28] O-2A progenitors and immature oligodendrocytes are also A2B5$^+$,[11, 21] and so are some cells not of the O-2A lineage; for example, many neurones are A2B5$^+$.[29, 30] Monoclonal antibody A4 is a more generally useful reagent which labels all CNS cells derived from the neural tube, but not cell types with other embryological origins.[31, 32] Thus, astrocytes, oligodendrocytes, neurones and ependymal cells are all A4$^+$, while microglia, meningeal cells, brain endothelial cells, and cells of all other tissues are A4$^-$. The properties of these antibodies are summarized in Table 3.1.

Table 3.1 Antibodies used in this work

Antibody	Antigen recognized
Polyclonal antisera	
Rabbit anti-GFAP	Glial fibrillary acidic protein, a 55 kD intermediate filament protein specific for astrocytes within the CNS[26-28]
Rabbit anti-FN	Fibronectin, a 239 kD extracellular matrix component, found on the surface of many cell types, but not normally on CNS glia. Also in plasma (for review see ref. 44).
Mouse monoclonal antibodies	
A2B5	Cell surface glycolipid found on neurons and some glial populations[28-30]
A4	Cell surface antigen found on all cells derived from the neural tube[31, 32]
anti-FN	Fibronectin[45]

Glioma-derived cells can be divided into two superfamilies on the basis of antigen expression

128/149 (85.9) per cent) primary (passage 1 to 3) glioma-derived cultures which we have examined were labelled only with antibodies to fibronectin (FN). Cell surface fibronectin expression was not seen in 17 of 149 (11.4 per cent) of the cultures tested, and cultures which did not express fibronectin were generally GFAP$^+$ (82 per cent) or A2B5$^+$ (12 per cent). Monoclonal antibody A4 labelled cultures which were GFAP$^+$ or A2B5$^+$, but not cultures that expressed fibronectin. Thus, 85.9 per cent of glioma-derived cultures were A4$^-$/FN$^+$, and 11.4 per cent were A4$^+$/FN$^-$, FN + cultures were derived from tumours in all histological classes with no apparent prevalence, while 65 per cent of A4 + cultures were derived from grade 4 gliomas. This observation directly contradicts the standard interpretations of morphological analysis of the astrocytomas, which predict a decrease in astrocytic characteristics (such as GFAP expression) with increasing malignancy. In addition, none of the 12 oligodendrogliomas examined expressed any oligodendrocyte-specific antigens. Most importantly, every gliomas which produced an A4$^+$ culture, whether GFAP$^+$ or A2B5$^+$, had morphologically identical counterparts which produced FN$^+$ cultures; thus, serological analysis revealed categories of gliomas which were not detected by traditional neuropathological analysis (Table 3.2). Confirmation that the FN$^+$ cells we saw were truly tumour cells, and not contaminating fibroblast-like cells of non-tumour origin, came with several observations. First the FN$^+$ glioma-derived cells were aneuploid, unlike normal human meningeal cells grown in culture. In addition, 22 of 25 tumours examined in sectioned biopsies contained FN$^+$ areas with no apparent morphological or antigenic relationship to blood vessels. Tumours which were clearly either FN$^+$ or A4$^-$ in section consistently gave rise to tissue culture populations with antigenic phenotypes like that of the tumour of origin. Similar sorts of observations have led other investigators to also conclude that the FN + cells derived from gliomas are correctly identified as tumour cells.[33]

Table 3.2 Antigen expression in human glioma-derived cell cultures, analysed by original tumour histology

Histological classification	Antigenic phenotype	
	FN$^+$	A4$^+$
Astrocytoma grade I	6/6	0/6
Astrocytoma grade II	12/13	1/13
Astrocytoma grade III	22/24	2/24
Astrocytoma grade IV	56/68	9/68
Oligodendroglioma	12/12	0/12
Ependymoma	3/3	0/3
Medulloblastoma	8/10	2/10
Other (2 chordoma, 4 mixed o/a, 1 PNET, 1 rhabdomyosarcoma, 4 gliomas not otherwise specified)	10/13	2/13
Total of all gliomas	128/149	17/149

Table does not include four cultures; three contained both A4$^+$ and FN$^+$ populations (mixed cultures), and one did not stain with any of the antibodies tested.

The most convincing demonstration that the FN$^+$ cells isolated from many gliomas are not only tumour cells, but are representative of the populations found within the tumour mass *in situ*, has come with molecular biological studies. In these studies we have used the recent observations that a high proportion of gliomas have lost genetic material from chromosome 10 as a basis for characterising FN⁺ cells.[34] We first identified patients whose lymphocyte-derived DNA showed the patient to be heterozygous at the position defined by the PLAU chromosome 10 probe,[35] whose tumour biopsy specimens showed that one of the two alleles for this locus had been lost during neoplastic development, and whose gliomas had given rise to FN⁺ tissue culture populations. In all cases evaluated thus far, the genetic aberration seen within the tumour *in situ* is accurately reflected in tissue culture, thus demonstrating unequivocally that the FN⁺ cells are bona fide tumour cells (manuscript in preparation).

The neoplasia-metaplasia feedback hypothesis and the control of tumour growth

A striking paradox for those studying human neoplasias has been the knowledge that these tumours grow effectively *in situ*, yet often grow poorly, or not at all, in tissue culture medium lacking serum or defined mitogens. Thus, human tumours are by and large not wholly growth factor independent. We have made similar observations with our glioma cultures, and these results suggested to us that glioma cells might be supplied *in vivo* with factors which they themselves were incapable of producing. Our other studies on mitogen secretion and mitogen response raised the possibility that these additional factors might be supplied from normal cells contained within the tumour mass.

It is clear that tumours growing *in situ* contain both tumour cells and endothelial cells. Our observations that most astrocytomas gave rise to FN⁺ GFAP⁻ cells in culture suggested to us that many of the GFAP⁺ cells seen within gliomas *in situ* might be normal astrocytes, growing within the tumour as a consequence of secretion of astrocytic mitogens by tumour cells and/or endothelial cells. Thus, we found it a reasonable hypothesis that many gliomas contain at least endothelial cells, normal astrocytes, and tumour cells and we therefore set out to determine whether either endothelial cells or astrocytes were able to promote the division of cells derived from gliomas.

Our studies have indicated that each of the three cell types which we think are found in tumours *in situ* are capable of stimulating DNA synthesis in the two other cell types. Thus, astrocytes stimulate DNA synthesis in endothelial cells and in many tumour populations, endothelial cells stimulate astrocytes and many tumour populations, and many tumour cells secrete growth factors which stimulate DNA synthesis in endothelial cells and/or astrocytes. These results suggest to us that a major factor controlling the growth of gliomas *in situ* might be the interplay between the tumour cells and the normal cells in the immediate microenvironment. Tumour cells could stimulate the growth of nearby normal cells, and these cells could in turn release mitogens which promote division of the tumour cells. Similar ideas have also been proposed by Westermark, Heldin and their colleagues.[36] It will now be of interest to identify specific mitogens which might contribute to such positive-feedback loops, and to determine whether it is possible to interrupt tumour growth with appropriate antibodies against externally-supplied mitogens. Interference of this nature has been used *in vitro*, to show that antibodies against platelet-derived growth factor inhibit the ability of type-1 astrocytes to promote division of O-2A progenitor cells.[9, 10]

Conclusions

By applying some of the tools of cellular and molecular biology to a study of the gliomas we have found that the families of tumours recognized by serological analysis are substantially different from those recognized by analysis of cytology. These findings are of particular interest when considered in light of the value of serological classification of the leukemias, where the use of biological classification systems has been associated with improvements in the ability to predict clinical prognosis and to assign patients to appropriate therapeautic regimes. Moreover, extensive analysis of lympoid tumour cells has led to the view that the pattern of antigens expressed by these cells is consistent with the antigenic phenotypes of normal lympoid cells.[37-39] By analogy with the experience of those who have studied antigen expression by leukemic cells, it will be of interest to determine whether expression of particular antigenic phenotypes by glioma-derived cells is of any prognostic value, either in respect to prediction of longevity or prediction of response to different therapeautic regimes. It will also be of interest to determine whether the fibronectin$^+$ cells derive from gliomas correspond with any cell-types found in the developing or mature CNS, of whether tumours of this tissue can evolve into cells with no detectable relationship with their tissue of origin.

As our knowledge about the different cell-types which make up the CNS continues to grow, and the number of useful molecular and serological markers increases, it will be of continued interest to apply these new tools to the study of gliomas. Although morphologically-based diagnosis, as currently practiced, is of obvious value to the clinician and the patient, it is likely that modifications to current neuropathological practice will enhance our ability to help afflicted individuals. Current experience in related fields suggests that useful modifications will revolve around detailed analysis of the expression of lineage-specific antigens and of the genetic aberrations associated with tumour progression.

References

1. Bailey P, Cushing H. *A classification of the Tumours of the Glioma Group On A Histogenic Basis With a Correlated Study of Prognosis*. Philadephia: Lippincourt, 1926.
2. Kernohan JK, Mabon RF, Svien J, Adson AW. A simplified classification of the gliomas. *Proceedings of the Mayo Clinic*. 1949; **24**, 71–5.
3. Zulch KJ. *Histological Typing of Tumours of the Central Nervous System*. Geneva: World Health Organization, 1979.
4. Small RK, Riddle P, Noble M. Evidence for migration of oligodendrocyte-type-2 astrocyte progenitor cells into the developing rat optic nerve. *Nature*. 1987; **328**, 155–157.
5. Noble M, Fok-Seang J, Cohen J. Glia are a unique substrate for the *in vitro* growth of central nervous system neurons. *Journal of Neuroscience*. 1984; **4**, 1892–1903.
6. Silver J, Sapiro J. Axonal guidance during development of the optic nerve: the role of pigmented epithelia and other intrinsic factors. *Journal of Comparative Neurology*. 1981; **202**, 521–538.

7. Janzer R, Raff MC. Astrocytes induce blood-brain properties in endothelial cells. *Nature.* 1987; **325**, 253-7.
8. Noble M, Murray K. Purified astrocytes promote the *in vitro* division of a bipotential glial progenitor cell. *The EMBO Journal.* 1984; **3**, 2243-7.
9. Noble M, Murray K, Stroobant P, Waterfield M, Riddle P. Platelet-derived growth factor promotes division and motility and inhibits premature differentiation of the oligodendrocyte-type-2 astrocyte progenitor cell. *Nature.* 1988; **333**, 560-2.
10. Raff MC, Lillien LE, Richardson WD, Burne JF, Noble M. Platelet-derived growth factor from astrocytes drives the clock that times oligodendrocyte development in culture. *Nature.* 1988; **333**, 562-5.
11. Raff MC, Miller RH, Noble M. A glial progenitor cell that develops into an astrocyte or an oligodendrocyte depending on the culture medium. *Nature.* 1983; **303**, 390-6.
12. Miller RH, David S, Patel ER, Raff MC. A quantitative immunohistochemical study of macroglial cell development in the rat optic nerve: *in vivo* evidence for two distinct astrocyte lineages. *Developmental Biology.* 1985; **111**, 35-43.
13. French-Constant C, Raff MC. The oligodendrocyte-type-2 astrocyte cell lineage is specialized for myelination. *Nature.* 1986; **323**, 335-8.
14. Miller RH, Fulton B, Raff MC. A novel type of glial cell associated with nodes of Ranvier in rat optic nerve. *European Journal of Neuroscience.* 1989; **1**, 172-80.
15. Wolswijk G, Noble M. Identification of an adult-specific glial progenitor cell. *Development.* 1989; **105**, 387-400.
16. Wolswijk G, Noble M. Co-existence during development of the rat optic nerve of perinatal and adult forms of a glial progenitor cell. (submitted)
17. Noble M, Wolswijk G, Wren D. The complex relationship between cell division and the control of differentiation in oligodendrocyte-type-2 astrocyte progenitor cells isolated from perinatal and adult rat optic nerves. *Progress in Growth Factor Research.* 1989; in press.
18. Price J. Retroviruses and the study of cell lineage. *Development.* 1987; **101**, 409-19.
19. Turner D, Sepko C. Cell lineage in the rat retina: a common progenitor for neurons and glia persists late in development. *Nature.* 1987; **328**, 131-6.
20. Watanabe T, Raff MC. Retinal astrocytes are immigrants from the optic nerve. *Nature.* 1988; **332**, 834-7.
21. Price J. Thurlow L. Cell lineage in the rat cerebral cortex: a study using retroviral-mediated gene transfer. *Development.* 1988; **104**, 473-82.
22. Raff MC, Williams BP, Miller R. The *in vitro* differentiation of a bipotential glial progenitor cell. *The EMBO Journal.* 1984; **3**, 1857-64.
23. Kennedy PGE, Watkins BA, Thomas DGT, Noble M. Antigenic expression by cells derived from gliomas does not correlate with morphological classification. *Neuropathology and Applied Neurobiology.* 1987; **13**, 327-47.
24. Schachner M, Schoonmaker G, Hynes RO. Cellular and subcellular localisation of LETS protein in the nervous system. *Brain Research.* 1978; **158**, 149-58.
25. Stewart GR, Pearlman AL. Fibronectin - like immunoreactivity in the developing cerebral cortex. *Journal of Neurosciences.* 1987; **7**, 3325-33.
26. Bigman A, Eng LF, Dahl D, Uyeda CT. Localisation of the glial fibrillary acidic protein in astrocytes by immunofluorescence. *Brain Research.* 1972; **43**, 429-35.
27. Dahl D, Bignami A. GFAP from normal and gliosed human brain. Demonstration of multiple and related polypeptides. *Biochemica et Biophysica Acta.* 1975; **386**, 41-51.
28. Raff MC, Abney ER, Cohen J, Lindsay R, Noble M. Two types of astrocytes in cultures of developing rat white matter: differences in morphology, surface gangliosides and growth characteristics. *Journal of the Neurosciences.* 1983; **3**, 1289-300.
29. Eisenbarth GS, Walsh FS, Nirenberg M. Monoclonal antibody to a plasma membrane antigen of neurons. *Proceedings of the National Academy of Science of the United States of America.* 1979; **76**, 4913-7.

30. Schnitzer J, Schachner M. Cell type-specificity of neural cell surface antigen recognised by monoclonal antibody A2B5. *Cell and Tissue Research*. 1982; **224**, 625–36.
31. Cohen J, Selvendren SY. A neuronal cell-surface antigen is found in the CNS but not in peripheral neurons. *Nature*. 1981; **291**, 421–3.
32. Miller RH, Williams BP, Cohen J, Raff MC. A4: An Antigenic marker of neural tube-derived cells. *Journal of Neurocytology*. 1984; **13**, 329–38.
33. McKeever PE, Smith BH, Taren JA, Wahl RL, Kornblith PL, Chronwall BM. Products of cells cultured from gliomas. IV; Immunofluorescent, morphometric and ultrastructural characterisation of two different cell types growing from explants of human gliomas. *American Journal of Pathology*. 1987; **127**, 358–72.
34. James CD, Carlbom E, Dumanski JP, Hansen M, Nordenskjold M, Collin VP, Cavaenee WK. Clonal genomic alterations in glioma malignancy stages. *Cancer Research*. 1988; **48**, 5546–5561.
35. Pearson PL, Kidd KK, Willard HF, Human gene mapping by recombinant DNA techniques. *Cytogenetics and Cell Genetics*. 1987; **46**, 390–566.
36. Westermark B, Nister M, Heldin C-H. Growth factors and oncogenes in human malignant glioma. *Neurologic clinics*. 1985; **3**, 785–99.
37. Greaves MF, Janossy G, Peto J, Kay H. Immunologically defined subclasses of acute lymphoblastic leukaemia in children: their relationship to presentation features and prognosis. *British Journal of Haematology*. 1981; **48**, 179–97.
38. Greaves MF. Analysis of the clinical and biological significance of lymphoid phenotypes in acute leukaemia. *Cancer Research*. 1981; **41**, 4752–66.
39. van Eys J, Pullen J, Head D, Boyett J. Crist W, Falletta J, Humphery B, Jackson J, Riccardi V, Brock B. The French-American-British classification of leukaemia – the pediatric oncology group experience with lymphocytic leukaemia. *Cancer*. 1986; **57**, 4752– .
40. Lillien LE, Sendtner M, Rohrer H, Hughes SM, Raff MC. Type-2 astrocyte development in rat brain cultures is initiated by a CNTF-like protein produced by type-1 astrocytes. *Neuron* 1988; **1**, 485–494.
41. Hughes S, Lillien LE, Raff MC, Rohrer H, Sendtner M. Ciliary neurotrophic induces type-2 astrocyte differentiation in culture. *Nature*. 1988; **335**, 70–73.
42. Anderson D. New roles for PDGF and CNTF in development of the nervous system *Trends in Neurosciencce*. 1988; **12**, 83–85.
43. Raff MC. Glial cell diversification in the rat optic nerve. *Science*. 1989; **243**, 1450–1455.
44. Hynes RO, Yamada KM. Fibronectins: multifunctional modular glycoproteins. *Journal of Cell Biology*. 1982; **95**, 369–77.
45. Walsh FS, Moore SE, Dhut S. Monoclonal antibody to human fibronectin: production and characterisation using human muscle cultures. *Developmental Biology*. 1981; **84**, 121–32.

4 Pathology of experimental brain tumours

Geoffrey J Pilkington and Peter L Lantos

Experimental animal brain tumour models which closely resemble human neoplasms histologically and biologically are few. These models are important in cancer research; they enable not only studies on the growth characteristics and basic cell biology of cerebral tumours, but also provide a valuable means for assessing the therapeutic potential of various chemical, immunological and radiological regimens.

The progressive, diffusely invasive nature of gliomas in man makes the study of the early pathogenesis of brain tumours impossible, since by the time the patient presents with the signs of such a lesion it is inevitably well established and large in size. Consequently, a further aim of experimental models is to provide a system in which the early stages of tumour development can be followed. Experimental tumours fall into two categories which carry both distinct advantages and disadvantages: (1) tumours induced by oncogenic agents; (2) transplantable tumours.

Tumours induced by oncogenic agents

There are three major types of oncogenic agents used in the induction of experimental brain tumours: chemical carcinogens, oncogenic viruses, and radiation.

Chemical carcinogens

Polycyclic aromatic hydrocarbons and nitrosocompounds are the two most widely used chemical carcinogens for the induction of brain tumours. Seligman and Shear first reported the induction of experimental brain tumours in mice by polycyclic aromatic hydrocarbons, following the implantation of pellets of compacted crystals of 20'-methylcholanthrene.[1] Subsequently, other compounds, including 1, 2, 5, 6-dibenzanthracene and 3, 4-benzpyrene, were seen to produce tumours in rats and mice;[2, 3] however, guinea pigs, rabbits, ferrets, cats and monkeys appeared to be resistant. The latent period – the time between administration of the carcinogen and the onset of neurological signs of neoplasia – was also variable, according to species, but usually exceeded 200 days.[4] The site of implantation of polycyclic aromatic hydrocarbons also determined the histological type of the tumours formed;[5] chemicals implanted into the cerebral meninges of rats gave rise to only a low incidence of sarcomas while implantation into the paraventricular region consistently resulted in the production of gliomas, the majority of which showed mixed cell populations. The importance of the implantation site for tumour production was confirmed by Hopewell and Wright who implicated the subependymal plate – a layer of undifferentiated cells beneath the ependymal lining of the lateral ventricles – in the formation of pleomorphic gliomas.[6]

The major drawback of polycyclic aromatic hydrocarbons lies in the fact that they are generally not absorbed into the circulation and only dimethylbenzanthrene has been shown to produce neural tumours on systemic administration. In order, therefore, to induce a high incidence of neoplasms, these compounds must be directly implanted into the brain. As a consequence, the chronic inflammatory response resulting from implantation of the chemical masks the early stages of tumour growth. In addition, this system does not yield any information on the natural distribution of neoplasms of the central nervous system.

The discovery of the carcinogenic action of nitrosocompounds by Magee and Barnes in 1956[7] and their subsequent introduction into the field of experimental neuro-oncology, largely through the work of Druckrey and his colleagues, greatly increased the possibilities for the study of the pathogenesis of neural tumours. Nitrosocompounds (nitrosamides and nitrosamines) are formed by the interaction of nitrites and secondary amines.[8] Enzymic metabolic activation is required for the decomposition of nitrosamines, whereupon they yield reactive intermediates.[9, 10] Nitrosamides, however, decompose in the absence of enzymic activity, sulphydryl compounds catalysing the process in some cases (Fig. 4.1). In assessing the carcinogenic potential of 65 nitrosocompounds, Druckrey and his co-workers discovered their organotropic action; they induce tumours in high incidence in a particular organ with a high degree of predictability.[10] The formation of reactive intermediates in the target cells was thought to be responsible for this organotropic action; indeed the production of alkylating metabolites during the breakdown of nitrosocompounds correlated well with their ability to produce tumours. Nitrosamides are neurotropic, inducing tumours preferentially in the nervous system. Two simple nitrosamides, N-methyl-N-nitrosourea (MNU) and N-ethyl-N-nitrosourea (ENU) have proved to be the most potent of neurocarcinogens and produce tumours with morphological and biological similarities to naturally occurring neural neoplasms in man and animals. These compounds may also carry an environmental risk, since they are present in small quantities in various foods. There is, however, no direct evidence that they can cause tumours in the human brain. Certain nitrosamines are present in food such as cured meats, to which preservaties, in the form of nitrites, have been added. Nitrosamides, however, appear to be absent from foodstuffs, but can be manufactured in the body from nitrites and amine precursors. Such nitrites may not only be taken into the body as food preservatives, but also with green vegetables, which contain relatively large amounts of these substances. Nitrates from drinking water can also be converted to nitrites in the body.

Nitrosamide carcinogenesis is influenced by both dose and mode of application as well as the species, age and sex of the experimental animals.[11, 12] Neural neoplasms induced by nitrosamides are not distributed at random, but develop at certain

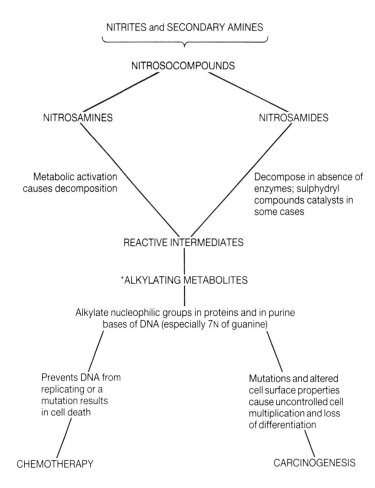

Fig. 4.1 Action of nitrosocompounds

preferential sites within the nervous system; the subcortical white matter and areas adjacent to the lateral ventricles in the brain (Fig. 4.2) and the trigeminal nerves and spinal roots are most commonly affected. In addition, it is not unusual for multiple tumours to arise in a single animal, indeed abnormal cell clusters, microtumours and macroscopic neoplasms may frequently be located in the same brain. The tumours produced are generally gliomas of the central nervous system and schwannomas of the cranial and peripheral nerves.[12, 13] Although neuroblasts have been described in these tumours,[14] neuronal tumours and teratomas are rare.

Since both MNU and ENU have a short half-life and are deactivated rapidly by exposure to alkylating solutions, they can be handled safely. They also have the advantage of the route of administration causing no mechanical trauma to the brain

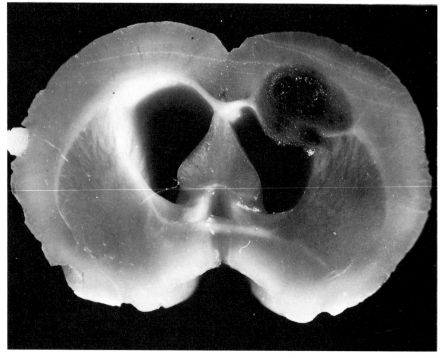

Fig. 4.2 A large haemorrhagic tumour is seen adjacent to and compressing the left lateral ventrice in an ENU-treated rat brain.

and of producing tumours which bear a histological and cell kinetic similarity to human tumours. However, the latency is long, the site of tumour localization not constant and the histological type of the tumour variable.

Both these nitrosoureas induce a high incidence of neoplasms. However, in order to achieve maximal effect, repeated doses of MNU must be given to adult animals, while transplacental or neonatal administration of a single dose of ENU produces a virtually 100 per cent tumour yield.[15, 16] ENU-induced tumourigenesis has been recently reviewed (Lantos 1986; Wechsler 1987).[17, 18]

Tumour induction by ENU provides an ideal system for the examination of the sequential pathogenesis of cerebral neoplasms, since the carcinogen rapidly decomposes *in vivo*[19] and its interaction with the relevant macromolecules can be accurately determined. In order to elucidate the origin of gliomas such studies of pre-neoplastic changes in the early part of the latent period are of paramount importance to the experimental neuro-oncologist.

In vitro analysis of ENU carcinogenesis established that cells endowed with malignant potential were already present in the brains of carcinogen-treated animals during the latent period.[20-22] A preliminary study of rat brains treated transplacentally with ENU revealed small foci of cell proliferations from the eight week post-natally. These lesions consisted chiefly of undifferentiated cells of the subependymal plate type. Moreover, they occurred in the areas in which gliomas predominantly develop and were thought to represent the earliest, histologically detectable changes in the development of brain tumours.[23] Fine structural examination of these early cell proliferations revealed that the cells showed the features of undifferentiated subependymal plate cells: high nuclear–cytoplasmic ratio, scarcity of cell organelles and dominance of free over membrane-bound ribosomes.[24] In the first comprehensive sequential light- and electron-microscopical study of the brains of rats treated transplacentally with ENU, animals were examined at two-weekly intervals between 2 and 20 weeks of age. The first pathological changes in these brains – collections of abnormal, undifferentiated subependymal plate-type cells – were identified from 8 weeks of age onwards, well before the manifestation of neurological signs of neoplasia which generally occur at around 245 days postnatally. These early lesions most commonly occurred at the angle of the lateral ventricles between the corpus callosum and caudate nucleus, the lateral aspect of the lateral ventricles and in the subcortical white matter adjacent to the hippocampus. These clusters of cells were frequently seen around neurones and blood vessels (Fig. 4.3) and were thought to represent the earliest morphologically detectable

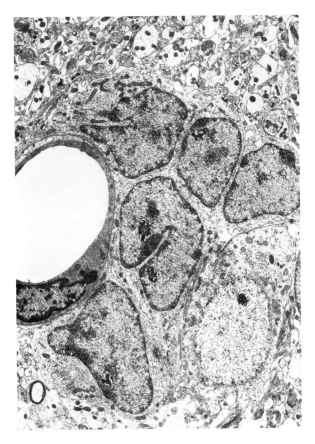

Fig. 4.3 A cluster of poorly differentated subependymal plate cells is seen adjacent to a neuron and a small blood vessel.

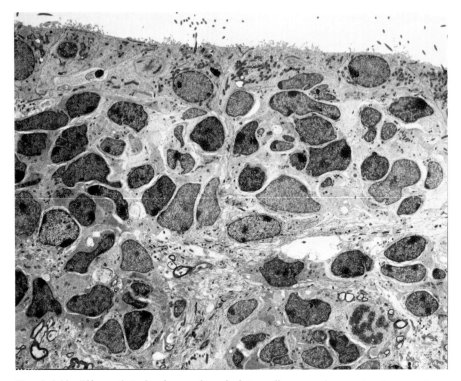

Fig. 4.4 Undifferentiated subependymal plate cells comprise a microtumour in an 18-week-old ENU-treated rat. (Reproduced by permission of Springer Verlag GmbH & Co. from Pilkington and Lantos. *Acta Neuropathologica* (Berlin), 1979; **45**: 177–85.)

changes in the development of cerebral gliomas.[25] In addition, focal cellular hyperplasia was often detected in the subependymal plate region itself. Between 16 and 20 weeks of age microtumours (detectable only upon microscopical examination) composed of subependymal plate cells, glioblasts and various glial cells at different stages of maturation were found.[26] Electron microscopy confirmed that not only were the abnormal cell clusters composed chiefly of subependymal plate-type cells, but that microtumours also contained a considerable proportion of these stem cells. In some microtumours subependymal plate cells and glioblasts predominated (Fig. 4.4); however glial differentiation was generally evident and astrocytic, ependymal and mixed oligodendrocytic–astrocytic maturation were all encountered. A considerable degree of cellular pleomorphism was, therefore, apparent and the invasive nature of the tumours was never in question. The high mitotic rate, haemorrhage, destruction of normal structures and cell necrosis proved that ENU-induced gliomas were already malignant at an early stage of their development.

The morphology of gliomas arising from the subependymal plate is seen to be determined by the diverging processes of anaplasia and differentiation which results in a pleomorphic cell population (Fig. 4.5). The pathogenesis of ENU-induced

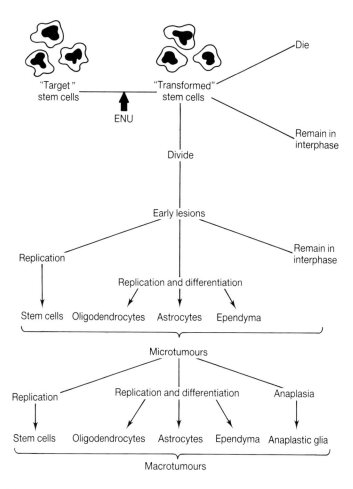

Fig. 4.5 Theoretical scheme for the cellular pathogenesis of ENU-induced brain tumours.

gliomas, therefore, is compatible with the hypothesis that tumours arising from stem cells are composed of various subpopulations of cells which retain the potential to differentiate and may simulate the normal cellular maturation sequence.[27, 28] An alternative view, however, suggests that experimentally induced brain tumours originate from differentiated cells by dedifferentiation.

In the brains of rats and rabbits treated with MNU, a proliferation of oligodendrocytes appeared to be the initial step in the pathogenesis of gliomas; these cells showed a more rapid response to the carcinogenic stimulus than did other glial cells[29] which became numerous only in larger tumours.[30] As foci of oligodendrocytes have been reported in the cortex and basal ganglia of rats treated transplacentally with ENU,[31] a dual pathogenesis for ENU-induced gliomas seems to be the most plausible explanation.[32] Oligodendrogliomas thus develop from these early oligodendrocytic proliferations whilst all other gliomas owe their origins to the subependymal plate cells.

The subependymal plate, with its mitotically active cells also exists in man and, although its cell population decreases throughout life, some of its undifferentiated cells still persist, even in adult human brains.[33] Moreover, tumours thought to have originated from the subependymal plate have been described.[34-36] There are, however, differences between human and ENU-induced gliomas. In particular, while multiple neoplasms at different stages of development can, and frequently does, occur in rats, gliomas in man are generally solitary lesions. In addition, some experimental tumours, notably ependymomas, are often less well differentiated than their human counterparts.

The interaction between the carcinogen and the subependymal plate cells may take place around the time of birth, when mitotic activity (a prerequisite for carcinogenesis) is at its peak, or in later life. Transformed cells may either die, remain in interphase or divide after a latency of varying length. This mitotic activity will result in small groups of abnormal cells which may become stationary or further mitotic activity will result in the formation of microtumours and macrotumours. The dividing stem cells may either follow a single line of maturation to give rise to astrocytomas, oligodendrogliomas or ependymomas or they may retain their potential to differentiate into the various types of glia and thereby produce mixed gliomas. This hypothesis for the pathogenesis of experimental gliomas suggests that some, if not all, human gliomas originate from the subependymal plate. In addition, it highlights the vulnerability of the developing nervous system to carcinogens and supports the view that foetuses carried by mothers exposed to environmental carcinogens may be at particular risk. Morever, it may be extrapolated from the long latency of ENU-induced gliomas that some human gliomas manifested during adult life may be the result of intrauterine exposure to carcinogens.

Tumour induction by nitrosourea compounds has contributed to the understanding of the molecular mechanisms underlying the development of malignancy. The formation and retention, as a result of a deficient repair mechanism, of O^6-alkylguanine in DNA have been associated with tumour induction in rats (for recent review see ref. 37). Molecular biology of ENU-induced rat brain tumours identified a new oncogene, *neu*, which is detectable by transfection into mouse NIH 3TC cells.[38, 39] This oncogene is related to, but distinct from, the gene encoding the EGF receptor (c-erb-B).[40, 41] It is not known whether the activation of *neu* is an early or late event in tumourigenesis, but recent results indicate that *neu* encodes for the receptor for an as yet unidentified growth factor.[42] The molecular genetics of nervous system tumours, including those induced by chemicals and viruses, have been recently reviewed.[43] Tumourigenesis in the central nervous system by nitrosourea compounds has lent support to the hypothesis that malignant transformation is a multi-step process. Structural alteration, in this case alkylation of the DNA molecule of target cells, is likely to be the initiating step, whilst subsequent stages of transformation are influenced by promoting and inhibiting factors. Further studies on oncogene abnormalities, growth factors and immunological mechanisms will shed light on changes occurring during latency which culminate in the appearance of clinically overt neoplasia.

Oncogenic viruses

Cerebral neoplasms have been induced by both intracranial and subcutaneous inoculation of viruses in a number of different species.[44] Both RNA and DNA viruses can be used to induce neural neoplasia,[45, 46] the neoplastic transformation of glial cells differing according to the nature of the nucleic acid.

Polyoma virus can produce tumours in 70 per cent of hamsters with a latency of 30 days or less, while Rous sarcoma virus produces tumours as soon as two weeks post-inoculation in 75 per cent of experimental dogs. The latter virus has become widely used in the production of neural neoplasia. Bucciarelli et al.[47] induced gliomas in hamsters and Bigner et al.[48] induced astrocytic tumours in puppies using the Schmidt–Ruppin strain of Rous sarcoma virus (SR-RSV). However, when chicken sarcoma cells producing SR-RSV were inoculated into the brains of mice they produced gliomas and "huge round cell tumours".[49-51] The "huge round cell tumours" occurred earlier and were more frequent than the gliomas (glioblastomas and astrocytomas) but, since they frequently produced reticulin fibres, their glial nature proved to be controversial.

Vick et al.[52] have also produced gliomas in neonatal dogs with subgroup C Bratislava-77 Avian sarcoma virus by intracerebral inoculation and a high incidence in inbred Fischer[53] and random-bred Sprague–Dawley rats[54] using the same virus.

Among the DNA viruses, adenovirus 12 has been used to produce brain tumours in mice, rats and hamsters while the JC strain of papovavirus has successfully induced medulloblastomas and glioblastomas in hamsters. The neuro-oncogenicity of human viruses, particularly three DNA viruses (adenovirus 12, polyoma virus JC and BK) has been recently reviewed.[55] Both JC and BK viruses penetrate the blood–brain barrier and produce a high tumour yield after a latency of several months. JC polyoma virus produced a wide spectrum of intrinsic tumours, including medulloblastomas, neuroblastomas, ependymomas, high-grade astrocytomas, choroid plexus papillomas and pineocytomas. The central nervous system was extensively involved and the tumours tended to grow diffusely. In contrast BK virus-induced growths were more restricted to the ventricular lining and choroid plexus. Tumours produced by adenovirus 12 arose around the ventricular system and were similar histologically to primitive childhood tumours, such as medulloblastomas and medulloepitheliomas. Interestingly, none of these viruses induced oligodendrogliomas or low-grade astrocytomas.

Virus-induced tumours have four advantages over other model systems: they have a predictable latency, their cell cycle time is similar to that of human gliomas, the small needle used for inoculation causes minimal mechanical trauma to the brain, and the resulting autochthonous cerebral tumours have a blood supply similar to that of spontaneous tumours.

Brain tumour models induced by oncogenic viruses have mainly been used in the study of viral tumourigenesis and tumour immunology. However chemotherapeutic trials have also been carried out on such systems.

Radiation

Although radiation has been shown to induce neural neoplasms in a range of mammals, including monkeys, rabbits, guinea-pigs and mice, it is still a relatively poorly documented method. Although the central nervous system has been damaged by X-rays, protons, neutrons, radioactive cobalt (^{60}C) and radioactive gold (^{198}Au), the incidence of neural tumours has been disappointingly low. The major problem is that the dose given to the animal is critical: high doses give rise to malformations while low doses fail to produce tumours. The latency of neoplasms induced by radiation is much longer (up to five years after treatment) than that of chemically or virally induced tumours. The long latency and low incidence reported suggest that some of these tumours might be naturally occurring gliomas. Therefore experimental data for radiation-exposed animals should be carefully examined.

Despite these difficulties of experimental models, radiation remains an important cause of cerebral neoplasia. Iatrogenic induction of gliomas, although rare, has been convincingly demonstrated in man. Radiation-induced human gliomas have been recently reviewed: histologically these neoplasms are astrocytomas or glioblastomas.[56]

Transplantable tumours

Transplanted brain tumour models include any neural neoplasm – irrespective of its original mode of induction – which is capable of serial passage in an animal host. Such tumours can be divided into two groups.

Syngeneic tumours

These are tumours which may be of spontaneous origin or may be chemically or virally induced and are subsequently transplanted intracerebrally, subcutaneously or intramuscularly into an animal of the same species and strain.

Heterotransplanted tumours

These may be defined as tumours which are transplanted from one species or strain of animal to another. Transplantation in this case is either into an immunodeficient animal or into an "immunologically privileged site" (e.g. brain, cheek pouch or anterior chamber of the eye) of an immunocompetent animal.

Neoplasms may be transplanted into host brains either directly in the form of tumour explants or cellular homogenates of tumour tissue which has been disaggregated by treatment with a suitable protease such as collagenase, the former retaining some degree of histoarchitectural stability for a period, while the latter may permit more satisfactory invasion of the host brain by neoplastic cells. In addition, tumour material may be removed from the donor and maintained as monolayer tissue cultures, then trypsinized, brought into suspension and injected into the host. In this case selection for the most malignant, tumourigenic cells may take place *in vitro*. Cells at later *in vitro* passage are generally more tumourigenic and faster growing than those at earlier passage. However, the former carry the disadvantage of their rapid growth resulting in a transplanted tumour which grows by expansion rather than invasion (Fig. 4.6). In addition, some workers have chosen to inject cells which have been maintained in three-dimensional tissue culture as multicellular tumour

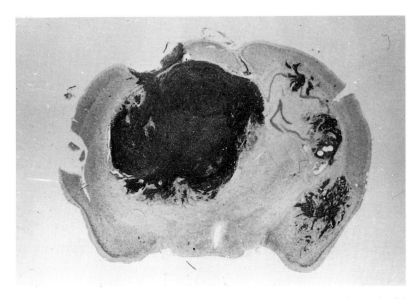

Fig. 4.6 Injection of rapidly growing VMDk P497 cells into the left cerebral hemisphere of a VM mouse has produced a large tumour which has grown by expansion rather than invasion. Cords of neoplastic cells from the main tumour mass have given rise to three lesions in the right hemisphere. (Reproduced by permission of Elsevier Science Publishers B.V., from Pilkington, et al. Journal of the Neurological Sciences, 1985: 71: 145-64.)

spheroids;[57] inoculation of such groups of cells may facilitate improved tumour "take" rates with certain cell lines. Cells may be inoculated by stereotaxic means rather than by "free" injection on the basis that dissimilar growth patterns may result from implantation into different regions of the brain (Fig. 4.7). However, variations in growth patterns have been noted for several cloned cell lines implanted stereotaxically[58] and this, together with the length of the procedure, when large numbers of animals are to be injected, has led to "free" injection being the method of choice for most experimenters.

Although syngeneic transplantable brain tumours of viral and spontaneous origin have been described, reports have been concentrated around the chemically induced transplantable models which fall into two main groups; mouse tumours originally induced by polycyclic hydrocarbons and rat tumours originally induced by nitrosoureas.

The predictability of site, latency and histology render syngeneic transplanted brain tumours particularly suitable for testing therapeutic regimens. Although by the late 1960s a number of animal brain tumour models were in use for drug testing, these were systems in which glial tumours were grown subcutaneously or non-glial tumours, such as the L1210 mouse leukaemia cell line, grown intracerebrally. Mouse leukaemia cell lines, however, have been shown to exhibit different chemosensitivities from glioma cell lines and therefore have proved to be a poor model for chemotherapy studies in relation to brain tumours. It was not until the development

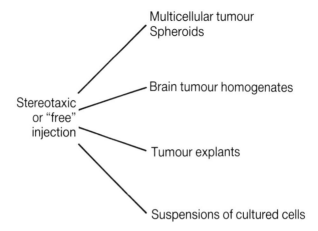

Fig. 4.7 Transplantation methods for brain tumours

of the transplantable murine ependymoblastoma[59] that an intracerebrally transplantable glial neoplasm was available for chemotherapy screening.

The murine ependymoblastoma was originally induced by implantation of a methylcholanthrene pellet into the brain of a mouse.[2] From this tumour a transplantable model was developed and a sub-line (ependymoblastoma A) was established.[59] Two further models, glioma 261 and glioma 26, also derived from methylcholanthrene-induced tumours[1, 60] were serially transplanted by Ausman and his co-workers. They found that the median survival following inoculation of ependymoblastoma cells in 26 groups of C57BL/6 mice was 29 ± 3 days. This consistent latent period led to its use as a chemotherapy screen[61] and in the study of the different effects of chemotherapy regimens on DNA.[62]

Muller et al.[63] concurred that the growth pattern and survival times of the ependymoblastoma implanted both peripherally and intracranially in non-nude C57Bl/6J mice were both consistent and predictable. They also found that a greater cell dose was required to generate peripheral tumours than brain tumours; a feature which may result from a greater immunological response to tumour implanted peripherally than that implanted into the "immunologically privileged" brain.

Chemotherapeutic agents can be tested against the ependymoma at both intracerebral and peripheral sites in order to establish whether the location of the tumour or its cellular sensitivity influences the efficacy of the drug. After extensive use of the model for drug screening trials the results have generally been consistent with the findings of human clinical brain tumour trials.[64] The model is economical, predictable and reproducible, has a statistically amenable latency and, unlike many other systems, has remained histologically stable. However, the ependymoblastoma is a rare tumour in man and cells of the murine ependymoblastoma lack many of the fine structural features of ependymal cells.[65] Moreover, the cell kinetics are also unlike those of human tumours[66] and murine mammary tumour virus particles and murine C-type viral structural antigens, thought to be endogenous retroviruses, have been detected in the cells of this tumour line.[67, 68]

Of the cell lines derived from nitrosourea-induced tumours, which have been successfully transplanted, the best characterized is the C6 clone.[69] This clone was originally obtained from a MNU-induced tumour in a random-bred Wistar-Furth rat. This non-inbred origin, however, has resulted in a lack of predictability in its propensity for transplantation. Although the C6 clone has been shown to express the "brain-specific" proteins S-100[70] and glial fibrillary acidic protein (GFAP)[71] in culture systems, it has been reported to undergo sarcomatous degeneration on serial transplantation and therefore its use as an *in vivo* system has been restricted. However, Auer *et al.*[72] produced a 100 per cent incidence of brain tumours, with a dose-dependent mean latency of 16–27 days, following intracerebral injection of newborn rats with C6 cells and classified them histologically as glioblastoma multiforme.

The 9L rat gliosarcoma is another transplantable tumour which was originally derived from an MNU-induced tumour. Benda *et al.*[73] established several cloned cell lines from gliomas which resulted from transplantation experiments with the original chemically induced tumour.[74] Although these clones were reported to maintain an astrocytic morphology and stable growth response in serial passage, 9L (produced by injection of one of these clones) has shown a sarcomatous nature on subsequent *in vivo* passage.[75] The transplantable 9L system, however, is reproducible and has, in consequence, been used extensively for chemotherapeutic and cell kinetic studies.

Ethylnitrosourea-induced tumours have also proved to be transplantable. One such tumour – glioma RG2 – was induced by ENU in inbred CD Fischer 344 rats and serially transplanted in syngeneic animals.[76] This tumour also retains various glial characteristics, including the presence of S-100 protein, on continued transplantation.

A further cell line – A15 A5 – cloned at the 28th passage from a parent culture (A15), was also derived from an ENU-induced pleomorphic glioma in a BDIX rat.[77] This clone has been extensively characterized *in vitro* and shows a number of glial features including the presence of 10 nm intermediate filaments and expression of the astrocytic markers, GFAP and glutamine synthetase.[78]

Davaki and Lantos[79, 80] injected the A15A5 clone into the brains of syngeneic BDIX rats and produced a 100 per cent tumour incidence at a dose of 5×10^5 cells. Malignancy was related to the *in vitro* passage of the cells: earlier passages produced less malignant tumours, containing better differentiated astrocytes than later passages. A sequential fine structural study also revealed that small tumours (one to two weeks post-inoculation) contained numerous fibrillary astrocytes, while in larger tumours (three to four weeks post-inoculation) the ratio of undifferentiated astrocytes to fibrillary astrocytes increased substantially. Variations in differentiation between cells of tumours produced by cells at different passages have also been detected immunocytochemically. Saggu and Pilkington[81] reported an inverse relationship between the expression of the astrocytic markers, GFAP and glutamine synthetase at low (10th) and high (40th) passage: GFAP decreased with increasing passage, while glutamine synthetase increased. This anaplastic change in the tumours may not correlate with the pathogenesis of human glial tumours and therefore this feature must be considered a disadvantage of such a model for chemotherapeutic studies.

Anaplastic change is, in fact, a common feature of transplanted tumour systems. This was well demonstrated by Yoshida and Cravioto[82] who compared two neural tumours which had been serially passaged *in vitro* and *in vivo*. The transplanted tumours, EA-652, a schwannoma originally induced by ENU and EA-285, a glioma originally induced by MNU, were both developed in CDF rats. Although these were easily distinguishable neoplasms, following serial *in vivo* passage the tumours appeared histologically identical. Similarly, after 20 *in vitro* passages cultured cells became indistinguishable by light microscopy, although fine structural examination revealed differences between the two lines, even after 87 passages.

Virus-induced tumours have rarely been transplanted into syngeneic animals successfully. Two models, however, have been developed which deserve further consideration.

The cultured line S69-C_5 derived from an avian sarcoma virus-induced anaplastic astrocytoma in an inbred F344 rat has been shown to transplant well, but reports on its stability on serial passage have not been forthcoming.[83]

Wodinsky *et al.*[84] produced an 87 per cent incidence of leptomeningeal sarcomas and cerebral gliomas after intracerebral inoculation of Rous sarcoma virus (S-R strain) in neonatal beagle dogs. A malignant glioblastoma was serially transplanted with cell suspensions or fragments of tissue from one of these virus-induced tumours. Histologically the tumour was composed of swollen, round, polygonal to stellate-shape astroblasts and gemistocytic astrocytes and showed a high mitotic index. Four cell lines derived from these tumours were subsequently established in culture. Although this model has the advantage of providing a larger brain for study, serial *in vivo* passage has resulted in the production of highly malignant tumours with an extremely short latency. The tumours also reverted to a sarcomatous pattern on microscopical examination.[66]

Reports of serially transplantable spontaneous animal brain tumours are also scarce. Fraser[85] described anaplastic astrocytomas in the inbred VM mouse strain, which could be serially transplanted into syngeneic mice by inoculation of cell homogenates.[86-88] A series of 85 transplantations into syngeneic mice was carried out from a spontaneous astrocytoma in a 168-day-old female VM mouse by intracerebral injection by tumour-bearing brain homogenates (Fig. 4.8). Injection of homogenates into other strains (C57BL and C3H) of mice failed to induce tumours.

In Fraser's series of experiments tumour-bearing mouse brain was trypsinized and suspended in culture medium, then injected subcutaneously or intracerebrally into syngeneic mice. Subcutaneous injections failed to produce tumours, but intracerebral injection gave rise to tumours at a latency up to 176 days. This latent period varied, but was reduced with serial passage (mean incubation time over 85 serial passages was 25-30 days). Long-term survivors, however, still existed and there was no obvious relationship between tumour take, latency and number of cells injected. Long-term survivors of both intracranial and subcutaneous injections were further challenged by intracerebral injection. Animals which had previously received intracerebral injections of cells were resistant to this second challenge but those which had previously been injected subcutaneously developed brain tumours. This subcutaneous inoculation did not confer immunity on the mice, but those which were resistant to the first intracerebral injection proved to be resistant also to further intracerebral challenge.

Serano *et al.*[89,90] have derived a number of tumourigenic cell lines from the spontaneous VM astrocytoma model. Three of these cell lines, VMDk P560, P540 and P497, have been exhaustively characterized *in vitro* and *in vivo*. Although electron

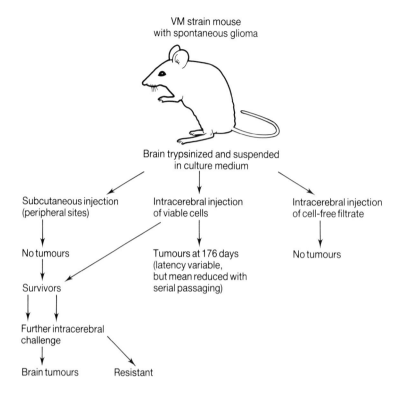

Fig. 4.8 Derivation of Fraser's (1975) spontaneous, transplantable, murine astrocytoma.

microscopy revealed differences in the number and ratio of 10 nm intermediate filaments and 24 nm microtubules in the three lines, a feature related to the degree of cellular differentiation,[91] they all displayed astrocytic features, including the presence of GFAP and glutamine synthetase and showed an enhanced arborization of cell processes on exposure to dibutyryl adenosine-3', 5'-cyclic monophosphate (dbcAMP).[92] *In vitro* growth properties of the cells correlated well with the extent of their differentiation.[93] When VMDk cells were injected intracerebrally into syngeneic mice the best differentiated cell line (P560) failed to produce gliomas while transplantation of the least well differentiated cell line (P497) resulted in a 100 per cent tumour incidence and line P540, intermediate in its level of differentiation, caused only a 5 per cent incidence.[94] The latent period in each case was related to the number of cells injected; the greater the cell number used, the shorter the latency. Although tumours produced by P497 have a consistent, short latency, they possess two disadvantages; intracerebral growth tends to be by expansion rather than invasion and the number of brain tumours with accompanying extracranial components is high. P540, however, although showing limited tumourigenicity *in vivo* produces invasive astrocytomas and may, therefore, by selective propagation *in vitro*, provide the best of these murine glioma models.

Light- and electron-microscopical studies of the tumours confirmed their glial nature; features such as invasiveness, high mitotic index, and pseudopalisading around areas of necrosis, determined the diagnosis as either anaplastic astrocytoma or glioblastoma multiforme.[94] Some tumours showed a pilocytic pattern of fusiform cells, some of which stained positively for PTAH: however immunocytochemical staining for the astrocytic markers GFAP and glutamine synthetase and for vimentin (the intermediate filament protein which predominates in immature and poorly-differentiated glia) suggest that the tumours are composed chiefly of poorly-differentiated neoplastic glial cells. A fine reticulin pattern – frequently seen to surround individual neoplastic cells – throughout the tumours (Fig. 4.9) and the expression of the basal lamina proteins, fibronectin and laminin, confirm the potential of neoplastic glia to express inappropriate proteins following *in vitro* propagation and subsequent *in vivo* passaging and highlights the plasticity of neoplastic cells. The P497 cell line has recently been cloned[95] and five of the six resultant clones possess tumourigenic potential.[96]

The syngeneic transplanted brain tumour models outlined above have a number of advantages.

(i) The transplantation procedure promotes selection of cells which are most resistant to host defences and therefore produces quite rapidly-growing, consistent tumours.
(ii) The simplicity of the technique permits the use of large numbers of animals at relatively low expense.
(iii) *In vitro* propagaton of cells may be carried out in parallel to *in vivo* passaging.

There are, however, several disadvantages inherent in the technique.

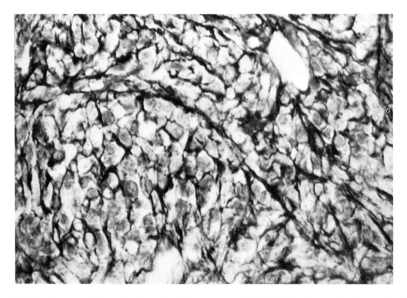

Fig. 4.9 A fine meshwork of reticulin surrounds individual neoplastic cells in a tumour produced in the mouse brain by transplantation of VMDK cells.

(i) Trauma to the brain caused by the injection or implantation procedure results in damage to the brain parenchyma and its vascular system, leading to breakdown of the structural blood–brain barrier.
(ii) Tumour lines often show a tendency to develop a more sarcomatous and less glial appearance on serial passage.
(iii) Glial-specific antigens expressed by cells *in vitro* are frequently absent from resulting tumours.
(iv) When chemotherapy is started soon after transplantation the tumour lacks its own vasculature and the neoplastic cells are nourished by extracellular fluid at the site of implantation; therefore a false environment is likely to be assessed.
(v) There is a questionable similarity between experimentally induced, transplantable animal brain tumours and spontaneous human gliomas.

The last problem has concerned scientists for many years. In order to study human rather than animal gliomas *in vivo* heterotransplantation into host animals has been carried out. The xenogeneic nature of the tumour, however, causes a host immune response which, together with differences in the nature of the supporting stroma, normally prevents successful tumour take.

This problem has long been recognized and attempts have been made to implant human tumours into the brains of animals since the late nineteenth century. The first successful heterografts of human brain tumours were reported in 1944 by Freeman and Zimmerman,[97] who carried out implants into the anterior chamber of the eye of mice and guinea pigs. Extended growth of such tumours could, however, only rarely be achieved. More recently Gluszcz *et al.*[98] reported the growth of 10 out of 54 gliomas which had been transplanted into the anterior eye chamber of guinea pigs. The hamster cheek pouch, however, has not proved to be a suitable site for the growth of human gliomas.

Although the brain, along with the anterior chamber of the eye and the cheek pouch, is considered to be an "immunologically privileged" site, attempts at heterotransplantation of human gliomas into the animal brain initially met with little success.[99-100] Nevertheless, Manuelidis[102] successfully transplanted human glioblastomas into both the guinea pig eye and brain and examined them histologically at a series of sequential passages. At early passage the tumours resembled the human neoplasms from which they were derived but at later passages their pleomorphic cell population changed to give rise to a predominantly spindle-shaped cell population. He also found that although a tumour, when transplanted into both eye and brain, retained its histological similarity, it showed differences in growth rate and chromosome number.

The next stage in the development of satisfactory brain heterotransplantation involved the irradiation and thymectomy of hamsters[103, 104] and mice.[105-108] These animals became immunodeficient and showed a greater propensity to accept heterotransplants. However, the complexities and expense involved in irradiating and thymectomizing large numbers of animals rendered this method less than ideal. The advent of the athymic nude mouse – a congenitally immunodeficient animal – was therefore of some singificance.[109]

The potential of the nude mouse as a host for heterotransplants was first realized with the acceptance of a rat skin graft.[110] Numerous further heterotransplants were made from a variety of animal species and subsequently a human colonic tumour was transplanted; this grew and was then serially passaged.[110]

The nude mouse tumour system offers three specific functions: (i) testing the sensitivity of individual patient's tumours against various antineoplastic drugs; (ii) screening of new drugs against a wide range of human tumours; (iii) the possible remedy of immunodeficient syndromes associated with malignant disease by immunopotentiation methods.

Extensive studies, in which a wide range of human tumours and human tumour-derived cell lines were implanted into nude mice, took place during the last decade. Fogh and Hajdu[111] carried out the subcutaneous inoculation of nude mice with 169 cell lines derived from 169 different human tumours and established 103 tumour-producing lines including a three out of 10 take for glioblastoma, one out of one for meningioma and one out of three for neuroblastoma.

Rana et al.[112] also reported the successful subcutaneous transplantation and growth of a human glioblastoma and meningioma in nude mice, and retention of their unique histological features. Both tumours, however, contained scattered A-type virus particles and mature C-type particles. Their assumption was that these were xenotropic viruses of the mouse, i.e. viruses which cannot be shown to multiply in mouse cells but which grow freely in transplanted cells from other species.[113]

Wara et al.[114] established cultures of various brain tumours, including glioblastoma multiforme, malignant glioma and medulloblastoma, and injected these into the flanks of nude mice. These tumours were subsequently transplanted over several passages with no change in histological appearance. Bradley et al.,[108] having successfully propagated 13 gliomas as subcutaneous xenografts in immuno-deprived or nude mice, concurred that the tumours remained histologically stable even after several serial passages. These tumours were from both children and adults: two out of 30 (6.7 per cent) paediatric tumours grew (a medulloblastoma and a grade III astrocytoma), while 11 out of 25 (44 per cent) adult tumours grew (mainly grade III astrocytomas).

Normally the growth rate of tumours transplanted into nude mice remains constant, irrespective of the number of in vivo passages. However, some tumours, including a grade IV astrocytoma, have shown a gradual increase in growth rate as selection for the fastest growing neoplastic cells occurs.[115] The growth rates of seven human brain tumours which had been transplanted, both subcutaneously and intracerebrally, into nude mice[116] also increased during serial transplantation after explant. The tumours, however, generally paralleled those in patients in their growth rates, but only gliosarcomas developed into long-term serial lines.

Kindred and Wechsler compared the growth of a series of xenogeneic rat tumour clones of the nervous system in nude mice and in syngeneic rats.[117] These tumour clones of the central and peripheral nervous systems were derived from primary and transplantable neurogenic tumours experimentally induced in inbred BDIX and Fischer CDF rats by transplacental administration of ENU. Cells were injected subcutaneously into syngeneic rats and BALB/c nude mice and tumour growth was monitored by measurement of tumour diameter. The latent period (period between injection and appearance of tumour) was related to the number of cells injected in both syngeneic rats and nude mice; the fewer cells injected, the longer the latency. However, in nude mice, producing a tumour was not simply a matter of the number of cells injected and the growth rate; the period between the appearance of tumour and its reaching a diameter of 10 mm changed only in the most rapidly growing tumours, thereby indicating that, once established, the tumours grew at approximately the same rate.

Although early reports suggested that human tumours retained their morphological stability on serial passaging in athymic mice, more recent studies have indicated that not only the histological pattern of the tumours, but also their antigenic characteristics may undergo change.

In a study of the morphology and GFAP content of 16 malignant astrocytic brain tumours which had been grown subcutaneously in nude mice Jones et al. concluded that while these gliomas retained some features of the tumours from which they were derived, they varied from one another morphologically.[118] They also continued to evolve, often raising or lowering their GFAP levels and showing an increased cellularity with serial passage.

Of 21 attempts at the heterotransplantation of malignant glial tumours into nude mice, Horten et al.[119] achieved 16 successful takes with a further tumour being transplanted into the brain following subcutaneous propagation. These xenografts generally grew as diffusely infiltrating tumours in the hemispheric white matter. The histological heterogeneity of the human gliomas was noted to disappear in serial passage, giving rise to tumours composed to a generally uniform cell type.

When injected into nude mice, established cell lines derived from human gliomas remained morphologically stable, but although a consistent latency and growth rate developed, the tumours became morphologically less distinct at later passages.[120]

Bigner et al.[121] used morphological, immunological and biochemical criteria to assess whether four permanent cell lines, derived from human gliomas and found to be tumourigenic in nude mice, could be distinguished from 11 other similarly derived cell lines which showed an inability to grow in athymic hosts. Although they concluded that the *in vitro* criteria of transformation are not synonymous with nude mouse tumourigenicity among human glioma-derived cell lines, they suggested that it may be possible to preselect tumourigenic cultures from both early passage and established lines for developing tumours in athymic mice by assessment of their cell biological characteristics.

Although the advent of the nude mouse provided the neuro-oncologist with a potent and reliable means of heterotransplantation, the technique has not been without its problems. Since the nude mouse is unable to recognize non-self, it is much more likely to succumb to infection and under conventional conditions its lifespan is short; perhaps four to six months. Animal husbandry is consequently much more demanding and even specific pathogen-free conditions only increase the life expectancy to about 10 months.

It is a fact that not all human implants will grow in nude mice: the determining factor for tumourigenicity remains unclear. There is often a lag period prior to the initiation of tumour growth which may be due to the inability of the implanted tumour to obtain adequate vascularization from its new host. The selection of certain cell populations or transplantation and serial passage also results in a modification of cell kinetics which may distort the information obtained from this model. The system is also limited in that human tumours are growing in a mouse stroma and the metabolic processes of the environment in which they proliferate are those of the mouse and not of man.[122] Thus a reproducible, transplantable spontaneous glial neoplasm in a small mammal which can be propagated *in vitro* and transplanted syngeneically may offer a more suitable model for the study of human gliomas.

References

1. Seligman AM, Shear MJ. Studies in carcinogenesis. VIII. Experimental production of brain tumors in mice with methylcholanthrene. *American Journal of Cancer.* 1939; **37**, 364–5.
2. Zimmerman HM, Arnold H. Experimental brain tumors: I. Tumors produced with methylcholanthrene. *Cancer Research.* 1941; **I**, 919–38.
3. Zimmerman HM, Arnold H. Experimental brain tumours. II. Tumours produced with benzpyrene. *American Journal of Pathology.* 1943; **19**, 939–55.
4. Janisch W, Schreiber D. *Experimentelle Geschwulste des Zentralnervensystems.* Jena: Gustav Fischer Verlag, 1969: 25–34.
5. Zimmerman HM. Brain tumors: their incidence and classification in man and their experimental production. *Annals of the New York Academy of Sciences.* 1969; **159**, 337–59.
6. Hopewell JW, Wright EA. The importance of implantation site in cerebral carcinogenesis in rats. *Cancer Research.* 1969; **29**, 1927–31.
7. Magee PN, Barnes HJM. The production of malignant primary hepatic tumours in the rat by feeding dimethylnitrosoamine. *British Journal of Cancer.* 1956; **10**, 114–22.
8. Ivankovic S, Preussmann R. Transplazentare Erzeugung maligner Tumoren nach oraler Gabe von Athylharnstoff und Nitric an Ratten. *Naturwissenschaften.* 1970; **57**, 460.
9. Magee PN, Barnes HJM. Carcinogenic nitroso compounds. *Advances in Cancer Research.* 1967; **10**, 163–246.
10. Druckrey H, Preussmann R, Ivankonic S, Schmahl D. Organotrope carcinogene Wirtkungen bei 65 verschiedenen *N*-Nitroso-Verbindungen an BD-Ratten. *Zeitschrift für Krebsforschung.* 1967; **69**, 103–201.
11. Janisch W, Schreiber D. In: Bigner DD, Swenberg JA, eds. *Experimental Tumours of the Central Nervous System.* Kalamazoo: Upjohn, 1977.
12. Kleihues P, Lantos PL, Magee PN. Carcinogenesis in the nervous system. *International Reviews of Experimental Pathology.* 1976; **15**, 360–408.
13. Wechsler W, Kleihues P, Matsumoto S, Zulch KL, Ivankovic S, Preussmann R, Druckrey H. Pathology of experimental neurogenic tumors chemically induced during prenatal and postnatal life. *Annals of the New York Academy of Sciences.* 1969; **159**, 360–408.
14. Lantos PL, Pilkington GJ. Neuroblasts in cerebral tumours induced by ethylnitrosourea in rats. A fine structural study. *Virchows Archiv B: Cell Pathology.* 1977; **25**, 243–59.
15. Druckrey H, Landschutz C, Ivankovic S. Transplacentare Erzeugung maligner Tumoren des Nervensystems. II. Athyl-nitrosoharnstoff an 10 genetisch definierten Rattenstammen. *Zietschrift für Krebsforschung.* 1970; **73**, 371–86.
16. Druckrey H, Schagen B, Ivankovic S. Erzeugung neurogener Malignome durch einmalige Gabe von Athyl-nitrosoharnstoff (ANH) an neugeborene und junge BD IX-Ratten. *Zeitschrift für Krebsforschung.* 1970; **74**, 141–61.
17. Lantos PL. Development of nitrosourea-induced brain tumours – with a special note on changes occurring during latency. *Food and Chemical Toxicology* (Oxford). 1986; **24**, 121–7.
18. Wechsler W. Experimental malignant gliomas: pathology and transplantation biology of ENU-induced rat tumours. In: Grundmann E, ed. *Cancer Campaign.* Vol. 10, Experimental Neurooncology, Brain Tumor and Pain Therapy. Stuttgart-New York: Gustav Fischer, 1987: 145–68.
19. Swann PF, Magee PN. Nitrosamine-induced carcinogenesis. The alkylation of N-7 of guanine of nucleic acids of the rat by diethylnitrosamine, *N*-ethyl-*N*-nitrosourea and ethyl methanesulphonate. *Biochemical Journal.* 1971; **125**, 841–7.

20. Laerum OD, Rajewsky MF. Neoplastic transformation of fetal rat brain cells in culture after exposure to ethylnitrosourea *in vivo*. *Journal of the National Cancer Institute*. 1975; **55**, 1177-87.
21. Roscoe JP, Claisse PJ. A sequential *in vivo-in vitro* study of carcinogenesis induced in the rat brain by ethylnitrosourea. *Nature*. 1976; **262**, 314-6.
22. Roscoe JP. *In vivo-in vitro* analysis of ethylnitrosourea-induced brain carcinogenesis in the rat. *British Medical Bulletin*. 1980; **36**, 33-8.
23. Lantos PL, Cox DJ. The origin of experimental brain tumours: a sequential study. *Experimentia*. 1976; **32**, 1467-8.
24. Lantos PL. The distribution and role of microtubules and filaments in the neoplastic astrocytes of experimental gliomas. *Neuropathology and Applied Neurobiology*. 1977; **3**, 281-96.
25. Lantos PL, Pilkington GJ. The development of experimental brain tumours: a sequential light and electron microscope study of the subependymal plate. 1. Early lesions (abnormal cell clusters). *Acta Neuropathologica* (Berlin). 1979; **45**, 167-75.
26. Pilkington GJ, Lantos PL. The development of experimental brain tumours: a sequential light and electron microscope study of the subependymal plate. 2. Microtumours. *Acta Neuropathologica* (Berlin). 1979; **45**, 177-85.
27. Pierce GB. Differentiation of normal and malignant cells. *Federation Proceedings*. 1970; **29**, 1248-54.
28. Dustin P, Jr. Cell differentiation and carcinogenesis: a critical review. *Cell and Tissue Kinetics*. 1972; **5**, 519-33.
29. Janisch W, Schreiber D, Warzok R, Osske G. Early stages in tumours in the central nervous system. Experimental studies on morphology. *Experimental Pathology*. (Jena), 1970; **4**, 60-8.
30. Swenberg JA, Koestner A, Wechsler W. The induction of tumours of the nervous system with intravenous methylnitrosourea. *Laboratory Investigations*. 1972; **26**, 74-85.
31. Schiffer D, Giordana MT, Pezzotta S, Lechner C, Paoletti P. Cerebral tumours induced by transplacental ENU: study of the different tumoral stages, particularly of early proliferations. *Acta Neuropathologica* (Berlin). 1978; **41**, 27-31.
32. Lantos PL. The fine structure of periventricular pleomorphic gliomas induced transplacentally by N-ethyl-N-nitrosourea in BDIX rats – with a note on their origin. *Journal of the Neurological Sciences*. 1972; **17**, 443-60.
33. Opalski A. Studien zur allgemeinen Histopathologie der Ventrikelwande. *Zeitschrift für Neurologie*. 1934; **150**, 42-74.
34. Smyth GE, Stern K. Tumours of the thalamus. *Brain*. 1938; **61**, 339-74.
35. Globus JH, Kuhlenbeck H. Tumors of the striatothalamic and related regions, their probable source of origin and more common forms. *Archives of Pathology*. 1942; **34**, 674-734.
36. Globus JH, Kuhlenbeck H. The subependymal cell plate (matrix) and its relationship to brain-tumors of the ependymal type. *Journal of Neuropathology and Experimental Neurology*. 1944; **3**, 1-35.
37. Kleihues P, Meer L, Wiestler OD, Bamberg M. Formation and repair of O-alkylated DNA bases: role in neuro-carcinogenesis and chemotherapy. In: Grundmann E, ed.: *Cancer Campaign*. Vol. 10, Experimental Neurooncology, Brain Tumor and Pain Therapy. Stuttgart-New York: Gustav Fischer, 1987: 1-17.
38. Shih C, Padhy LC, Murray M, Weinberg RA. Transforming genes of carcinomas and neuroblastomas introduced into mouse fibroblasts. *Nature*. 1981; **290**, 261-4.
39. Schubert D, Heinemann S, Carlisle W, Tarikas H, Kimes B, Patrick J, Steinbach JH, Culp W, Brandt BL. Clonal cell lines from the rat central nervous system. *Nature*. 1974; **249**, 224-7.
40. Schechter AL, Stern DF, Vaidyanathan L, Decker SJ, Drebin JA, Greene MI, Weinberg RA. The neu oncogene: an erb-B-related gene encoding a 185,000-M_r tumour antigen. *Nature*. 1984; **312**, 513-6.

41. Schechter AL, Hung M-C, Vaidyanathan L, Weinberg RA, Yang-Feng TL, Franke U, Ullrich A, Coussens L. The neu gene: An erbB-homologous gene distinct from and unlinked to the gene encoding the EGF receptor. *Science.* 1985; **229**, 976-8.
42. Bargmann CI, Hung M-C, Weinberg RA. The neu oncogene encodes an epidermal growth factor receptor-related protein. *Nature.* 1986; **319**, 226-30.
43. Schmidek HH. The molecular genetics of nervous system tumors. *Journal of Neurosurgery.* 1987; **67**, 1-16.
44. Grove AS, Jr, Di Chiso G, Rabotti GF. Experimental brain tumors with a report on those induced in dogs by raw sarcoma virus. *Journal of Neurosurgery.* 1967; **26**, 465-77.
45. Rabotti GF. Experimental intracranial tumours of viral etiology. In: Kirsch WM, E Grossi-Paoletti E, Paoletti P, eds. *The Experimental Biology of Brain Tumors.* Springfield: C.C. Thomas, 1972: 148-80.
46. Yohn DS. Oncogenic viruses: expectations and applications in neuropathology. *Progress in Experimental Tumour Research.* 1972; **17**, 74-92.
47. Bucciarelli E, Rabotti GF, Dalton AJ. Ultrastructure of gliomas in hamsters induced with Rous sarcoma virus. *Journal of the National Cancer Institute.* 1967; **38**, 865-89.
48. Bigner DD, Odom GL, Mahaley MS, Jr, Day ED. Brain tumors induced in dogs by the Schmidt-Ruppin strain of Rous sarcoma virus. *Journal of Neuropathology and Experimental Neurology.* 1969; **28**, 648-70.
49. Kumanishi T, Yamamoto T. Brain tumors induced with Rous sarcoma virus, Schmidt-Ruppin strain 2. Rous tumor specific transplantation antigen and subcutaneously passaged mouse brain tumors. *Japanese Journal of Experimental Medicine.* 1970; **40**, 79-86.
50. Kumanishi T, Ikuta F, Nishida K, Ueti K, Yamamoto T. Brain tumors induced in adult monkeys by Schmidt-Ruppin brain of Rous sarcoma virus. *Gann.* 1973; **64**, 641-3.
51. Kumanishi T, Ikuta F, Yamamoto T. Brain tumors induced by Rous sarcoma virus, Schmidt-Ruppin strain III. Morphology of brain tumors induced in adult mice. *Journal of the National Cancer Institute.* 1973; **50**, 95-109.
52. Vick NA, Lin M-J, Bigner DD. The role of the subependymal plate in glial tumorigenesis. *Acta Neuropathologica* (Berlin). 1977; **40**, 63-71.
53. Bigner DD, Robinson SC, Self DJ. In *Proceedings, International Symposium on Experimental Brain Tumours 1973.* Halle, GDR, 1974.
54. Swenberg JA, Bigner DD, Hall TL. Experimental chemotherapy of virally induced brain tumours. *Proceedings at the American Association for Cancer Research.* 1974; **15**, 43.
55. Zu Rhein GM. Human viruses in experimental neuro-oncogenesis. In: Grundmann E, ed. *Cancer Campaign.* Vol. 10, Experimental Neurooncology, Brain Tumor and Pain Therapy. Stuggart-New York: Gustav Fischer, 1987: 19-46.
56. Liwnicz BH, Berger TS, Liwnicz RG, Aron BS. Radiation-associated gliomas: a report of four cases and analysis of postradiation tumors of the central nervous system. *Neurosurgery.* 1985; **17**, 436-45.
57. Stewart PA, Hayakawa K, Hayakawa E, Farrell CL, Del Maestro RF. A quantitative study of blood-brain barrier permeability ultrastructure in a new rat glioma model. *Acta Neuropathologica.* 1985; **67**, 96-102.
58. Hossmann K-A, Mies G, Paschen W, Szabo L, Dolan E, Wechsler W. Regional metabolism of experimental brain tumors. *Acta Neuropathologica* (Berlin). 1986; **69**, 139-47.
59. Ausman JI, Shapiro WR, Rall DP. Studies on the chemotherapy of experimental brain tumors: development of an experimental model. *Cancer Research.* 1970; **30**, 2394-2400.
60. Sugiura K. Tumor transplantation. In: Gay WI, ed. *Methods of Animal Experimentation.* Vol. 2 New York: Academic Press, 1969: 171-222.

61. Shapiro WR, Ausman JI, Rall DP. Studies on the chemotherapy of experimental brain tumors: evaluation of 1, 3-bis(2-chloroethyl)-1-nitrosourea, cyclophosphamide, mithramycin, and methotrexate. *Cancer Research.* 1970; **30**, 2401-13.
62. Shapiro WR. The effect of chemotherapeutic agents on the incorporation of DNA precursors by experimental brain tumors. *Cancer Research.* 1982; **32**, 2178-85.
63. Muller PJ, Shin KHN, Shin DH. The murine ependymoblastoma: growth pattern and survival in C57B1/6J mice. *Canadian Journal of Neurological Science.* 1983; **10**, 105-9.
64. Geran R, Congletan GF, Dudeck LE, Vendetti J, Abbott BJ, Gargus JL. A mouse ependymoblastoma as an experimental model for screening potential anti neoplastic drugs. *Cancer Chemotherapy Reports.* 1974; **4**, 53-87.
65. Rubin R, Sutton CH, Zimmerman HM. Experimental ependymoblastoma (fine structure). *Journal of Neuropathology and Experimental Neurology.* 1968; **27**, 421-438.
66. Swenberg JA. Animal models for brain tumour research. In: *Progress in Neurological Surgery.* Ser. No. 320. Amsterdam: Excerpta Medica, 1974: 116-22.
67. Rubin RC, Ames RP. Mammary tumour virus in experimental ependymoblastoma. In: Zimmerman M, ed. *Progress in Neuropathology.* Vol. II New York and London: Ervine and Stratton, 1973: 335-49.
68. Manuelidis L, Manuelidis EE. Amount of satellite DNA in four experimentally induced tumors of the central nervous system. Quantitative changes in a glioblastoma producing C-type particles. *Journal of the National Cancer Institute.* 1976; **56**, 43-50.
69. Benda P, Lightbody J, Sato G, Levine L, Sweet W. Differentiated rat glial cell strain in tissue culture. *Science.* 1968; **161**, 370-1.
70. Moore BW, Perez VJ, Gehnig M. Assay and regional distribution of a soluble protein characteristic of the nervous system. *Journal of Neurochemistry.* 1968; **15**, 265-72.
71. Bissell MG, Rubinstein LJ, Bignami A, Herman MM. Characteristics of the rat C-6 glioma maintained in organ culture systems. Production of glial fibrillary acidic protein in the absence of gliofibrillogenesis. *Brain Research.* 1974; **82**, 77-89.
72. Auer RN, Del Maestro RF, Anderson R. A simple and reproducible experimental *in vivo* glioma model. *Canadian Journal of Neurological Science.* 1981; **8**, 325-31.
73. Benda P, Someda K, Messer J, Sweet WH. Morphological and immunochemical studies of rat glial tumors and clonal strains propagated in culture. *Journal of Neurosurgery.* 1971; **34**, 310-23.
74. Schmidek HH, Nielsen SL, Schiller SL, Messer J. Morphological studies of rat brain tumors induced by *N*-nitrosomethylurea. *Journal of Neurosurgery.* 1971; **34**, 335-40.
75. Barker M, Hoshino T, Gurcay O, Wilson CB, Nielsen SL, Downie R, Eliason J. Development of an animal brain tumour model and its response to therapy with 1, 3-bis-(2-chloroethyl)-1-nitrosourea. *Cancer Research.* 1973; **33**, 976-86.
76. Wechsler W, Ramadan MA, Gieseler A. Isogenic transplantation of ethylnitrosourea-induced tumors of the central and peripheral nervous systems in two different inbred rat strains. *Naturwissenschaften.* 1972; **59**, 474.
77. Lantos PL, Roscoe JP, Skidmore CJ. Study of the morphology and tumorigenicity of experimental brain tumours in tissue culture. *British Journal of Experimental Pathology.* 1976; **57**, 95-104.
78. Pilkington GJ, Martin JM, Lantos PL. Cloned neoplastic cells from a chemically-induced rat glioma: immunocytochemical characterization. *British Journal of Experimental Pathology.* 1985; **66**, 561-6.
79. Davaki P, Lantos PL. The development of brain tumours produced in rats by the intracerebral injection of neoplastic glial cells: a fine structural study. *Neuropathology and Applied Neurobiology.* 1981; **7**, 49-61.
80. Davaki P, Lantos PL. Morphological analysis of malignancy: a comparative study of transplanted brain tumours. *British Journal of Experimental Pathology.* 1980; **61**, 655-60.
81. Saggu H, Pilkington GJ. Immunocytochemical characterization of the A15 A5

transplantable brain tumour model *in vivo*. *Neuropathology and Applied Neurobiology*. 1986; **12**, 291–303.
82. Yoshida J, Cravioto H. Nitrosourea-induced brain tumors: an *in vivo* and *in vitro* tumor model system. *Journal of the National Cancer Institute*. 1978; **61**, 365–74.
83. Bigner DD. Appropriate viral-induced, chemical-induced and spontaneous brain tumor models for immunotherapy. In: *Proceedings of Neurologen*. Columbia: Abstract, 1978.
84. Wodinsky I, Kensler CJ, Rall DP. The induction and transplantation of brain tumors in neonatal beagles. *Proceedings of the American Association for Cancer Research*. 1969; **10**, 99.
85. Fraser H. Astrocytomas in an inbred mouse strain. *Journal of Pathology*. 1971; **103**, 266–70.
86. Fraser H. Spontaneous astrocytomas in inbred mice – serial transmissions studies with intact cells. In: Kornyey S, Trariska S, Gosztonyi G, eds. *Proceedings of the 7th International Congress of Neuropathology*. Amsterdam: Excerpta Medica, 1975; 491–4.
87. Fraser H. Spontaneous astrocytoma in mice and its transmission with viable cells. In: Clifford-Rose F, Behan PO, eds. *Animal Models of Neurological Disease*. London: Pitman, 1980: 393–404.
88. Fraser H. Brain tumours in mice with particular reference to astrocytoma. *Food and Chemical Toxicology (Oxford)*. 1986; **24**, 105–11.
89. Serano RD, Pegram CN, Fraser H, Dickinson AG, Bigner DD. Established tumorigenic cell lines from a spontaneous VM/Dk murine astrocytoma (SMA). *Journal of Neuropathology and Experimental Neurology*. 1978; **37**, 689.
90. Serano RD, Pegram CN, Bigner DD. Tumorigenic cell cultures from a spontaneous VM/Dk murine astrocytoma (SMA). *Acta Neuropathologica* (Berlin). 1980; **51**, 53–64.
91. Pilkington GJ, Lantos PL, Darling JL, Thomas DGT. Three cell lines from a spontaneous murine astrocytoma show variation in astrocytic differentiation. *Neuroscience Letters*. 1982; **34**, 315–20.
92. Pilkington GJ, Darling JL, Lantos PL, Thomas DGT. Cell lines (VMDk) derived from a spontaneous murine astrocytoma. Morphological and immunocytochemical characterization. *Journal of Neurological Sciences*. 1983; **62**, 115–39.
93. Pilkington GJ, Darling JL, Lantos PL. Evaluation of a transplantable mouse brain tumour: a model for the study of human glioma. In: Walker MD, Thomas DGT, eds. *Biology of Brain Tumour*. Boston: Martinus Nijhoff, 1984: 153–60.
94. Pilkington GJ, Darling JL, Lantos PL, Thomas DGT. Tumorigenicity of cell lines (VMDk) derived from a spontaneous murine astrocytoma. Histology, fine structure and immunocytochemistry of tumours. *Journal of Neurological Sciences*. 1985; **71**, 145–64.
95. Koppel H, Martin JM, Pilkington GJ, Lantos PL. Heterogeneity of a cultured neoplastic glial line. Establishment and characterisation of six clones. *Journal of the Neurological Sciences*. 1986; **76**, 295–315.
96. Koppel H, Pilkington GJ, Lantos PL. Tumorigenicity of six clones of a cultured neoplastic cell line derived from a spontaneous murine astrocytoma: morphology and immunocytochemistry of tumours. *Journal of the Neurological Sciences*. 1988; **83**, 227–42.
97. Freeman H, Zimmerman HM. Experimental brain tumors. V. Behaviour in intraocular transplants. *Cancer Research*. 1944; **4**, 273–8.
98. Gluszcz A, Alwasick J, Papierz W, Lach B. Morphological observations of gliomas in the course of repeated transplantations in guinea pigs. *Neuropatologia Polska*. 1973; **11**, 11–21.
99. Greene HSN. The transplantation of tumors to the brains of heterologous species. *Cancer Research*. 1951; **11**, 529–34.
100. Greene HSN. The transplantation of human brain tumors to the brains of laboratory animals. *Cancer Research*. 1953; **13**, 422–6.

101. Yablonovskaya LY. *Experimental Brain Tumors Through Heterotransplantation and Induction.* Leningrad: Meditsina, 1967.
102. Manuelidis EE. Experiments with tissue culture and heterologous transplantation of tumors. *Annals of the New York Academy of Science.* 1969; **159**, 409-31.
103. Cobb LM. Metastatic spread of human tumor implanted into thymectomized antithymocyte serum treated hamsters. *British Journal of Cancer.* 1972; **26**, 183-9.
104. Cobb LM. The hamster as a host for the growth and study of human tumor cell populations. *Cancer Research.* 1974; **34**, 958-63.
105. Cobb LM. The behaviour of carcinoma of the large bowel in man following transplantation into immune-deprived mice. *British Journal of Cancer.* 1973; **28**, 400-11.
106. Cobb LM, Mitchley BCV. The growth of human tumors in immune-deprived mice. *European Journal of Cancer.* 1974; **10**, 473-6.
107. Kopper L, Steel G. The therapeutic response of three human tumour lines maintained in immune-suppressed mice. *Cancer Research.* 1975; **35**, 2704-13.
108. Bradley NJ, Bloom HJG, Davies AJS, Swift SM. Growth of human gliomas in immune-deficient mice: a possible model for pre-clinical therapy studies. *British Journal of Cancer.* 1978; **38**, 263-72.
109. Pantelouris EM. Absence of a thymus in a mouse mutant. *Nature.* 1968; **217**, 370-1.
110. Rygaard J, Povlsen CO. Heterotransplantation of a human malignant tumor to the mouse mutant "Nude". *Acta Pathologica et Microbiologica Scandinavica.* 1969; **77**, 758-60.
111. Fogh J, Hajdu SI. The nude mouse as a diagnostic tool in human tumor cell research. *Journal of Cell Biology.* 1975; **67**, 117a.
112. Rana MW, Pinkerton H, Thornton H, Nagy D. Heterotransplantation of human glioblastoma multiforme and meningioma to "nude" mice. *Proceedings of the Society for Experimental Biology and Medicine.* 1977; **155**, 85-8.
113. Levy JA. Xenotrophic viruses: murine leukemia viruses associated with NIH Swiss, NZB, and other mouse strains. *Science.* 1973; **182**, 1151-3.
114. Wara WM, Begg A, Phillips TL, Rosenblum ML, Vasquez D, Wilson CB. Growth and treatment of human brain tumors in nude mice-preliminary communication. In: Houchens DP, Ovejera AA, eds. *Proceedings of the Symposium on the Use of Athymic (Nude) Mice in Cancer Research.* New York, Stuttgart: Gustav Fischer, 1978: 251-6.
115. Reid LM, Holland J, Jones C, Wolf B, Niwayana G, Williams R, Kaplan NO, Sato G. Some of the variables affecting the success and transplantation of human tumors into the athymic nude mouse. In: Houchens DP, Ovejera AA, eds. *Proceedings of the Symposium on the Use of Athymic (Nude) Mice in Cancer Research.* New York, Stuttgart: Gustav Fischer, 1978: 107-21.
116. Shapiro WR, Basler GA, Chernik NL, Posner JB. Human brain tumor transplantation into nude mice. *Journal of the National Cancer Institute.* 1979; **62**, 447-53.
117. Kindred B, Wechsler W. Comparison of rat nervous system tumor clones grown in syngeneic rats and mice. In: Houchens HP, Ovejera AA, eds. *Proceedings of the Symposium on the use of Athymic (Nude) Mice in Cancer Research.* 1978.
118. Jones TR, Bigner SH, Schold SC, Jr, Eng LF, Bigner DD. Anaplastic human gliomas grown in athymic mice. Morphology and glial fibrillary acidic protein expression. *American Journal of Pathology.* 1981; **105**, 316-27.
119. Horten BC, Baster GA, Shapiro WR. Xerograft of human malignant glial tumors into brains of nude mice. A histopathological study. *Journal of Neuropathology and Experimental Neurology.* 1981; **40**, 493-511.
120. Bullard DE, Schold SC, Jr, Bigner SH, Bigner DD. Growth and chemotherapeutic response in athymic mice of tumors arising from human glioma-derived cell lines. *Journal of Neuropathology and Experimental Neurology.* 1981; **40**, 410-27.
121. Bigner SH, Bullard DE, Pegram CN, Wilkstrand CJ, Bigner DD. Relationship of *in*

vitro morphologic and growth characteristics of established human glioma-derived cell lines to their tumorigenicity in athymic nude mice. *Journal of Neuropathology and Experimental Neurology.* 1981; **40**, 390–409.
122. Giovanella BC, Stenlin JS. Experimental chemotherapy of human tumors heterotransplanted in nude mice. In: Evans AE, ed. *Advances in Neuroblastoma Research.* New York: Raven Press, 1980: 299–307.

5 The classification of intracranial tumours

RO Barnard

The chief object of any scheme of classifying tumours is to enable communication to take place. Words are used to specify the nature of the process under consideration so that accumulated knowledge can be readily exchanged. In the present day, tumours of the brain and its coverings are classified according to their light-microscopical appearances. The recent contributions of electron microscopy and of immunohistochemistry have not been reflected in new proposals for classification, and, by and large, existing nomenclature works reasonably well. Yet the evolution of classification is a continuous process; perceptives in neuro-oncology change and new data must gradually be assimilated when their value is confirmed.

Tumours of neuroepithelial tissue

Nineteenth-century landmarks in the development of brain tumour classification from the time of the discovery of the cell in the 1830s have been detailed by Zülch.[1] The pace of research into brain tumours accelerated, in keeping with the rapid strides made in neurosurgery from the time of Rickman Godlee's pioneer operation for the removal of an intrinsic glial tumour of the brain in 1884. Soon after the turn of the century it was obvious that a tumour must be investigated simultaneously both from a neurosurgical and a pathological standpoint; the value of such an approach was exemplified in Cushing's early monographs on the disorders of the pituitary and the acoustic nerve tumours. Gliomas, and the confusing variety of appearances that they display, had to wait until 1926 when Bailey and Cushing's monograph was published. *A Classification of Tumors of the Glioma Group*[2] was probably the most influential publication in this field for many years. It was the attempt of two surgeons, both skilled in pathology, to produce an orderly structure containing a place for every glioma variety, determined by a comparison of its constituent cells with cells in the course of development showing different degrees of differentiation (Table 5.1).

Many of these tumour entities survive to the present day. "Medulloepithelioma" is still used to connote a very primitive type of malignant tumour of infancy

Table 5.1 Bailey and Cushing's original classification

1. Medulloepithelioma
2. Medulloblastoma
3. Pineoblastoma
4. Pinealoma
5. Ependymoblastoma
6. Ependymoma
7. Neuroepithelioma
8. Spongioblastoma
   (a) Multiforme
   (b) Unipolare
9. Astroblastoma
10. Astrocytoma
    (a) Protoplasmic
    (b) Fibrillary
11. Oligodendroglioma
12. Neuroblastoma
13. Ganglioneuroma
14. Choroid plexus papilloma

showing a pattern of tubules and canals resembling the original medullary tube. "Medulloblastoma" denotes a malignant tumour located in the cerebellum composed of primitive cells with bi-potential differentiation: in at least some examples the ability to proceed along neuronal and/or glial lines can be demonstrated. "Pineoblastoma" remains the accepted title for malignant, poorly differentiated neoplasms of pineal cells, but for the more differentiated tumours the term "pineocytoma" is generally employed since "pinealoma" has been used in an imprecise fashion for other lesions at this site. "Ependymoblastoma" has been revived recently to denote the malignant primitive tumour of childhood showing unmistakeable features of ependymal differentiation. Ependymoma is still a current and well-defined term. "Neuroepithelioma" is confusing: it has been used for well-differentiated ependymomas and also for brain tumours of a primitive character that should be regarded as medulloepitheliomas. In the peripheral nervous system rare examples of malignant tumours showing the appearances of a primitive central nervous system tumour have also been called neuroepithelioma.

"Spongioblastoma" has been replaced by "glioblastoma" as the accepted term for the common, malignant, multiform tumour that frequently occurs in adults. Confusingly, "spongioblastoma" has also been employed for the relatively benign pilocytic astrocytoma. A rare infantile tumour with a distinctive palisading pattern is the true polar spongioblastoma defined by Russell and Cairns.[3] Astroblastoma may exist in a pure form, identified by the perivascular arrangement of processed cells, and as such is rare, but other gliomas may contain astroblastomatous foci.

Astrocytomas are, of course, very common tumours and since Bailey and Cushing's day the "piloid" or "pilocytic" astrocytoma has been separated off as it has been recognized that many cerebellar astrocytomas are of this type and carry a relatively favourable prognosis. The oligodendroglioma, described in detail by Bailey and Bucy[4] is a well-known and distinct type of glioma, but the classification is unhelpful when mixed forms containing both astrocytic and oligodendrocytic elements are encountered. The terms "neuroblastoma", "ganglioneuroma" and choroid plexus papilloma are current, and clearly defined.

Following Bailey and Cushing's work the main tendency was towards simplification of the classification and to place more emphasis on anaplasia. But the whole concept of a cytogenetic classification based on pure cell morphology was not without its critics. During the 1930s HJ Scherer made several fundamental contributions towards understanding the way in which gliomas grow and behave, based upon the study of large brain sections embedded in celloidin, and deplored the idea of diagnosis made on individual cell morphology. Scherer's emphasis on the diffuseness of glioma growth and on the presence of "secondary structures" (perivascular and subpial aggregates of cells) remain important observations but do not invalidate attempts at cellular classification. Pio del Rio-Hortega, on the other hand, based his classification[5] entirely on cytogenesis without reference to clinical experience; the metallic impregnation methods, of which he was the undoubted master, revealed to him a much greater variety of morphological detail than would otherwise have been available, but led to the use of accurate but cumbersome terminology such as "astroblast-oligodendrocytoma". Rio-Hortega's pupils, especially Polak[6] continued to rely on his techniques and maintain his classification.

Kernohan and his co-workers applied the principles of numerical grading on a scale of I to IV to the study of gliomas.[7] Their scheme was extremely popular with clinicians and with general pathologists: it was apparently simple to use, discarded difficult entities, and related directly to prognosis. Neurosurgeons may like to grade a tumour in terms of a number rather than a description, but the limitations of the Kernohan scheme become apparent when it is used for the grading of small tumour biopsies. In the overall assessment of a brain tumour the age of the patient, the site, the length of symptoms are all factors that carry considerable prognostic import and there is little doubt that microscopical "grading" may sometimes be less helpful a criterion than these others. The astrocytomas show the best correlation between microscopical appearances and clinical behaviour, while the oligodendrogliomas and ependymomas show greater variation. The Kernohan group based their grades upon cellular differentiation and anaplasia, but in practice it became obvious that additional factors such as the presence of necrosis, mitotic figures and vascular proliferation had to be carefully evaluated. Clearly a reasonable assessment can be made only when adequate samples of material are available, and the careful pathologist will study details of the clinical and radiological findings, and the age, sex and family history of the patient, before venturing on prognosis. It must also be remembered that the natural history of many gliomas is in the direction of increased anaplasia, and sequential biopsy and ultimately post-mortem studies of gliomas often establish a degree of progressive malignancy that could not have been predicted earlier.

Further criticism of the proposals of the Kernohan school was directed chiefly at the loss of rare, but well defined, tumour entities such as the astroblastoma and the ependymoblastoma.

The World Health Organization decided to make an attempt to obtain international agreement for the criteria on which cancer should be classified and established 23 reference centres involving pathologists from over 50 countries. The monograph *Histological Typing of Tumours of the Central Nervous System*[8] was the result of several years' work on the problem of establishing a reasonable consensus following discussions within a group of 10 neuropathologists.

The broad outlines of the WHO classification of tumours of neuroepithelial tissue are given in Table 5.2.

The concepts underlying this classification are essentially those established by Bailey and Cushing. The most valid criticism of the arrangement lies in the grouping of the glioblastomas, many of which are the end-products of anaplasia in the astrocytoma group with the medulloblastomas which, in essence, are embryonal tumours

Table 5.2 The WHO classification of tumours of neuroepithelial tissue

I. TUMOURS OF NEUROEPITHELIAL TISSUE
  A. Astrocytic tumours
    1. Astrocytoma
      (a) Fibrillary
      (b) Protoplasmic
      (c) Gemistocytic
    2. Pilocytic astrocytoma
    3. Subependymal giant-cell astrocytoma (ventricular tumour of tuberous sclerosis)
    4. Astroblastoma
    5. Anaplastic (malignant) astrocytoma
  B. Oligodendroglial tumours
    1. Oligodendroglioma
    2. Mixed oligo-astrocytoma
    3. Anaplastic (malignant) oligodendroglioma
  C. Ependymal and choroid plexus tumours
    1. Ependymoma
      Variants:
      (a) Myxopapillary ependymoma
      (b) Papillary ependymoma
      (c) Subependymoma
    2. Anaplastic (malignant) ependymoma
    3. Choroid plexus papilloma
    4. Anaplastic (malignant) choroid plexus papilloma
  D. Pineal cell tumours
    1. Pineocytoma (pinealocytoma)
    2. Pineoblastoma (pinealoblastoma)
  E. Neuronal tumours
    1. Gangliocytoma
    2. Ganglioglioma
    3. Ganglioneuroblastoma
    4. Anaplastic (malignant) gangliocytoma and ganglioglioma
    5. Neuroblastoma
  F. Poorly differentiated and embryonal tumours
    1. Glioblastoma
      Variants:
      (a) Glioblastoma with sarcomatous component (mixed glioblastoma and sarcoma)
      (b) Giant-cell glioblastoma
    2. Medulloblastoma
      Variants:
      (a) Desmoplastic medulloblastoma
      (b) Medullomyoblastoma
    3. Medulloepithelioma
    4. Primitive polar spongioblastoma
    5. Gliomatosis cerebri

Table 5.3 Revised classification of tumours of neuroepithalial tissue by Russell and Rubinstein[9]

A. Tumours of neuroglial cells
   I. Astrocytic group
      1. Astrocytoma
      2. Astroblastoma
      3. Polar spongioblastoma
   II. Oligodendroglia
      Oligodendroglioma
   III. Ependymoma
      1. Ependymoma
      2. Subependymoma
      3. Ependymoblastoma
   IV. Anaplastic
      Glioblastoma multiforme
B. Tumours of neuronal cells and primitive bipotential precursors
   I. Medulloepithelioma
   II. Medulloblastoma and cerebellar neuroblastoma
   III. Cerebral neuroblastoma
   IV. Gangliocytoma and ganglioglioma
C. Tumours of specialized tissues of central neuroepithelial origin
   I. Neuroepithelial tumours of the retina
      1. Retinoblastoma
      2. Medulloepithelioma
      3. Adult glioma (astrocytoma)
   II. Glioma of the optic nerve and chiasm
   III. Tumours of the neurohypophysis
      1. Astrocytoma
      2. Granular cell tumour
   IV. Tumours of the parenchymal and glial cells of the pineal body
      1. Pineoblastoma
      2. Pineocytoma
      3. Glioma
         (a) Astrocytoma
         (b) Glioblastoma
   V. Tumours of the choroid plexus epithelium
      1. Papilloma
      2. Carcinoma

capable of divergent differentiation. Russell and Rubinstein[9] depart from the WHO classification as shown in Table 5.3.

By this means the glioblastoma is placed in more appropriate surroundings and the neuronal and bi-potential tumours kept together. The range of the true tumours of the pineal is also displayed.

Russell and Rubinstein[9] enlarged the detailed classification of astrocytomas as follows:

(1) Protoplasmic
(2) Fibrillary (a) diffuse, (b) circumscribed
(3) Pilocytic

(4) Gemistocytic
(5) Subependymal giant-cell
(6) Pleomorphic xanthoastrocytoma
(7) Desmoplastic cerebral astrocytoma of infancy
(8) Anaplastic

The first four categories refer to descriptive cell types. The fifth, the subependymal giant cell tumour, has a distinctive appearance and in a fair proportion of cases is associated with tuberose sclerosis. In the pleomorphic xanthoastrocytoma the appearances are paradoxical: it is a superficially sited tumour in the younger age-group, with a pleomorphic cellular composition including lipid-filled cells. It is usually much more benign in behaviour than might be expected from its appearances. Category (7) refers to a recently defined group of infantile gliomas characterized by intense desmoplasia (see ref. 10). The anaplastic astrocytoma (Group (8)) is the common malignant glioma of adults overlapping with glioblastoma, but the prognosis in some cases is possibly slightly more favourable. The anaplastic astrocytoma corresponds broadly with the "grade III" used by many neuropathologists. The WHO investigators stressed that "many neuroepithelial tumours contain mixtures of different neoplastic cells". An astrocytoma may often contain several different types of astrocytic cell, arranged in different patterns, while an oligodendroglioma frequently contains some astrocytic cells which may, in some foci, dominate the scene. In general, terminology allows for some latitude in the precise cellular composition of a tumour: no name can ever express completely every cytological variation which a tumour is capable of expressing. The mixed tumours can be subdivided further into those containing two or more types of glial cell, e.g. astroblast-oligodendroglioma and those with a fundamental variety of tissues present such as the mixed glioblastoma and sarcoma. Sarcoma arising within the prolific vascular endothelium of a glioblastoma is usually a fibrosarcoma but as a rare curiosity chondroid or muscular elements may be found.

In the classification proposed by Rorke et al.[11] the mixed gliomas are subdivided and each given a separate category (e.g. oligoastroependymoma). Such nomenclature may be precise, but only at the expense of a certain clumsiness.

The vexed question of to what extent a histological classification should be based on cell appearances only, and to what extent the site of origin should be included, was considered by Burger and Vogel[12], who point out that any classification is prone to complexity and controversy. These authors decided to deal with astrocytic neoplasms both from the viewpoint of the anatomical localization and that of the cell of origin, enabling the particular features at each site to receive attention.

A more fundamental criticism of the classification established by the WHO group, and to a large extent followed by Russell and Rubinstein, concerns the identity of the various poorly differentiated or embryonal tumours of infancy. Tumours "previously diagnosed as medulloblastoma, ependymoblastoma, central neuroblastoma and pineoblastoma should be reclassified", it was proposed, under the general heading of "primitive neuroectodermal tumour (PNET)". However, the separate category of medulloepithelioma, surely the most fundamental of the primitive tumours, was to be retained. This proposal described by Rorke et al.[11] and by Rorke[13] has also been discussed in detail by Rubinstein,[14] who urges the importance of the precise definition of the various tumours of embryonal type since the majority can be classified with accuracy on a scheme to correlate each neoplasm with the stages of neurocytogenesis.

At present it certainly appears ill-advised to try to replace well-established terms such as "medulloblastoma" when an important and universally understood message can be conveyed, relevant to the site of the tumour, its treatment and prognosis. Since the general category of "PNET" contains both well-defined, and ill-defined entities at a lower stage of classification, the nature of the information conveyed by its use is not sharply focussed. From a genetic viewpoint, the "PNET grouping" is essentially heterogeneous.

The most striking advances in diagnostic neuro-oncology in the 1980s have come from the application of immunoperoxidase histochemistry. A large literature has recently accumulated about the demonstration of antibodies and the ways in which they can be regarded as specific markers (see ref. 15). Glial fibrillary acidic protein is probably the most popular and widely used of these and is of great value in revealing the astrocytic nature of controversial neoplasms. Its presence can readily be demonstrated in normal, reactive or neoplastic astrocytes, certain ependymal cells, some neoplastic oligodendrocytic cells and in the stroma of haemangioblastomas and in the epithelial elements of choroid plexus papilloma.

S100 protein, first isolated in the nervous system, is localized in glial and Schwann cells, but can also be found in a wide variety of tissues. Neuron-specific enolase has been proposed as a marker for cells of neuronal origin, but in practice proved to be of limited utility since it could be demonstrated in neoplastic elements of varied origin. Markers for normal oligodendrocytes such as carbonic anhydrase C have not proved of much consistent value in the demonstration of neoplastic cells of oligodendrocytic origin. The monoclonal antibody HNK-1 (anti-leu 7) is useful in the identification of peripheral nerve sheath tumour and also is likely to yield positive results in astrocytomas, oligodendrogliomas and other neuroglial tumours. There are many other potential "markers" under test.

At present this field of study is advancing so rapidly that it is impossible to predict how the results of immunocytochemistry may improve the classification of brain tumours in future and make existing categories better defined or, alternatively, render them obsolete. The future value of "markers" may well be in their application in groups which together cover a wide range of tissue components rather than as individual entities.

Tumours of nerve sheath cells

The WHO classification of nerve sheath tumours (Table 5.4) is on familiar lines, drawing a clear distinction between the neurilemmoma or schwannoma, a well-defined mass of highly cellular tumour situated on a nerve, with interlacing bundles of spindle cells whose nuclei are often arranged in parallel, alternating with semi-cystic looser-textured areas, and the neurofibroma, as seen in multiple neurofibromatosis, where there is a more diffuse enlargement of a nerve and where axons are incorporated and often surrounded, in a mass of collagenous fibres, mucoid material, and Schwann cells. The malignant variants are rare except in multiple neurofibromatosis.

Table 5.4 The WHO classification of tumours of nerve sheath cells

II. TUMOURS OF NERVE SHEATH CELLS
  A. Neurilemmoma (schwannoma, neurinoma)
  B. Anaplastic (malignant) neurilemmoma (schwannoma, neurinoma)
  C. Neurofibroma
  D. Anaplastic (malignant) neurofibroma (neurofibrosarcoma, neurogenic sarcoma)

Meningiomas

The meningioma group is unique, in that the tumours are named from a tissue, not from a cell. Several elaborate pathological classifications have been proposed, but these variants do not reflect essential differences in clinical performance, with a few exceptions such as the haemangiopericytic type. Indeed the complexity and variety of cell appearances seen in the meningiomas reflect the polyblastic nature of the meningeal cell; when tumours are derived from it you would expect to find epithelioid, angiomatous, pericytomatous and sarcomatous forms and this in practice is indeed what is found.

For the most part the WHO classification of meningiomas (Table 5.5) is not a controversial matter. Groups I to VI are regarded as benign, while the haemangiopericytic (7) and papillary (8) types tend toward more malignant characteristics, and group (9) includes tumours with clearly malignant features, while not purely sarcomatous. The remarkable variety that meningiomas can display is not fully reflected in the WHO classification. Osteoblastic and chondroblastic areas may be found; xanthomatous and lipomatous changes are well-recognized; microcystic (or "humid") meningiomas (as described by Michaud and Gagne),[16] may raise special diagnostic problems as they can mimic astrocytomas or even schwannomas. Some meningiomas are heavily pigmented with melanin.

It is in the definition of the haemangioblastic type of meningioma that some difficulties arise. There is general agreement that such tumours display a more aggressive mode of behaviour, and therefore they must be clearly distinguished from those meningiomas containing conspicuous groups of dilated blood vessels, resulting in an angiomatous appearance (WHO group V). The two types of haemangioblastic meningioma under consideration are (1) a tumour identical to the capillary haemangioblastoma of the cerebellum (WHO group VI) and (ii) a tumour which, in at least some areas, is similar to the haemangiopericytoma that occurs in other organs of the body (WHO group VII). The appearances of the latter have prompted some authors to remove such tumours from the meningioma group altogether and call them "haemangiopericytoma of the meninges". While it is agreed that in many cases the appearances – highly cellular masses, without whorls, and with a wealth of fine reticulin fibres which may outline small vascular spaces – are unlike those familiar in more typical meningiomas, the existence of transitional forms as described by Horten et al.[17] links the haemangiopericytic tumours with the meningiomas in general and justifies their retention within this group.

The development of a papillary pattern in a meningioma is rare, and is often accompanied by enhanced cellular anaplasia and a degree of invasiveness.

Table 5.5 The WHO classification of meningiomas

III. TUMOURS MENINGEAL AND RELATED TISSUE
  A. Meningioma
    1. Meningotheliomatous (endotheliomatous, syncytial, arachnotheliomatous)
    2. Fibrous (fibroblastic)
    3. Transitional (mixed)
    4. Psammomatous
    5. Angiomatous
    6. Haemangioblastic
    7. Haemangiopericytic
    8. Papillary
    9. Anaplastic (malignant) meningioma
  B. Meningeal sarcomas
    1. Fibrosarcoma
    2. Polymorphic cell sarcoma
    3. Primary meningeal sarcomatosis
  C. Xanthomatous tumours
    1. Fibroxanthoma
    2. Xanthosarcoma (malignant fibroxanthoma)
  D. Primary melanotic tumours
    1. Melanoma
    2. Meningeal melanomatosis
  E. Others

Russell and Rubinstein[9] put forward a simpler classification. They favour three main groups: the first to include the usual types of classical meningioma – the meningothelial (or syncytial) type, the transitional type, and the fibroblastic type. Included in this category are a number of histological variants: the psammomatous, the microcystic or "humid", the myxomatous, the xanthomatous, the lipomatous, the granular, the secretory, the chondroblastic, the osteoblastic and the melanotic, together with the giant-celled meningiomas and those with lymphoid- or plasma-celled infiltration. All these are regarded as benign. The second main group includes the angioblastic meningiomas, divided into the haemangioblastic and haemangiopericytic variants. The third group comprises the malignant meningiomas, including the papillary type.

For further discussion of meningiomas and their variable appearance the reader may be referred to the recent book by Kepes,[18] and to the classical volume by Cushing and Eisenhardt.[19]

Primary malignant cerebral and spinal lymphomas form a group possessed of many features of special interest. Their association with all types of immunodeficiency, including AIDS, their multifocal perivascular and diffuse distribution, are distinctive. In recent years it has been shown that the majority are B-cell lymphomas. There is some current evidence pointing to a possible association with EB virus. Secondary lymphoma should be classified with the other metastatic tumours.

Of blood vessel tumours, the haemangioblastomas affecting the cerebellum and, less commonly, the pial covering of the medulla and spinal cord is the most common.

86 *The classification of intracranial tumours*

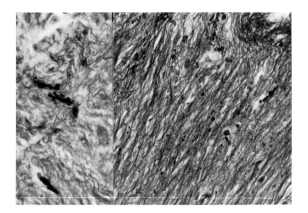

Fig. 5.1 Pilocytic astrocytoma. A dense meshwork of fine hair-like processes. Insert: Irregular dark staining Rosenthal fibres. PTAH × 320

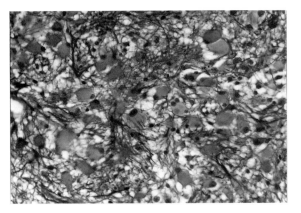

Fig. 5.2 Gemistocytic astrocytoma. The cells have rounded or oval masses of cytoplasm and there is an extensive background of glial fibrils. HE × 500

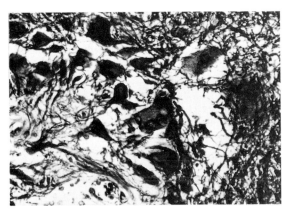

Fig. 5.3 Astrocytoma showing the variety of cell forms and abundance of fibrils. PTAH × 300

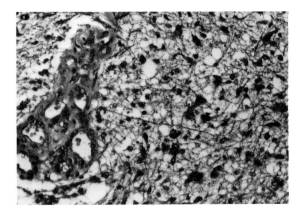

Fig. 5.4 Astrocytoma with a mass of abnormal hyperplastic capillaries – an important sign of malignancy. PTAH × 300

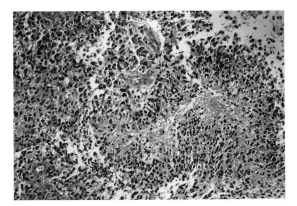

Fig. 5.5 Glioblastoma. A highly cellular small-celled example with a small central necrotic zone surrounded by prolific cells – a "pseudo-palisade". HE × 140

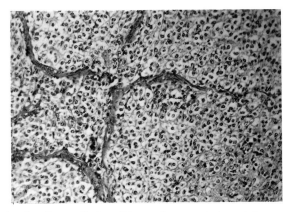

Fig. 5.6 Oligodendroglioma. Cells with regular rounded nuclei surrounded by clear unstained cytoplasm are arranged in groups contained within a fibrovascular network. HVG × 160

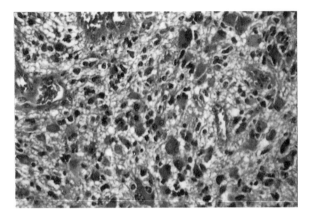

Fig. 5.7 Mixed glioma. An assortment of oligodendroglial and astrocytic cells. The capillary hyperplasia is moderate. HE × 250

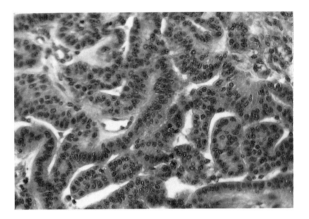

Fig. 5.8 Papillary ependymoma. HE × 275

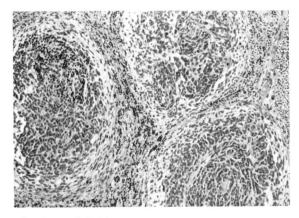

Fig. 5.9 Desmoplastic medulloblastoma with a lobular pattern of mainly neuroblastic cells enclosed within connective tissue. HE × 180

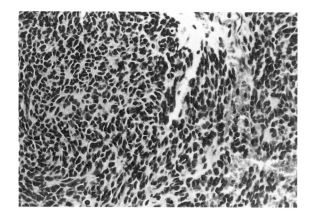

Fig. 5.10 Medulloblastoma of classical type showing a tendency to rosette formation. HE × 100

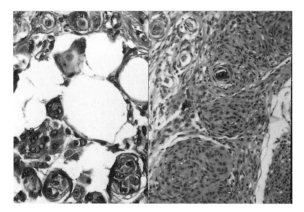

Fig. 5.11 (a) Lipomatous meningioma, HE × 300. (b) Typical meningioma of syncytial type with whorls. HE × 170

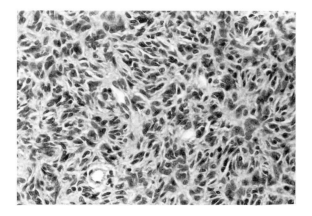

Fig. 5.12 Meningioma of haemangiopericytic type. The cells are orientated around slit-like blood-spaces. HE × 500

Table 5.6 Other categories in the WHO histological classification of tumours of the central nervous system

---

IV. PRIMARY MALIGNANT LYMPHOMAS
V. TUMOURS OF BLOOD VESSEL ORIGIN
    A. Haemangioblastoma (capillary haemangioblastoma)
    B. Monstrocellular sarcoma
VI. GERM CELL TUMOURS
    A. Germinoma
    B. Embryonal carcinoma
    C. Chorion carcinoma
    D. Teratoma
VII. OTHER MALFORMATIVE TUMOURS AND TUMOUR-LIKE LESIONS
    A. Craniopharyngioma
    B. Rathke's cleft cyst
    C. Epidermoid cyst
    D. Dermoid cyst
    E. Colloid cyst of the third ventricle
    F. Enterogenous cyst
    G. Other cysts
    H. Lipoma
    I. Choristoma (pituicytoma, granular cell myoblastoma)
    J. Hypothalamic neuronal hamartoma
    K. Nasal glial heterotopia (nasal glioma)
VIII. VASCULAR MALFORMATIONS
    A. Capillary telangiectasia
    B. Cavernous angioma
    C. Arteriovenous malformation
    D. Venous malformation
    E. Sturge-Weber disease
XI. TUMOURS OF THE ANTERIOR PITUITARY
    A. Pituitary adenomas
        1. Acidophil
        2. Basophil (mucoid cell)
        3. Mixed acidophil–basophil
        4. Chromophobe
    B. Pituitary adenocarcinoma
X. LOCAL EXTENSIONS FROM REGIONAL TUMOURS
    A. Glomus jugulare tumour (chemodectoma, paraganglioma)
    B. Chordoma
    C. Chondroma
    D. Chondrosarcoma
    E. Adenoid cystic carcinoma (cylindroma)
    G. Others
XI. METASTATIC TUMOURS
XII. UNCLASSIFIED TUMOURS

Table 5.7 Revised classification of the germ-cell tumours by Walter and Kleinert[20]

A. Germinoma, embryonal and extraembryonal tissue teratoma
   1. Germinoma
      (a) Classical
      (b) Spermatocytic
      (c) Anaplastic
   2. Embryonal carcinoma
      (a) Classical
      (b) Polyembryoma
   3. Endodermal sinus tumours (yolk sac tumour)
   4. Choriocarcinoma
   5. Mixed
      (a) Germinoma with syncytiotrophoblastic giant cells
      (b) Choriocarinoma and any other type
      (c) Teratocarcinoma
      (d) Other combinations
B. Adult tissue teratoma
   1. Monodermoma
      (a) Epidermoid cyst
      (b) Enterogenous cyst
      (c) Colloid cyst of the third ventricle
      (d) Lipoma
      (e) Craniopharyngioma
      (f) Rathke's cleft cyst
   2. Didermoma
      (a) Dermoid cyst
   3. Tridermoma
      (a) Mature teratoma
      (b) Immature teratoma
      (c) Teratoma with malignant transformation
C. Neuroectodermal malformative tumours and tumour-like lesions
   1. Cysts
      (a) Arachnoid
      (b) Ependymal-lined
      (c) Neuroglial-lined
   2. Choristoma
   3. Hypothalamic neuronal hamartoma
   4. Nasal glial heterotopia (nasal glioma)
D. Tumours of the phakomatoses
   1. Neurofibromatosis of von Recklinghausen
   2. von Hippel-Lindau disease
   3. Sturge-Weber disease
   4. Tuberous sclerosis of Bourneville-Pringle
   5. Melanocytic tumours
      (a) Neurocutaneous melanosis
      (b) Primary meningeal melanomatosis
      (c) Retinal anlage tumour (melanocytoma of infancy)

The inclusion of other tumours within the blood vessel group is more controversial. The monstrocellular sarcoma (Zulch)[1] is considered by many authorities to include anaplastic examples of glioblastoma and glioblastoma–sarcoma. Perhaps there should be included in this category those malignant tumours of the angiosarcoma and angio-endotheliosis group while Kaposi's sarcoma clearly belongs with the metastatic lesions.

The germ-cell tumours have been subdivided in more detail by Walter and Kleinert,[20] who propose the term "dysonto-genetic brain tumours" for the group shown in Table 5.7. Whether this arrangement will prove to be more helpful in practice remains to be assessed.

The inclusion of vascular malformations in the WHO scheme can be criticized on the grounds that they are not true tumours. However, the borderlines of neoplasia in the nervous system cannot always be sharply drawn. Similarly the inclusion of anterior pituitary tumours may be regarded as out of place and in any event these adenomas are now classified on the basis of hormone production, not on tinctorial characteristics.

Classification is not a static process. Gradually as new understanding is accumulated, changes are made to established concepts, and the validity of any classification reflects the quality of the scientific information upon which it is based. From a practical viewpoint the value of a classification can only be judged by the accuracy with which it can be used to transmit information and by the ease with which it can be used by different people.

Acknowledgement

The author wishes to thank Dr LJ Rubinstein for help with the preparation of this text and Mr Trevor Scott FIMLT for the preparation of the pictures.

References

1. Zulch KJ. *Brain Tumours, their Biology and Pathology*. 3rd edn. Berlin: Springer-Verlag, 1986.
2. Bailey P, Cushing H. *A Classification of the Tumors of the Glioma Group on a Histogenetic Basis*. Philadelphia: Lippincott, 1926.
3. Russell DS, Cairns H. Polar spongioblastoma *Arch. Histo.* (Buenos Aires) **3**: 423–41.
4. Bailey P, Bucy PC. Oligodendrogliomas of the brain. *Journal of Pathology*. 1929; **32**, 735–51.
5. Rio-Hortega P del, (1934), translated as *The Microscopic Anatomy of Tumours of the Central and Peripheral Nervous System* by Pineda, Russell and Earle. Springfield: CC Thomas, 1962.
6. Polak M. *Blastomas del Sistema Nervioso Central y Periferico. Patologia y Ordenacion Histogenetica*. Buenos Aires; Lopez, 1966.
7. Kernohan JW, Sayre GP. *Tumours of the Central Nervous System*. Washington: Armed Forces Institute of Pathology, 1952.
8. Zulch KJ. *Histological Typing of Tumours of the Central Nervous System*. Geneva: World Health Organization, 1979.
9. Russell DS, Rubinstein LJ. *Pathology of Tumours of the Nervous System*. 5th edn revised by *LJ Rubinstein*. London: Edward Arnold, 1989.

10. VandenBerg SR, May EE, Rubinstein LJ, Herman MM, Perentes E, Vinores SA, Collins P, Park TS. Desmoplastic supratentorial neuroepithelial tumours of infancy with divergent differentiation potential ("desmoplastic infantile gangliogliomas") *Journal of Neurosurgery.* 1987; **66**, 58–71.
11. Rorke LB, Gilles FH, Davis RL, Becker LE. Revision of The World Heath Organization classification of brain tumours for childhood brain tumours. *Cancer.* 1985; **56**, 1869–86.
12. Burger PC, Vogel FS. *Surgical Pathology of the Nervous System and its Coverings. Second edition.* New York: John Wiley and Sons, 223–301; 1982.
13. Rorke LB. Editorial. *Journal of Neuro-Oncology.* 1987; **5**, 95–7.
14. Rubinstein LJ. A commentary on the proposed revision of World Health Organization Classification of brain tumours for childhood brain tumours. *Cancer.* 1985; **56**, 1887–8.
15. Perentes E, Rubinstein LJ. Recent applications of immunoperoxidase histochemistry in human neuro-oncology. *Archives of Pathology and Laboratory Medicine.* 1987; **111**, 796–812.
16. Michaud J, Gagné F. Microcystic meningioma. Clinico-pathologic report of 8 cases. *Archives of Pathology and Laboratory Medicine.* 1980; **107**(2), 75–80.
17. Horten BC, Urich H, Rubinstein LJ, Montague SR. The angioblastic meningioma: a reappraisal of a nosological problem. Light, electron microscopic, tissue, and organ culture observations. *Journal of Neurological Science.* 1977; **31**, 387–410.
18. Kepes JJ. *Meningiomas, Biology. Pathology and Differential Diagnosis.* New York; Masson, 1982.
19. Cushing H, Eisenhardt L. *Meningiomas.* Springfield: CC Thomas, 1938.
20. Walter GF, Kleinert R. Dysontogenetic tumours–proposal for an improved classification. *Neuropathology and Applied Neurobiology.* 1987; **13**, 273–87.

6 Neuroradiological imaging of brain tumours

DPE Kingsley

Diagnostic imaging relies heavily on computed tomography (CT) and magnetic resonance imaging (MRI) in the diagnosis and follow up of intracranial tumours. Other investigations, apart from angiography, provide little useful information not already obtained from CT and MRI, and if relied upon when normal to exclude pathology may lull the physician with a false sense of reassurance.

Modern imaging is a very powerful diagnostic tool. CT and MRI are sometimes complementary but in general the useful information can be obtained with either modality; the use of both procedures is unwarranted and adds to the cost of treatment. Which of the two is likely to provide the most useful information is difficult to predict in an individual case but without a knowledge of the uses and limitations of each procedure, the choice may lead to an unsuitable procedure being performed.

Computed tomography

Despite the recent flood of literature on MRI, modern CT is still likely to continue to play a large part in imaging in most radiological departments for the foreseeable future. At present, good CT scanners are much cheaper than corresponding MRI equipment with respect to both capital (purchase price and installation) and revenue costs. Most reasonably sized hospitals will probably have CT whereas MRI is likely to be less widely available. The conduct of the examination depends on what is required from the scan and such questions as whether a simple axial scan is adequate for diagnosis and management or whether reformatted images are required and whether the patient is co-operative or confused will have a bearing on the technique used and the results obtained.

Axial scans with and without intravenous contrast are sufficient to provide the essential information in a majority of cases. However third- or fourth-generation scanners are provided with a wide variety of facilities which allow extensive manipulation of data. This may be of great value in the marginal case where an uncooperative patient is too restless to allow an adequate study using standard protocols. Short scanning times (1–3 s) or scan segmentation may be necessary and, although reducing the quality below that achievable under optimal conditions, nevertheless will often produce a result adequate for management. Another technique which can be used to reduce scan-time when reformatting is necessary is to use overlapping 5 mm slices rather than thinner (1.5 or 2 mm) sections. The examination can be undertaken in less time than would otherwise be the case and the final image is more tolerant of patient movement. Despite a lower overall resolution in the reformatted plane the advantages of shortened scanning time often outweigh the disadvantages of suboptimal quality.

Patient movement and sedation

The quality of any scan will ultimately depend upon patient cooperation and prior assessment is essential. In the majority of cases voluntary movement can usually be adequately controlled by sedation and even if the examination is of suboptimal quality sufficient information may be obtained to influence further management. Involuntary movements on the other hand are frequently either quite unpredictable or the repeat rate may be within the scanning time; furthermore these patients respond poorly to sedation. If sufficiently frequent such movements may prevent a satisfactory scan being performed without anaesthesia.

The scanning of children is more of an art than a science. In departments used to the scanning of young patients many relatively uncooperative children can be "talked" through the examination by the staff or an accompanying parent. The most difficult age is between 18 months and 5 years when the child is often unable to understand what is required and is frequently frightened; retarded children of any age are also difficult to scan and in both these groups sedation is usually necessary. The exact dosage of sedation should be agreed with the neuroanaesthetist responsible. In infants scanning may be attempted following a feed since a full stomach or the act of suckling often causes the child to sleep. If contrast is thought likely to be required a dummy is preferable in case vomiting occurs.

Intravenous contrast (CT)

Most intravenous contrast agents used in CT contain three atoms of iodine in each molecule. Enhancement results from the increased X-ray attenuation caused by the high atomic number of iodine. In the normal patient contrast only outlines normal vascular structures (1 mg/ml of iodine raises the average attenuation by 24–30 Hounsfield Units.[1,2] The intact blood–brain barrier results in insignificant extravasation of contrast medium across the tight capillary junctions.[3] However, normal cerebral parenchyma shows slight overall enhancement amounting to 4–5 per cent[4] due to the distribution of iodine in the blood vascular pool in the brain and resulting in an average increase of 1.9 Hounsfield Units for grey matter and 1.4 units for white matter, the difference being due to the more richly vascularized grey matter.[5]

Intrathecal contrast

CT cisternography is occasionally used to image small lesions in the basal cisterns not revealed by standard CT since it still provides the best anatomical delineation of structures at the base of the brain and around the brain stem. However it is an invasive procedure and indications for its use are decreasing particularly when MRI is available. Its main role is now in the demonstration of the site of a CSF leak.[6]

Dynamic Tomography

Routine CT scanning provides morphological information only and in order to obtain a functional study it is necessary to undertake repeated scans of the same plane over a period of time. By selecting a region of interest, using either the cursor or light pen facility, information of the wash-in and wash-out phases of contrast agents is set out in histogram form providing a time–density curve. The earliest studies using second-generation scanners with scan times of 30–60s per slice providing sequential information over periods of up to 2 h[7] showed some correlation between enhancement patterns of different types of tumour and between tumours and other vascular lesions. Rapid scanning times available on third- and fourth-generation scanners provide more points on the early part of the curve. Although useful in blood flow studies[8,9] and in the investigation of pituitary microadenomas, they do not really contribute to the routine investigation of cerebral tumours.

These studies appear to separate gliomas from meningiomas[8,9] and can provide some help in the grading of gliomas[7] but since tumour tissue is seldom homogeneous the information from small regions of interest is relatively inaccurate and there is too much variation in sampling to make this procedure clinically useful.

Magnetic resonance

In X-ray CT the image is directly proportional to the attenuation of X-rays by the structure being scanned. This gives an attenuation coefficient to any volume element (voxel) in the scan slice which can only be changed by altering the physical characteristics of the X-ray beam, which in practice are usually standardized and constant for a particular procedure. By assigning a colour or a shade on a grey scale to different degrees of X-ray absorption a colour or tonal image can be produced.

MRI is similar to CT only in so far as it uses a grey scale or colour system to denote the physical state of each voxel and computes the information obtained during the scan into a two-dimensional image. However, the physical state is far more complex. Although any atom with an unequal number of protons and neutrons can be made to resonate, conventional MRI is concerned with the imaging of the naturally abundant hydrogen nucleus – the proton – and one characteristic of this state is the number of protons in each voxel (proton density). The physical state can also be altered by changing a number of variables in the MR system and by sampling at different points along the decay curves produced during the process of magnetic resonance. These decay curves occur once the protons have been raised to a higher energy level by applying a radiofrequency pulse for a certain length of time. The subsequent rate of decay depends on the physical characteristics of the different tissues being examined. There are decay curves for two time constants – T_1 and T_2. When protons are placed in a homogeneous magnetic field of high strength their axes become aligned parallel or antiparallel to the main magnetic field although they spin about their own axes in random phase. By applying a pulse of radiofrequency energy, at a frequency (larmor frequency) specific for the field strength, for a set period of time at right angles to the main field the protons will be flipped out of the plane of the magnetic field though an angle which depends on the length of time for which the pulse is applied. This RF pulse will also result in the individual spins becoming in-phase about their own axes.

The T_1 decay curve (spin lattice relaxation curve) follows the application of an RF pulse of sufficient length to flip the protons by 180° and depends on the ability of protons to give up energy to their environment. Since signal is only received at right angles to the main field a 90° pulse is subsequently applied and the signal is collected immediately from protons that have not relaxed completely at the time of data collection. Water either in the form of liquid or as oedematous tissue has widely dispersed molecules and therefore the ability of the water protons to impart energy to their environment is relatively poor and the T_1 decay curve is long. More compact tissues and those with a lower water content give up energy more quickly and therefore have a shorter T_1 decay curve. A high signal (white image) will be produced when the decay is rapid (short T_1) and a low signal (black) when the decay is slow. Examples of tissue having a short T_1 decay curve are fat and shed blood, which in the latter is caused by conversion of oxy- to methaemoglobin. Most cerebral tumours and the surrounding oedema contain a high concentration of water molecules and are therefore of low signal intensity.

The T_2 decay curve is called the spin spin relaxation curve. An RF pulse is applied sufficient to flip the protons by 90°. Once the RF pulse has been switched off the signal which is initially maximal will begin to decay because the rate of spin of each proton differs from each of its neighbours due to the local magnetic effects from the surrounding protons; the protons will therefore gradually move out of phase with one another. Eventually when the phases become random no signal will be detected. Some tissues have a more homogenous local field so neighbouring protons remain longer in phase with each other, i.e. dephasing is slower. The protons in solid tissues dephase quickly and lose signal more rapidly than the more mobile protons of liquids and tissues of high water content such as tumours. The latter have a long T_2 relaxation time and therefore are bright on T_2 weighted sequences. Both relaxation curves are exponential.

In order to provide sufficient signal to produce an image, a set of radiofrequency pulses termed a sequence are repeated for a sufficient number of times (over periods ranging between 5 and 25 min) to give a good enough sample. The most commonly used sequence is the spin echo (SE). The main variables are: (i) the repeat time (TR) which is the time in milliseconds (ms) between each set of 90° RF pulses and (ii) the echo time (TE), the time between the initial RF pulse and the beginning of the signal sampling period. In inversion recovery sequences the interval between the initial 180° and the 90° pulse is termed TI time. Altering the TR and the TE will increase or decrease the effect of the T_1 or T_2 relaxation time on the received signal. The signal intensity (contrast) in a particular voxel is a product of proton density and T_1 and T_2 relaxation rates. In general in spin echo (SE) sequences the shorter the TR the more T_1 weighted the image and the longer the TE the more T_2 weighted it is, since the signal due to proton density and TE is low at short TR times and that due to proton density and TR is also low at long TE times. The effects on contrast of altering TR, TE and TI are shown in Fig. 6.1. Therefore a short TR short TE sequence will be T_1 weighted, a long TR, long TE sequence will be T_2 weighted and a long TR, short TE sequence will be neither T_1 nor T_2 weighted (the signal being mainly dependent on

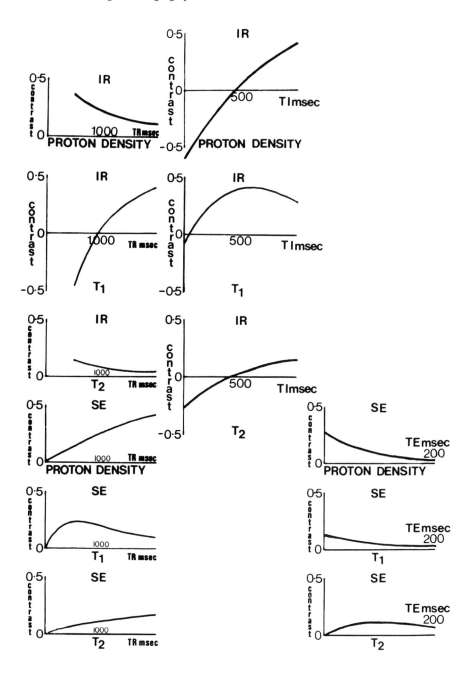

Fig. 6.1 Effects on contrast of altering TR, TI and TE.

proton density). The image is also affected by flow and movement within or through the slice which usually results in a low (black) signal with fast flow states and a high signal (flow-related enhancement) in slow flow states. This feature is of little direct importance in tumours although signal void in neighbouring vessels demonstrates vascular displacement of major vessels. The position of these arteries and their relation to the altered signal indicates the anatomical extent of the pathology and may be of considerable value in the differentiation of intra- from extra-axial masses.

Since T_1, T_2 and proton density affect all sequences to a certain extent the scan appearance of a pathological structure will depend on the relative dominance of each of these parameters and the proportionate effect each has on the signal. Many other sequences have been devised but in routine imaging, apart from spin echo sequences, only the inversion recovery, which is a strongly T_1 weighted sequence, is commonly used.

Tissue characteristics

Most pathological tissue has a different water content from normal tissue; usually it is increased, resulting in long T_1 and T_2 relaxation times. This causes low and high intensity changes respectively in most tumours and ischaemic or inflammatory processes, with no useful differentiation between these conditions on the basis of differential signal intensity.

Blood and fat behave differently. Fat has short T_1 and relatively normal T_2 relaxation times and appears bright on T_1 weighted sequences. Haemorrhage evolves through certain well-defined stages. Early haemorrhage is hypointense on T_1 sequences due to oxyhaemoglobin but after the first few days becomes of high intensity once methaemoglobin has been formed. These changes persist for many months,[10] unlike CT where the high density rapidly becomes iso- and then low-density. A similar bright intensity occurs in T_2 weighted sequences at the same time corresponding to the haematoma and surrounding low density seen on CT; later, a ring of low intensity representing the enhancing capsule on CT appears and persists indefinitely due to deposition of haemosiderin.[10, 11]

Scanning protocol sequences

Since the two most significant variables affecting the signal are the T_1 and T_2 relaxation times it is necessary to undertake sequences which separately reflect the effects of each. The patient is usually first scanned in the axial plane using a T_2 weighted sequence with a TR of 2000–2500 ms and a TE of about 80–100 ms. This sequence is particularly sensitive to small changes in water content and so will detect the smallest volume of pathological tissue. Unfortunately, using this sequence, differentiation of tumour from oedema and brain from CSF is poor so that a second sequence, usually T_1 weighted, is undertaken in one of the other orthogonal planes, i.e. coronal or sagittal. Since short TR, short TE sequences are only mildly T_1 weighted we prefer the inversion recovery sequence, which provides good anatomical localization with high contrast between normal grey and white matter, CSF and pathological tissue.

The scan time for each of the above sequences is 17–23 min during which a number of contiguous slices are obtained, sufficient to cover the whole of the cranial cavity in the axial plane.

Sedation

Patient co-operation is essential during the period of scanning so that the need for sedation will have to be assessed beforehand. Similar sedation regimes can be used as in CT but because of the constraints of the magnetic field and the long scanner tunnel, patient monitoring is not as easy and non-magnetic monitoring and anaesthetic equipment will be required. In the event of cardiac or respiratory arrest the patient should be removed immediately from the scanning room so that constraints are not placed on the type of resuscitation equipment used. Less than 5 per cent of examinations fail because of claustrophobia.

Intravenous contrast

The high inherent contrast produced by many sequences results in images which have a high sensitivity to pathology while allowing good spatial localization because of excellent demonstration of anatomy. Unfortunately discrimination of different pathological tissues is rather poor and it can be difficult to separate tumour edge from surrounding oedema without a contrast agent which differentially enhances tumour tissue.

The iodine-containing contrast agents which are used in CT and which produce their effect by increased absorption of X-ray photons are not suitable for MRI as they are not paramagnetic. For a contrast agent to be suitable for MRI it needs to alter the T_1 and T_2 relaxation times from that of normal surrounding tissue. Substances that produce useful increase in T_1 and T_2 values have not been identified and only those that are paramagnetic and mainly cause shortening of the T_1 relaxation time have been found useful. Salts of iron[12] and manganese,[13] and nitroxide free radicals[14] have been studied but are toxic in solution and are unsuitable for intravenous injection. Only the lanthanide series of rare earth elements has so far provided the optimal combination of the ability to shorten T_1 adequately while at the same time having a relatively non-toxic formulation. The most widely studied of these elements is gadolinium (Gd) which in its ionic form cannot be injected because it is too toxic.[15] However chelation with ethylenediaminetetraacetic acid (EDTA) or diethylenetriaminepentaacetic acid (DTPA) produces compounds with low toxicity warranting further study. Of the two DTPA is the safest; the gadolinium becomes almost completely bound with virtually none remaining in the ionic form. The binding is much stronger than with EDTA. Both are eliminated from the body in the same way as CT contrast agents, being excreted by glomerular filtration with a half-life of about 20 min[16] and almost complete elimination by 7 days. Gd DTPA is given in a dose of 0.1 mmol/kg body weight which is 1/100 of the LD_{50}.[17] At this concentration it causes marked shortening of T_1 relaxation time. The effects of a short T_1 and T_2 tend to cancel. In lower concentrations the T_1 effect is greater resulting in tissue enhancement but with higher concentrations the T_2 effect predominates. Paramagnetic contrast agents do not cross the intact blood–brain barrier but behave in a similar manner to CT contrast media in tumours and other pathology demonstrating the margins between lesion and oedema.[18] The distribution and uptake of gadolinium is similar to that in CT with time-dependent scanning.[19]

Safety factors

In vivo studies have been undertaken into the harmful efects of MR on biological tissues. In an extensive review of the subject[20] three sources have been identified as possible causes: (a) static magnetic fields; (b) changing magnetic fields; (c) radiofrequency heating. Static magnetic fields up to 2.0 T do not cause morphological or physiological changes nor do changing magnetic fields under 0.5 mT/s, such as are induced by gradient coils used in localization. Radiofrequency heating may occur under certain circumstances such as with large "metallic" prostheses and care should be exercised when scanning patients with these implants.

An absolute contraindication to MR exists in patients who have had aneurysm surgery or in whom a loose metallic foreign body could be present, e.g. in the orbit, because there is a risk that the static magnetic field could alter its position with harmful results.

Cerebral angiography

Indications for cerebral angiography in the management of the tumour patient have decreased since CT became widely available. Its role is now mainly limited to the demonstration of vascular anatomy prior to surgery, assessment of patency of venous sinuses in extracerebral tumours and the requirements of embolization.

Conventional angiography using cut film supplemented by subtraction techniques still provides the greatest radiographic detail and although this may provide information in the assessment of the degree of malignancy[21] it is usually a refinement which does not alter the management of the patient. The majority of procedures are undertaken by the transfemoral route with catheterization of selective cervical arteries. Complications of cerebral angiography are either related to the contrast used, to the clinical condition of the patient or as a direct result of the procedure itself.

General complications are rare in an adequately prepared patient. However, angiography is frequently required in ill patients who may deteriorate at any time and not all adverse changes are due to the procedure itself.[22] Minor contrast reactions are quite common but the incidence of severe reactions is much lower[23] particularly with the use of non-ionic contrast media.[24] Of the other serious complications acute renal failure is the most common. It is more frequent in the very young and in those suffering from diabetes, hypertension, myeloma and liver disease and is more common when high doses of contrast are used.[25]

Complications as a direct result of the procedure have become less common with the increased safety of contrast media and with increase in the skill of radiological staff with catheter techniques, but even in the most experienced hands identifiable deficits approach 1 per cent[26] and detailed examination of the patient immediately after the procedure suggests transient deterioration in the neurological state in up to 50 per cent.[27]

Recent advances in technology have resulted in the wider use of digital subtraction angiography (DSA). The fluoroscopic image of each frame of the angiogram run is converted from analogue to digital form and stored on disk with a matrix of at least 512 × 512. Immediate subtraction of one image from another (in practice from one of the masks prior to the contrast injection) provides real-time subtracted images considerably reducing the time spent on the procedure and potentially increasing safety.

There are currently two main methods of DSA – the intravenous and intra-arterial routes. The intravenous route has become popular because it is primarily an outpatient procedure and therefore reduces overall costs. Each run requires about 40 ml of non-ionic contrast injected as a bolus either through the antecubital fossa into the basilic vein or more commonly, and more satisfactorily, via a catheter with the tip close to the right atrium. The leading edge of the bolus reaches the basal cerebral arteries after passing through the lungs approximately 4–6 s after the injection commences, depending on the cardiac output. The quality of the image depends on the concentration of contrast. The bolus tends to break up and the concentration to decrease with increase in the heart rate and decrease in pulse volume. Because both of these are high in childhood, intravenous DSA frequently does not produce images of satisfactory quality in the very young. Intravenous angiography is also not vessel-selective since all cerebral arteries are filled simultaneously. Relatively, the basal intracranial arteries are poorly visualized even on a high-quality study and smaller vessels cannot be resolved at all. However, it produces good opacification of cerebral veins and venous sinuses because there is no washout effect by non-opacified blood. Intravenous DSA is therefore inappropriate for angiography in tumours other than to assess sinus patency.

Intra-arterial DSA provides similar information to conventional angiography. Although the resolution is lower (vessels smaller than 0.5 mm usually cannot be clearly seen) pathological vessels and early draining veins are well demonstrated. Since DSA is more contrast-sensitive than conventional radiographic film, lower concentrations of contrast are used resulting in a greater safety margin and a more comfortable procedure.

Complications of intra-arterial DSA are the same as with conventional angiography. Those of intravenous DSA are infrequent and of no lasting consequence. The general complications, already mentioned, apply to intravenous DSA as to conventional angiography. Local complications are limited to extravasation of contrast at the puncture site when only a short cannula is placed in the antecubital vein and rupture of a peripheral or mediastinal vein occurs, the latter causing some chest pain and occasional dyspnoea. However none of these effects persists.[28]

Imaging in tumour assessment

A description of the radiological features of even the most common intra- and extra-axial tumours is not possible in a chapter of this size and the wide variation in their appearance often results in a radiological diagnosis which depends as much on other factors, such as position of mass, age of patient, relevant clinical features, etc., as on the imaging appearances. The ultimate diagnosis, however, still rests with obtaining histological material. Investigations are requested for a number of reasons and because both CT and MRI usually give reasonably definite answers it is rarely necessary to request both procedures since the information obtained it frequently common to both.

Rather than consider tumours in general, the following comments refer mainly to intra-axial rather than to extra-axial tumours. With this in mind the role of imaging will be considered from the baseline of CT but MRI will be considered where appropriate in relation to the following features.

1. Tissue characterization (Tumour versus oedema)
2. Invasion and tumour margin
3. Rate of growth and grade of malignancy
4. Postoperative imaging (response to treatment, radiation effects, tumour recurrence etc.)

Tissue characterization

Skull radiographs play little part in the current investigation of tumours and although abnormal calcification will alert the radiologist to the presence of underlying pathology, such a feature is only seen in about 6 to 13 per cent of tumours,[29, 30] and may occur in other conditions. Abnormalities on the skull radiograph are generally non-specific and include signs of raised intracranial pressure which are of little localizing or diagnostic value. Such features as focal vault expansion or reactive changes due to local effects on bone are difficult to appreciate unless firmly established and their absence does not exclude underlying pathology.

With occasional exceptions, the hallmark of a tumour is a mass causing space occupation with displacement of neighbouring structures. However, this description can be applied to many other pathological processes during a particular phase of evolution, so that the initial assessment of a structural lesion must be aimed at differentiating tumour from other conditions. Sometimes the appearances are quite typical of tumour even when clinical features suggest otherwise but usually these typical radiological features are accompanied by typical clinical features of a progressive nature and can be diagnosed on CT in over 90 per cent of such cases.[31, 32]

Tumours commence as solid masses of cells. Subsequently areas of necrosis and calcification may develop but neither the presence nor absence of these is required to establish the diagnosis.

Solid components

On CT the density of solid components depends on the water content of the tissue but in general is either isodense with brain or close to it. The ability to separate mass from normal brain depends on surrounding vasogenic oedema which is of lower density and involves the white matter tracts. The nature of the tumour cannot be inferred from the density of the solid components of the mass alone. The attenuation of gliomas, ependymomas and many metastases may be similar; they are usually iso- or slightly hypodense and the solid components form only part of the tumour (Figs 6.2, 6.3). Hyperdense tumours most commonly encountered are meningiomas,[33] lymphomas,[34] and some metastases particularly melanomas[35] and those from the gastrointestinal tract. These are more likely to be homogeneous but the attenuation coefficients are rarely more than 40 Hounsfield Units (20 EMI Units).[35] Differentiation from haemorrhage is seldom a problem since in the acute stage the

104 *Neuroradiological imaging of brain tumours*

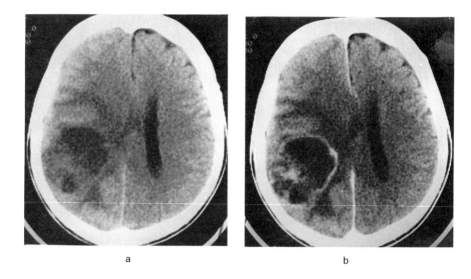

Fig. 6.2 Malignant glioma; (a) plain CT scan; (b) post-contrast. A typical mixed density partly necrotic mass with irregular enhancement and a variable thickness of tumour wall is accompanied by extensive vasogenic oedema and considerable mass effect.

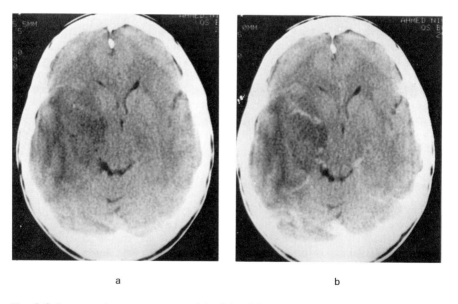

Fig. 6.3 Low-grade astrocytoma; (a) plain CT scan; (b) post-contrast. There is mixed but mainly low-density mass with little enhancement causing relatively minor mass effect. Differentiation between tumour and oedematous normal tissue is difficult to assess.

density coefficient of a haematoma measures about 80 Hounsfield Units, and although it gradually decreases with time its appearance also alters over a shorter period than does a tumour. The margins become less well-defined whereas hypodense tumours persist with time and are usually well-circumscribed masses.

Haemorrhage

Haemorrhage into a tumour is not uncommon and is particularly common in glioblastomas, medulloblastomas and metastases. It is detected on CT in about 3.6 per cent of tumours.[36] Haemorrhage within the tumour mass is suggestive of a glioma, but more solid haematomas and haemorrhagic infarction suggest underlying metastases.[36] The haematoma may extend to involve the subarachnoid space or break through into the ventricle.[37]

Haemorrhage associated with a tumour will also be demonstrated by MRI, using appropriate sequences if it is of a significant volume. The short T_1 of methaemoglobin and the short T_2 of haemosiderin which so characterizes blood products will usually be present within a larger area of long T_1 and T_2 due to the surrounding tumour and oedema than is normally present around a simple haematoma. However, absence of surrounding oedema and even lesions commonly labelled as occult vascular malformations do not exclude underlying primary or metastatic tumours.[38] Because of partial volume MRI is much less effective in demonstrating small amounts of blood within the region of pathology.

Differentiation from haemorrhage secondary to a ruptured aneurysm, hypertension etc., may be difficult although the presence of excessive vasogenic oedema in the acute phase suggests an underlying lesion (Fig. 6.4). Further scans will ultimately reveal the nature of the haematoma but angiography is necessary to exclude an angioma or aneurysm and may demonstrate pathological vessels.

Low-density components

These feature in most gliomas but their contribution to the whole mass largely conforms to the degree of malignancy. In low-grade gliomas low-density components generally form the major part but irregular isodense components may contribute to the mass resulting in an inhomogeneous appearance.

Another common appearance of low-grade gliomas, most of which prove to be grade I,[39] is of a virtually homogeneous rounded mass of low density below that of surrounding brain but often higher than CSF (Fig. 6.5). Some are cystic with a high protein content but many are gelatinous and apparently solid (microcystic). Diagnosis is usually not difficult since differentiation from other circumscribed low-density lesions is based on the anatomical site, response to contrast, and associated oedema. Superficial masses involving the cortex are unlikely to be confused with extra-axial lesions such as porencephalic or arachnoid cysts which are of CSF density but localization can be refined further by MRI using inversion recovery sequences in axial and coronal planes. Low-density components in high-grade tumours usually form a small part of the whole lesion representing areas of necrosis in an intially solid tumour. Not infrequently this results in a ring-shaped isodense mass, the centre of which forms the bulk of the tumour. Since the signal in magnetic resonance imaging depends mainly on the density of the mobile protons and there is increased water in

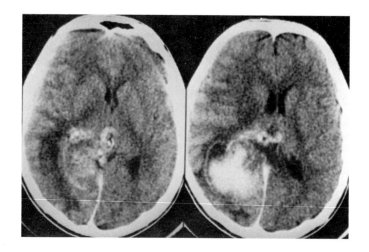

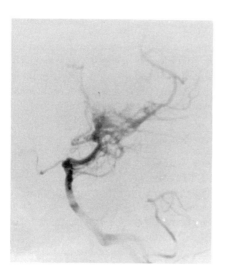 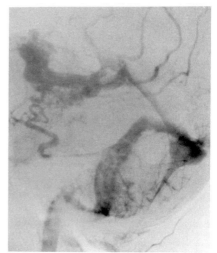

Fig. 6.4 Cerebral haematoma with associated angioma. (a) Post-contrast CT scans of adjacent slices demonstrate residual haematoma with surrounding granulation enhancement. Areas of more florid enhancement anterior to the mass are due to underlying pathology (vascular in this case) the appearances of which are non-specific. (b) Corresponding angiogram; arterial and venous phases demonstrate supply through perforating and posterior choroidal branches of the posterior cerebral artery with rapid drainage into ependymal veins.

all pathological tissues there is a similar difficulty in attempting to differentiate tumours on the basis of their signal characteristics alone. When using sequences which are not strongly T_1 or T_2 weighted (i.e. T_1 weighted spin echo – short TR, short TE), the effect on the signal of increase in T_1 recovery time will counteract that of increased in T_2 and result in tissue contrast (normal and pathological) close to that of the adjacent brain. Strongly T_2-weighted sequences are more sensitive than T_1 sequences for demonstrating small lesions such as metastases,[40] and very strongly T_1-and T_2-weighted sequences are more likely to demonstrate tissue structure in a tumour mass and allow the signal intensity to be compared with that of the surrounding grey and white matter and CSF. Nevertheless the only absolute indication of a cyst is a fluid level in the most dependent part (Fig. 6.6).

A number of studies have attempted to measure the T_1 and T_2 recovery times in the hope that this would provide discrimination between different pathological tissues. Comparison of these parameters between different machines even of the same static magnetic field strength is meaningless because recovery times are not absolute. Even in a particular scanner there is a wide variation of relaxation rates between tumours of different grades of malignancy and histology[41, 42] and between tumours and other pathologies;[43, 44] for example the T_1 and T_2 values of meningiomas are significantly shorter than those of other tumours[45] but not all neoplasms that have short T_1 or T_2 relaxation times are meningiomas. Also, CT attenuation is not related to T_1 recovery time but does appear to have an inverse relation to T_2.[46]

Oedema

Most focal pathology causes local effects on adjacent brain tissue, increasing the water content. Oedema may occur with intrinsic masses such as tumours and vascular and inflammatory lesions and may also be secondary to extrinsic pathology such as meningiomas. It is of two main types, vasogenic (associated with tumours, abscesses etc.) and cytotoxic (associated with ischaemia and infarction).[47] On CT, vasogenic oedema appears to involve only the white matter with finger-like processes of low density extending along the white matter tracts.[48] Low-grade gliomas usually have very little surrounding oedema but high-grade tumours, both primary and metastatic are commonly associated with extensive oedema[39] (Fig. 6.7) which in metastases[31] and some meningiomas, particularly those arising from the skull base and subfrontal region,[49] is often disproportionate to the size of the tumour.

Oedema increases the length of the T_1 and T_2 recovery times resulting in high signal on T_2-weighted and low signal on T_1-weighted sequences. This may be greater than the signal from the tumour itself and sometimes provides discrimination between tumour and oedema. The increased sensitivity of MRI indicates that vasogenic oedema is more widely distributed than that observed on CT. Not only is there extensive involvement of the white matter tracts but the cortex is also involved particularly on T_2-weighted sequences with a distribution similar to ischaemia on CT.[47] Some difficulty may be experienced in differentiating tumour from infarct if the extent of a tumour and its surrounding oedema is seen to occupy a particular vascular territory.

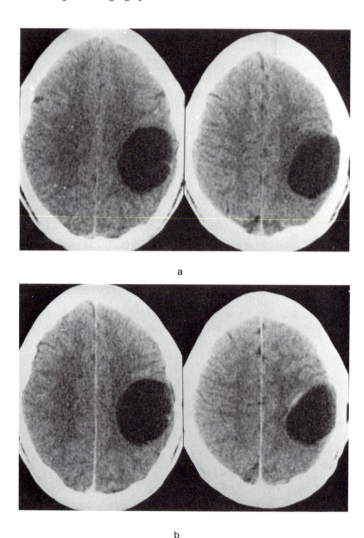

Fig. 6.5 Cystic astrocytoma; (a) plain CT scan; (b) post-contrast. There is a well-defined round low density mass of CSF attenuation with an enhancing wall. Many of these masses contain gelatinous material and are not fluid-containing.

Calcification

CT is very sensitive to the attenuating effects of calcification and even small and relatively poorly calcified regions can be identified. Although the density coefficients may be no different from that of blood, the extent and location is rarely likely to cause confusion. Significant calcification is obvious and may be due to many causes but it is the associated features such as mass, oedema, enhancement, etc., which indicate a tumour. The extent of the calcification provides little indication of the likely

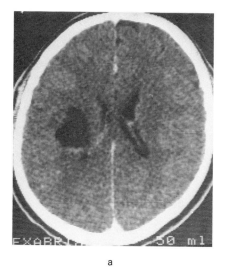

a

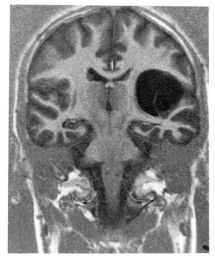

b

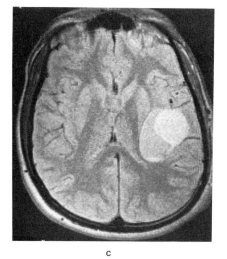

c

Fig. 6.6 Cystic glioma; (a) CT scan; (b) MRI scan coronal plane; (c) MRI scan axial plane. There is a fluid level on the axial CT and MRI scans in the most dependant region which is not present on the coronal MRI scan.

pathology. Tumour calcification is not uncommon. Approximately 10 per cent of astrocytomas and 50 per cent of oligodendrogliomas calcify, and since the former are more common, calcification in a brain tumour is most likely to indicate an astrocytoma.

Neither the presence nor extent of calcification provides any guide to the grade of tumour. Low-grade tumours can grow slowly for many years with the subsequent development of malignant change in one area of the tumour leading to rapid enlargement of the mass.

Calcification can be difficult to detect on MRI (Fig. 6.8). The protons in calcium

110 *Neuroradiological imaging of brain tumours*

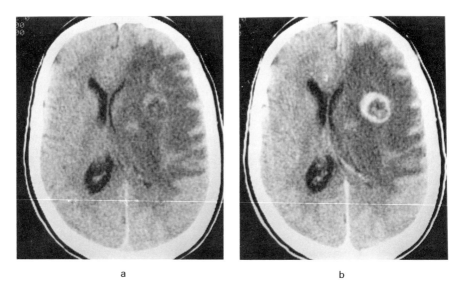

Fig. 6.7 Typical cerebral metastasis; (a) plain CT scan; (b) post-contrast. There is a relatively small densely enhancing mass with central necrosis and a large amount of vasogenic oedema displacing the ventricles to the right.

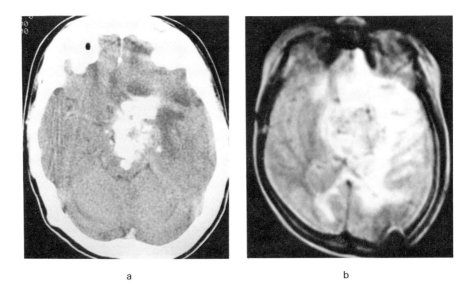

Fig. 6.8 Calcified tumour; (a) CT scan; (b) MRI scan. There is very dense calcification on CT which is only just visible on the MRI scan as a patchy area of low intensity within an extensive area of abnormal high intensity consisting of tumour and surrounding oedema.

are immobile and so give no signal. On T_2-weighted sequences foci should therefore be identified as areas of relatively low density. More often, however, viable tumour tissue in and around the calcification produces such high signal that the signal effects of the calcification are overshadowed within the partial volume.

Were MRI to supercede CT as the primary diagnostic investigation, as has been suggested, the inability to detect calcification unequivocally could limit its value in situations where the management of a patient depends on an accurate radiological diagnosis, and for this reason indications for CT will remain, particularly in the perisellar region where masses containing calcium (craniopharyngiomas, aneurysms etc.) need to be differentiated from chiasmal and pituitary tumours.

CT and MRI are complementary in regions such as the skull base where CT accurately identifies the minor and early changes of bone destruction. MRI does not demonstrate bone destruction but provides primary evidence of the tumour with high signal on T_2-weighted sequences and gadolinium-enhanced T_1 sequences.

Intravenous contrast

It is customary to give intravenous contrast in CT when focal masses are demonstrated on the plain scan. In neoplastic tissue, contrast usually enhances the isodense components. In high-grade gliomas the central necrotic area is commonly of irregular shape and the enhancing peripheral margin is of variable thickness which differentiates malignant tumours from cerebral abscesses and resolving haematomas. When the margins of the tumour are well-defined it is uncommon for the contrast to

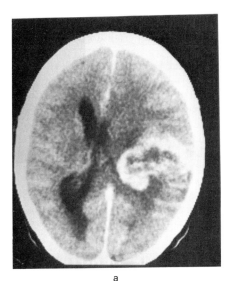 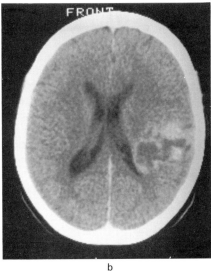

a b

Fig. 6.9 Effect of steroid treatment. Glioma; (a) post-contrast scan; (b) post-contrast scan two weeks later after treatment with steroids. Although the tumour remains the same size there is marked reduction in mass effect and virtually no oedema. There may also be some decrease in the amount of enhancement.

provide significant additional information. Under the influence of angiogenic factors[50] tumours cause the formation of abnormal capillaries which are more permeable than usual.[51] The more malignant the tumour the greater the effect on these capillaries; in low-grade gliomas the capillaries appear normal with preservation of the blood–brain barrier and so significant enhancement,[4] but in malignant tumours there tends to be increased permeability with marked contrast enhancement.[52, 53] Steroid therapy decreases this accumulation,[54, 55] and in some cases may reduce the volume of tumour[56] and surrounding oedema[57] (Fig. 6.9). Varying degrees of malignancy may be found even in the same tumour mass and enhancement appears to correlate best with histological evidence of vascularity and necrosis.[58] Loss of the blood-brain barrier is a gradual process which depends partly on the number of tumour cells and their local effects. Stereotactic biopsies demonstrate viable malignant cells in the surrounding vasogenic oedema at a distance from the main tumour mass[59] and areas of enhancement. Since the response of a tumour to gadolinium-DTPA is similar to iodine-containing contrast agents[60] the same information will be obtained on contrast-enhanced MRI as on CT so that the use of both procedures is unnecessary. With supratentorial intracerebral tumours contrast-enhanced CT which provides good anatomical localization of the tumour is therefore the investigation of choice in the majority of cases.

A mass close to the skull base can be localized prior to surgery by reference to adjacent bony landmarks. Tumours in the hemispheres, however, cannot be positioned in this manner and displacement of intracranial anatomy may contribute to false localization particularly in earlier scanners. This contributed to the persistence of isotope imaging long after its other uses had disappeared, since the lateral image superimposed on a lateral radiograph provided a simple means by which freehand localization could be undertaken prior to biopsy. Nevertheless the chosen site was sometimes some distance from the mass, resulting in inaccurate biopsies.

Modern scanners possess more sophisticated software which enable the position of a lesion to be transferred on to the scout image in sagittal or coronal planes by identifying its margins on each of the axial images which contain the tumour using a light pen or cursor (Fig. 6.10). This technique gives an accurate representation of the site of the tumour for planning the position of a small craniotomy or freehand burrhole biopsy and is useful in more superficial and larger but inoperable lesions when a formal craniotomy is not desirable. Morbidity and operative mortality of freehand biopsy are generally higher than with tumour excision[16] and multiple biopsies may be required to achieve a diagnosis.[62]

More accurate localization can only be provided by stereotactic techniques. The precise imaging of CT, and more recently MRI, has been combined with the accuracy of stereotactic procedures, and following the earlier pioneering work of Bergstrom and Greitz[63] CT-guided stereotactic biopsies have been reported in a large variety of intracranial tumours.[64] Adaptations of virtually all the common stereotactic frames have been made for use with CT, allowing a whole range of different therapies, such as aspiration, interstitial irradiation and the insertion of chemotherapeutic agents, to be undertaken as well as diagnostic biopsies.

The patient's head is held in a base ring attached to the scanner table or to a specially designed stereotactic apparatus by a number of pins inserted into the skull, sometimes penetrating the outer table. After contrast-enhanced CT the desired

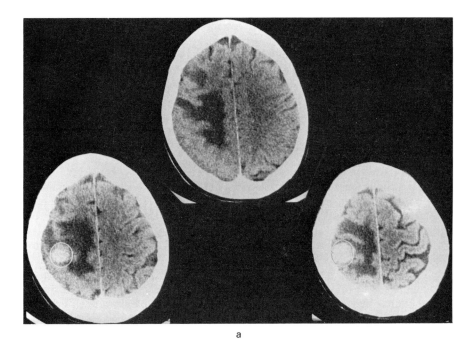

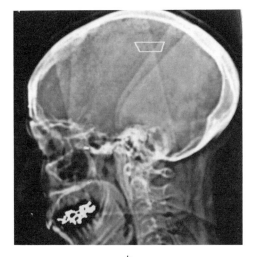

Fig. 6.10 Tumour localization; (a) CT scan; (b) scout image to show position of the tumour by identification of its margins on the axial scans and direct transfer on to the scout image using the computer software.

location for biopsy is identified in the three orthogonal planes $(X, Y, Z,)$ and the coordinates transferred on to the stereotactic apparatus using simple software facilities. A high degree of precision is claimed[65-67] with a similar incidence of positive histology in samples taken from the enhancing rim and central non-enhancing low density.[68, 69] The mortality is low, averaging 2 to 3 per cent.[70]

A similar technique has been applied to magnetic resonance imaging using non-magnetic materials,[71] and although an equally high degree of accuracy can be obtained, the system is prone to a greater variation of image distortion than with CT due to the incidental introduction of field inhomogeneities. Because in many cases the cause of these effects is uncertain and may be uncontrollable, there is a significant risk that the location chosen on the MR image may not correspond to the actual site of the tumour within the frame.

Tumour malignancy and rate of growth

There have been many attempts to characterize the degree of tumour malignancy particularly on the various CT appearances, but in general this has met with limited success since overall survival is dependent on more than just the aggressiveness of the tumour. Many relatively benign tumours eventually threaten life because of their critical location but one of the main indicators of malignancy is rate of growth.

Several reports have focussed on the false-negative CT scan[72–74] which occurs from time to time irrespective of which CT scanner is used. These studies have emphasized the need to repeat the radiological examination if clinical features indicate a structural lesion.[72] In one study using a second-generation scanner[74] approximately 1.5 per cent of gliomas were undetected on the first examination with a further 6.5 per cent of false-positives and another 6.5 per cent mis-diagnosed as benign lesions. The majority of these (27/40) proved to be high-grade tumours. Since tumour growth can be very rapid in glioblastomas with a doubling time, reported in one series of between 15 and 21 days irrespective of histological variation,[75] it is hardly surprising that patients may be investigated before structural lesions can be detected. As long as the tumour does not induce density changes, cause mass effect or affect the blood–brain barrier, CT will not reveal its presence.

In all cases where a normal CT is accompanied by a strong clinical indication of a developing structural lesion MRI should be undertaken if available using a T_2-weighted spin echo sequence. Alterations in local water content will allow even the smallest changes to be apparent where no lesion has been detected on CT.[76] Whether these early changes are due to tumour or to the altered surrounding brain with developing oedema cannot be inferred from MRI alone[77] and gadolinium-enhanced studies are unlikely to provide more specific information while the blood–brain barrier is still intact. Stereotactic biopsies however, have demonstrated viable tumour cells at this stage of development within the abnormal areas.

The size of a tumour when scanned will depend to a certain extent on whether it is situated in a critical position and whether it causes symptoms early on.[78] Frontal lobe tumours are notoriously silent. Since the growth rate of glioblastomas is rapid and appears to be exponential, only a short time may elapse before a small tumour reaches a much larger size. Furthermore, since there is little relation between the absolute volume of the tumour and the area of enhancement demonstrated, it is not surprising that in glioblastomas there is no significant correlation between tumour size (as defined by area of enhancement) and prognosis.[79]

Extent of tumour

It has been noted that the response of tumour to enhancement gives a reasonably accurate measure of malignancy, with high-grade tumours causing greater enhancement than those of lower grade and tumours of grade I and II causing insignificant enhancement.[80] However enhancement does not quantify the size of the mass for not only are large numbers of malignant cells often found in the non-enhancing central "necrosis" but numerous mitotic cells are also found in non-enhancing regions adjacent to enhancing tumour masses.

Evidence in support of this is provided by positron emission tomography (PET) scans. Metabolic studies using ^{18}F-labelled 2-deoxy-D-glucose in glioblastomas indicated close correlation between the grade of tumour and the uptake of this metabolite, and this relationship occurs irrespective of the state of the blood–brain barrier.[81] The prognostic significance of tumour enhancement is much less clear. There appears to be little relationship between enhancement and the long-term survival in patients with low-grade gliomas; in one series the four years actuarial survival was 58 per cent in patients whose tumours enhanced and 65 per cent in those that did not.[82]

The postoperative patient

Imaging in the postoperative period is complicated by the effects of surgery and subsequent radio- and chemotherapy so that CT and MR can often play only a relatively limited role in the difficult case. Usually patients are examined only when new symptoms occur or when there are complications of the surgical procedure and often there is only the preoperative scan on which to base a comparison.

In these cases the appearances often confirm the clinical suspicion, i.e. that there is tumour recurrence sufficient to explain the clinical features but at other times treatable complications such as hydrocephalus and extracerebral collections are demonstrated. During the early postoperative period appearances in and adjacent to the site of the surgery are particularly time-dependent. During the first few days CT demonstrates a mixed density pattern, in general low but with areas of high density due to blood products, Sterispon, etc., in the tumour bed and any enhancement will indicate residual tumour. Vascular proliferation into the tumour bed as a direct result of surgery does not develop until the end of the first postoperative week. For the next three to six weeks contrast enhancement may occur at the site of the surgery and tumour recurrence cannot be excluded on this basis alone. Vasogenic oedema gradually resolves but can remain for many months so that its persistence does not necessarily indicate persisting tumour. In the absence of any obvious mass only comparison with a study performed within a day or two of surgery enables a reasonable judgement to be made of tumour recurrence.

Routine scans however, are not to be encouraged as evidence suggests that neurological assessment is superior to CT as the first indicator of tumour recurrence.[83] This is in part due to the difficulty experienced in obtaining comparable slices and hence appreciating small changes in appearance.

Frequently surgery is followed by irradiation or chemotherapy. In the acute phase radiotherapy may be accompanied by an increase in symptoms sufficient to postpone further treatment. These are thought to be brought about by an increase in perivascular lymphocytic exudation;[84] CT changes have not been reported and insufficient evidence is as yet available from MRI.

A transient enlargement of residual tumour simulating regrowth may occur during the first three months after completion of radiotherapy[85] and reversible CT changes consisting of diffuse periventricular white matter low density have also been reported in the subacute stage.[86] More permanent features such as radiation necrosis,[87] neuronal loss resulting in cerebral atrophy and permanent white matter changes[88] are often delayed although they may become apparent within one month of the completion of radiotherapy.[89]

Enlargement of the ventricles and cortical sulci are commonly encountered in the elderly as the brain involutes and are not to be considered pathological. However, similar changes occur after radiotherapy in half the patients who have received doses of 30 to 60 Gy[90] and, particularly in the young patient, must be considered abnormal.

An increase in white matter low density is also encountered with increasing age on both CT[91] and MRI[92]. Following radiotherapy there is a generalized increase in the signal intensity of the deep periventricular white matter on T_2 weighted sequences.[88] Although more common with high doses these changes were encountered after doses as small as 24 Gy.

Radiation necrosis may develop as early as one month or be delayed as long as 14 years and is often accompanied by clinical features suggestive of tumour recurrence.[89] The incidence correlates reasonably well with the amount of radiation given, being most common with doses in excess of 50 Gy.[87] The most common appearance of a mass with or without abnormal enhancement[89, 93] is easily mistaken for tumour recurrence which may have important consequences for management. Neither CT nor MRI provide conclusive evidence as to the underlying pathology.

It appears that only PET can differentiate necrosis from tumour recurrence[94], oxygen uptake being significantly reduced in radionecrosis whereas it is elevated with tumour recurrence. Because of the very short half-life of many of the metabolites used and the necessity to be located within easy reach of a cyclotron these studies are not routinely practiced. Radiation necrosis which develops late in the course of the disease is usually free of tumour but similar changes developing within the first year of treatment almost invariably contain viable tumour cells in the peripheral ring of enhancement.[95]

References

1. Riding M, Bergström M, Bergvall U, Greitz T. Computer intravenous angiography. *Acta Radiologica*, (Suppl.) Stockholm. 1975; **346**, 82–90.
2. Kritcheff II, Lin J. Contrast enhancement in computed tomography. In: Caile J, Salamon G, eds. *Computerised Tomography*. Berlin: Springer, 1980: 163–5.
3. Phelps ME, Grubb RL, Jr, Ter Pogossian MM. *In vivo* regional cerebral blood volume by X-ray fluorescence. *Journal of Applied Physiology*. 1973; **35**, 741–7.
4. Caillé JM, Guilbert Tranier F, Calabet A, Billerey J, Piton J. In: Caille JJM, Salamon G, eds. *Abnormal Enhancements after Contrast Injection in Computerised Tomography*. Berlin: Springer, 1980: 166–71.
5. Arimitsu T, Di Chiro G, Brooks RA, Smith PB. White-grey matter differentiation in computed tomography. *Journal of Computer Assisted Tomography*. 1977; **1**, 437–42.
6. Manelfe C, Cellerier P, Sobel D, Prévost C, Bonafé A. Cerebrospinal fluid rhinorrhoea; evaluation with metrizamide cisternography. *American Journal of Roentgenology*. 1982; **138**, 471–6.
7. Lewander R, Bergström M, Bergvall U. Contrast enhancement of cranial lesions in computed tomography. *Acta Radiologica, Diagnosis*. 1978; **19**, 529–52.
8. Leonardi M, Biasizzo E, Calabo A. Application of dynamic CT or angio CT in neuroradiology; a disappointing experience. *Computerised Radiology*. 1985; **9**, 29–36.

9. Nakagomi T, Segawa H, Tanaka H. Dynamic computed tomography of the brain. *Neurosurgical Review.* 1985; **8**, 15-25.
10. Gomori JM, Grossman RI, Goldberg HI, Zimmerman RA, Bilanuik LT. Intracranial haematoma; imaging by high field MR. *Radiology.* 1985; 157, 87-92.
11. Enzmann DR, Butt RH, Lyons BE, Buxton JL, Wilson DA. Natural history of experimental intracerebral haematoma; sonography, computed tomography and neuropathology. *American Journal of Neuroradiology.* 1981; **2**, 517-26.
12. Block F, Hansen W, Packard M. The nuclear induction experiment. *Physics Reviews.* 1946; **70**, 474.
13. Lauterbur PC, Mendoça Dias M, Ruden AM. Segmentation of tissue water proton spin lattice relaxation rates by the *in vivo* addition of paramagnetic ions. In: Dutton PO, Leigh JS, Scarpa A, eds. *Frontiers of Biological Energetics.* New York: Academic Press, 1978.
14. Brasch RC, Nitecki DE, Brant-Zawadski M, Enzmann DR, Wesbey GE, Tozer TN, Tuck, Cann CE, Fike JR, Sheldon P. Brain nuclear magnetic resonance imaging enhanced by a paramagnetic nitroxide contrast agent: preliminary report. *American Journal of Roentgenology.* 1983; **141**, 1019-23.
15. Aruela P. Toxicity of rare earths. *Progress in Pharmacology.* 1979; **2**, 71-114.
16. Brant-Zawadski M, Berry I, Osaki L, Brasch RC, Murovic J, Norman D. Gd DTPA in clinical MR imaging of the brain. 1. Intraaxial lesions. *American Journal of Roentgenology.* 1986; **147**, 1223-30.
17. Brasch RC, Weinmann HJ, Wesbey GE. Contrast enhanced NMR imaging; animal studies using Gadolinium DTPA complex. *American Journal of Roentgenology.* 1984; **142**, 625-30.
18. Carr DH, Brown J, Bydder GM. Intravenous chelated gadolinium as a contrast agent in NMR imaging of cerebral tumours. *Lancet.* 1984; **1**, 484-6.
19. Schörner W, Laniado M, Niendorf HP, Schubert Ch, Felix R. Time dependent changes in image contrast in brain tumours after gadolinium DTPA. *American Journal of Neuroradiology.* 1986; **7**; 1013-20.
20. Budinger TF. Nuclear magnetic resonance (NMR) *in vivo* studies; known thresholds for health effects. *Journal of Computer Assisted Tomography.* 1981; **5**, 800-11.
21. Joyce P, Bentson J, Takahashi M, Winter J, Wilson G, Byrd S. The accuracy of predicting histological grades of supratentorial astrocytomas on the basis of computerised tomography and cerebral angiography. *Neuroradiology.* 1978; **16**, 346-8.
22. Baum S, Stein GN, Kuroda KK. Complications of "no arteriography". *Radiology.* 1966; **86**, 835-8.
23. Ansell G. Adverse reactions to contrast agents. *Investigative Radiology.* 1970; **5**, 374-84.
24. Skalpe IO, Anke IM. Complications in cerebral angiography. A comparison between non ionic contrast medium Iohexol and Meglumime metriozoate (Isopaque cerebral). *Neuroradiology.* 1983; **25**, 157-60.
25. Lang EK, Foreman J, Schlegel JV, Leslie C, List A, McCormick P. The incidence of contrast medium induced acute tubular necrosis following arteriography. *Radiology.* 1981; **138**, 203-6.
26. Mani RL, Eisenberg RL, McDonald EJ, Pollock JA, Mani JR. Complications of catheter cerebral angiography; analysis of 5000 procedures. I. Criteria and Incidence. *American Journal of Roentgenology.* 1978; **131**, 861-5.
27. Binnie CD, Bernstein DC, Booth AE, McCaul IR, Margerison JH, Scott JF. Clinical and electroencephalographic sequelae of carotid angiography. *Acta Radiologica, Diagnosis.* 1971; **11**, 626-40.
28. Pinto RS, Manuell M, Kitcheff II. Complications of digital intravenous angiography; experience in 2499 cervicocranial examinations. *American Journal of Roentgenology.* 1984; **143**, 1925-9.

29. Burrows EH. Calcification of intracranial gliomas. *Journal Belge de Radiologie.* 1973; **56**, 359–62.
30. Gilbertson EL, Good CA. Roentgenographic signs of tumours of the brain. *American Journal of Roentgenology.* 1956; **76**, 226–47.
31. Claveria LE, Du Boulay GH, Kendall BE. The diagnostic limitations of computerised axial tomography in hemispheric tumours. In: Boris J, ed. *The Diagnositic Limitations of Computerised Axial Tomography.* Berlin: Springer Verlag, 1978: 2–16.
32. Tans JTJ, de Jongh IE. Computed tomography of supratentorial astrocytoma. *Clinical Neurology and Neurosurgery.* 1978; **80**, 156–68.
33. Vassiloathis J, Ambrose J. Computerised tomography scanning appearances of intracranial meningiomas. *Journal of Neurosurgery.* 1979; **50**, 320–7.
34. Jack CR. Radiographic findings in 32 cases of primary CNS lymphoma. *American Journal of Roentgenology.* 1986; **146**, 271–6.
35. Steinhoff H, Kazner E, Lanksch W, Grumme T, Meese W, Lange S, Aulich A, Wende S. The limitations of computerised axial tomography in the detection and differential diagnosis of intracranial tumours. A study based on 1304 neoplasms. In: Boris J, ed. *The Diagnosis Limitations of Computerised Axial Tomography.* Berlin: Springer Verlag, 1978: 40–9.
36. Zimmerman RA, Bilanuik LT. Computed tomography of acute intratumoural haemorrhage. *Radiology.* 1980; **135**, 355–9.
37. Mandybur TI. Intracranial haemorrhage caused by metastatic tumours. *Neurology.* 1977; **27**, 650–5.
38. Sze G, Krol G, Olsen WL, Harper PS, Galicich JH, Heier LA, Zimmerman RD, Deck MDF. Haemorrhagic neoplasms: MR mimics of occult vascular malformations *American Journal of Neuroradiology.* 1987; **8**, 795–802.
39. Kazner E, Wende S, Grumme T, Lanksch WI, Stochdorph O. *Computed Tomography in Intracranial Tumours.* Berlin: Springer, 1982.
40. Smith AS, Weinstein MA, Modic M, Pavlicek W, Rogers LR, Rudd TG, Bukowski RM, Purvis JD, Weick JK, Duchesneau PM. Magnetic resonance with marked T_2 weighted images; improved demonstrations of brain lesions, tumour and oedema. *American Journal of Neuroradiology.* 1986; **6**, 691–7.
41. Brady TJ, Buonanno FS, Pykett IL, New PJF, Davis KR, Prohost GM, Kistler JP. Preliminary clinical results of proton (^{1}H) imaging of cranial neoplasms; *in vivo* measurements of T_1 and mobile proton density. *American Journal of Neuroradiology.* 1983; **4**, 225–8.
42. Araki T, Inuoye T, Suzuki H, Machida T, Iio M. Magnetic resonance imaging of brain tumours. Measurement of T_1. *Radiology.* 1984; **150**, 95–8.
43. Eggleston J, Saryan LA, Hollis DP. Nuclear magnetic resonance investigations of human neoplastic and abnormal non-neoplastic tissues. *Cancer Research.* 1975; **41**, 183–91.
44. Rinck PA, Meindl S, Higer HP, Bieler EV, Pfannensteil P. Brain tumours: detection and typing by use of CPMG sequences and *in vivo* T_2 measurements. *Radiology.* 1985; **105**, 103–6.
45. Komiyama M, Yagura H, Baba M, Yasui T, Hakuba A, Nishimura S, Inoue Y. MR Imaging: Possibility of tissue characterisation of brain tumours using T_1 and T_2 values. *American Journal of Neuroradiology.* 1987; **8**, 65–70.
46. Borello JA, Aisen AM, Gebarski SS. Comparison of MR relaxation times and X-ray attenuation coefficients of focal brain lesions. *Journal of Computer Assisted Tomography.* 1985; **9**, 1062–4.
47. Monajati A, Heggeness L. Patterns of oedema in tumours vs. infarcts: Visualisation of white matter pathways. *American Journal of Neuroradiology.* 1982; **3**, 251–5.
48. Drayer BP, Rosenbaum AE. Brain oedema defined by cranial computed tomography. *Journal of Computer Assisted Tomography.* 1979; **3**, 317–23.

49. Stevens JM, Ruiz JS, Kendall B. Observation on peritumoural oedema in meningioma Part 1. Distribution, spread and resolution of vasogenic oedema seen on computed tomography. *Neuroradiology*. 1983; **25**, 71-80.
50. Folkman J. Tumour angiogenesis; therapeutic implications. *New England Journal of Medicine*. 1971; **283**, 1182-6.
51. Bradbury M. *The Concept of a Blood-Brain Barrier*. New York: Wiley, 1979.
52. Steinhoff H, Aviles CH. Contrast enhancement response of intracranial neoplasms. Its validity for the differential diagnosis of tumour in CT. In: Lanksch W, Kazner E, edn. *Cranial Computerised Tomography*. Berlin Springer, 1976: 151-61.
53. Kormano M, Dean PB. Extravascular contrast material; the major component of contrast enhancement. *Radiology*. 1976; **121**, 379-82.
54. Crocker EF, Zimmerman RA, Phelps MD, Kuhl DE. The effects of steroids on the extravascular distribution of radiographic contrast material and technetium pertechnetate in brain tumours as determined by computed tomography. *Radiology*. 1976; **119**, 471-4.
55. Eisenberg HM, Barlow CF, Lorenzo AV. Effect of dexamethasone on altered brain vascular permeability. *Archives of Neurology*. 1970; **23**, 18-22.
56. Hatam A, Bergström M, Yu Zhao-Ying, Granholm L, Berggren BM. Effect of dexamethasone treatment on volume and contrast enhancement of intracranial neoplasms *Journal of Computer Assisted Tomography*. 1983; **7**, 295-300.
57. Hatam A, Yu Z-Y, Bergström M, Berggren BM, Greitz T. Effect of dexamethasone treatment on peritumoral brain oedema. *Journal of Computer Assisted Tomography*. 1982; **6**, 586-92.
58. Butler AR, Horii SC, Kritcheff II, Shannon MB, Budzilovich TN. Computed tomography in astrocytomas. *Radiology*. 1978; **129**, 433-9.
59. Munari C, Musolino A, Daumas Duport C, Mis ir O, Brunet P, Giallonardo AT, Chodkiewicz JP, Baucard J. Correlation between stereo EEG, CT-scan and stereotactic biopsy data in epileptic patients with low grade gliomas. *Applied Neurophysiology*. 1985; **48**, 448-53.
60. Clausssen C, Laniado M, Schörner W, Niendorf HJ, Weinmann H-J, Fiegler W, Felix R. Gadolinium DTPA in MR imaging of glioblastomas and intracranial metastases. *American Journal of Neuroradiology*. 1985; **6**, 669-74.
61. Hitchcock E, Sato F. Treatment of malignant gliomata. *Journal of Neurosurgery*. 1964; **21**, 497-505.
62. Shetter AG, Bertuccini TV, Pittmann HW. Closed needle biopsy in the diagnosis of intracranial mass lesions. *Surgical Neurology*. 1977; **8**, 341-5.
63. Bergström M, Greitz T. Stereotactic computed tomography. *American Journal of Roentgenology*. 1976; **127**, 167-70.
64. Lunsford LD, Maroon JC. CT localisation and biopsy of intracranial lesions. In: Shmidek HH, Sweet WH, eds. *Operative Neurosurgical Techniques; Indications, Methods and Results*. Vol 1. New York: Grune & Stratton. 1982: 403-18.
65. Levin AB. Experience in the first 100 patients undergoing computerised tomography guided steotactic procedures utilising the Brown-Roberts Wells guidance system. *Applied Neurophysiology*. 1985; **48**, 45-9.
66. Thomas DGT, Powell MP, Bradford R, Darling JL, Olney J, Barnard RO. Correlation of CT directed target site with histology and cell culture in cerebral glioma. *Applied Neurophysiology*. 1985; **48**, 460-2.
67. Thompson GSM, Kingsley DPE, Afshar F, Wylie IG. Stereotactic brain biopsy using a narrow aperture computed tomography scanner. *Clinical Radiology*. 1984; **35**, 209-14.
68. Boethius J, Collins VP, Edner G, Lewander R, Zajicek J. Stereotactic biopsies and computer tomography in gliomas. *Acta Neurochirugica*. 1978; **40**, 223-32.
69. Hitchon PW, Schelper RL, Barloon T. Accuracy of CT scans in identifying tumour tissue. *Applied Neurophysiology*. 1985; **48**, 463-6.

70. Ostertag CB, Mennel HD, Kiessling M. Stereotactic biopsies of brain tumours. *Surgical Neurology.* 1980; **14**, 275–83.
71. Thomas DGT, Davis CH, Ingram S, Olney JS, Bydder GM, Young IR. Stereotaxic biopsy of the brain under MR imaging control. *American Journal of Neuroradiology.* 1986; **7**, 161–3.
72. Bolender NF, Cromwell LD, Graues V, Margolis MT, Kerber CW, Wendling L. Interval appearance of glioblastomas not evident in previous CT examinations. *Journal of Computer Assisted Tomography.* 1983; **7**, 599–603.
73. Tentler RC, Palacios E. False negative computerised tomography in brain tumour. *Journal of the American Medical Association.* 1977; **238**, 339–40.
74. Kendall BE, Jakubowski J, Pullicino P, Symon L. Difficulties in diagnosis of supratentorial gliomas by CAT scan. *Journal of Neurology, Neurosurgery, and Psychiatry.* 1979; **42**, 485–92.
75. Yamashita T, Kuwabara T. Estimation of rate of growth of malignant brain tumours by computed tomography scanning. Surgical Neurology. 1983; **20**, 464–70.
76. Young IR, Hall AS, Pallis CA, Legg NJ, Bydder GM, Steiner RE. Nuclear magnetic resonance imaging of the brain in multiple sclerosis. *Lancet.* 1981; ii, 1063–6.
77. Gräfin von Einsiedel H, Löffler W. Nuclear magnetic resonance imaging of brain tumours unrevealed by CT. *European Journal of Radiology.* 1982; **2**, 226–34.
78. Onoyama Y, Abe M, Yabumoto E, Sakamoto T, Nishidai T, Suyama S. Radiation therapy in the treatment of glioblastoma. *American Journal of Roentgenology.* 1976; **126**, 481–92.
79. Reeves GI, Marks JE. Prognostic significance of lesion size for glioblastoma multiforme. *Radiology.* 1979; **132**, 469–71.
80. Lewander R, Bergström M, Boethius J, Collins VP, Edner G, Greitz T, Willems J. Stereotactic computer tomography for biopsy of gliomas. *Acta Radiological (Diagnosis).* 1978; **19**, 867–88.
81. Di Chiro G, Brooks RA, Patronas NJ, Bairamian D, Kornblith PL, Smith BH, Mansi L, Barker J. Issues in the *in vivo* measurement of glucose metabolism of human central nervous system tumours. *Annals of Neurology.* 198 ; **15** (suppl), S138–S146.
82. Silverman C, Marks JE. Prognostic significance of contrast enhancement in low grade astrocytomas of the adult cerebrum. *Radiology.* 1981; **139**, 211–3.
83. Mahaley MS, Mitchell WG, Whaley R, Dudka L, Symons MJ. The relative roles of neurological examination, functional abilities and computed tomography in the definition of treatment failure in patients with anaplastic gliomas. *Surgical Neurology.* 1983; **20**, 297–300.
84. Almqvist S, Dahlgren S, Dabilger S, Notter G, Sundbom L. Brain necrosis after irradiation of the hypophysis in Cushing's Disease. *Acta Radiologica* (Stockholm) 1964; **2**, 179–88.
85. Graeb DA, Steinbock P, Robertson WD. Transient early computed tomographic changes mimicking tumour irradiation. *Radiology.* 1982; **144;** 813–7.
86. Wendling LR, Bleyer WA, Di Chiro G, McIlvanie SK. Transient severe periventricular hypodensity after leukaemic prophylaxis with cranial irradiation and intrathecal methotrexate. *Journal of Computer Assisted Tomography.* 1978; **2**, 502–5.
87. Mikhael MA. Radiation necrosis of the brain; correlation between patterns on computed tomography and dose of radiation. *Journal of Computer Assisted Tomography.* 1979; **3**, 241–9.
88. Dooms GC, Hecht S, Brant Zawadski M, Berthiaume Y, Norman D, Newton TH. Brain radiation lesions. MR Imaging. *Radiology.* 1986; **158**, 149–55.
89. Kingsley DPE, Kendall BE. CT of the adverse effects of therapeutic radiation of the central nervous system. *American Journal of Neuroradiology.* 1981; **2**, 453–60.
90. Pay NT, Carella RJ, Lin JP, Kritcheff II. The usefulness of computed tomography

during and after radiation theraphy in patients with brain tumours. *Radiology.* 1976; **121**, 79–83.
91. George AE, de Leon MJ, Gentes CI, Miller J, Landon E, Budzilovick GN, Ferris S, Chase N. Leucoencephalopathy in normal and pathologic aging; CT of brain lucencies. *American Journal of Neuroradiology.* 1986; **7**, 561–6.
92. Bradley WG, Waluch V, Brant Zawadski M, Yadley RA, Wycoff R. Patchy periventricular white matter lesions in the elderly; common observation during NMR imaging. *Non-invasive Medical Imaging.* 1984; **1**, 35–41.
93. Littman P, James H, Zimmerman RA, States R. Radionecrosis of the brain presenting as a mass lesion. *Journal of Neurology, Neurosurgery, and Pschiatry.* 1977; **40**, 827–9.
94. Patronas NJ, Di Chiro G, Brooks RA, De la Paz RL, Kornblith PL, Smith BH, Rizzilo HV, Kessler RM, Manning, RG, Channing M, Wolf AP, O'Connor CM. Work in progress on ^{18}F fluorodeoxy-glucose and positron emission tomography in the evaluation of radiation necrosis of the brain. *Radiology.* 1982; **144**, 885–9.
95. Selker RG, Mendelow H, Walker M, Sheptak PE, Philips JG. Pathological correlation of CT ring in recurrent previously treated gliomas. *Surgical Neurology.* 1982 **17**, 251–4.

7 *In vivo* metabolism of human cerebral tumours

DJ Brooks

Introduction

An understanding of human tumour metabolism is of therapeutic importance for several reasons. Firstly, the pharmacological sensitivity of tumours to cytotoxic agents is proportional both to the tumour growth rate and to the fraction of a given tumour actively dividing.[1,2] Secondly, the state of oxygenation of tumours influences tumour response to radiotherapy, those tumours which are anoxic being less radiosensitive.[3] Thirdly, the regional pH of tumours influences the rate of uptake of acidic or basic cytotoxic agents by neoplasms.[4] Fourthly, the knowledge that carbohydrate or amino acid metabolism has become selectively increased in a tumour enables tracers to be specifically designed for imaging the extent of tumour invasion. Such tracers may well demonstrate more extensive tumour invasion than can be shown using conventional CT or MRI scanning.[5,6]

Until recently, tumour metabolism could only be studied using tissue slices, tumour homogenates, tissue cultures of transformed cells, or freeze-trapped tumour biopsies. The advent of positron emission tomography and surface-coil nuclear magnetic resonance spectroscopy has enabled the metabolism of human cerebral tumours to be studied relatively non-invasively in man. The purpose of this chapter is to review the results obtained using these two techniques.

Positron emission tomography

Examples of isotopes which are positron emitters include ^{15}O, ^{13}N, ^{18}F and ^{11}C. The half-lives of the above isotopes, which are generated using a cyclotron, range from two minutes to two hours. Naturally occurring organic substrates such as sugars and amino acids can be labelled with the above isotopes to form positron-emitting tracers. If such tracers are administered to subjects their regional distribution in tomographic slices of brain can be mapped out using positron emission tomography (PET).[14] PET can be used simply as a tracer imaging device, or alternatively to measure the kinetics of regional cerebral uptake of tracers. By comparing such kinetics with the time-

Table 7.1 Positron emitting tracers and their application to the measurement of regional cerebral function

Application	Labelled tracers
Cerebral blood flow	$C^{15}O_2$, $H_2{}^{15}O$, ^{11}C-alcohols, $^{13}NH_3$
Cerebral blood volume	^{11}CO, $C^{15}O$, ^{68}Ga-EDTA, ^{68}Ga-transferrin
Cerebral oxygen utilization	$^{15}O_2$
Cerebral glucose utilization	^{18}F-2-fluoro-2-deoxy-D-glucose (^{18}FDG)
	^{11}C-2-deoxy-D-glucose, ^{11}C-D-glucose
Amino-acid uptake	^{11}C-methionine, leucine, valine
Cerebral pH	^{11}C-dimethyl oxazolidinedione (^{11}C-DMO)
	$^{11}CO_2$
Blood–brain barrier integrity	$^{82}Rb^+$, ^{68}Ga-EDTA, ^{11}C-3-O-methyl-D-glucose,
	^{11}C-methyl albumin
Drug uptake	^{11}C-BCNU

course of the tracer in arterial plasma, functions such as regional cerebral blood flow, regional cerebral oxygen, glucose and amino acid metabolism, regional cerebral pH, and blood–brain barrier integrity can be computed.[7] Table 7.1 details some PET tracers in common use and their various biological applications:

The principle behind PET scanning is annihilation coincidence detection. When a positron-emitting isotope decays in any region of the brain, the positron released travels about 2 mm before being captured by a neighbouring electron and undergoing annihilation. The annihilation energy that results is emitted as two 511 keV energy gamma rays at 180° to each other. PET scanners consist of circular or hexagonal arrays of photomultiplier detectors which register the paired arrival of these 511 keV gamma rays at oppositely placed detectors as a 'coincident event'. By counting coincident events from a tomographic slice of brain, an image can be constructed which represents the true spatial distribution of positron-emitting tracer in the transaxial plane.[8] Current commercial PET scanners have a resolution of about 5 mm, though most of the published data to date are from lower resolution scanners.

Surface-coil nuclear magnetic resonance spectroscopy

Nuclear magnetic resonance (NMR) is based on the concept that certain atomic nuclei, for example ^1H, ^{19}F, ^{31}P, ^{13}C and ^{23}Na, have an inherent angular momentum or spin. This gives rise to a nuclear magnetic moment. In the presence of a static magnetic field these magnetic nuclei acquire nuclear spin-states with different discrete energy levels.[19] The nuclei can be induced to jump from their ground spin-states to the spin-states with a higher energy level by exposing them to electromagnetic radiation of the correct frequency directed at right angles to the static magnetic field. The nuclei subsequently drop back to their ground energy spin-state by emitting electromagnetic radiation at a rate determined by two relaxation times T_1 and T_2. T_1 is the spin–lattice and T_2 the spin–spin relaxation time. The emitted radiation is detected by a receiver coil and the various intensities and frequencies of this emitted radiation comprise the NMR spectrum.

In 1974 it was demonstrated that phosphorus ^{31}P-NMR spectroscopy could be used to measure the concentration of ^{31}P metabolites such as ATP, ADP, AMP, creatine phosphate, hexose-phosphates and inorganic phosphate in intact muscle fibres.[10] Later it was shown that using surface radiofrequency coils the concentrations of these same substrates could be estimated in the muscle and brain of intact rats.[11] The difference in the spectral frequencies of the creatine–phosphate and inorganic phosphate ^{31}P peaks is dependent on the intracellular pH of the organ being studied.[12] Surface-coil ^{31}P NMR spectra can now be obtained *in vivo* in man using a 60 cm bore superconducting magnet and 2.5–9 cm diameter radiofrequency surface coils.[13]

The oxygen and glucose metabolism of cerebral tumours

Historical aspects

The initial work on the respiration, aerobic fermentation, and anaerobic fermentation of both solid tumours and suspensions of ascitic cancer cells was carried out by Otto Warburg.[15] He observed that tumours had a much higher level of anaerobic glycolysis than normal tissue, the level of such glycolysis correlating with the degree of malignancy of the tumour. He also noted that tumours used aerobic glycolysis preferentially rather than respiration to generate ATP. Since his studies, a large amount of work on glucose transport and metabolism, and on levels of glycolytic and gluconeogenic enzymes in normal and transformed cells has been carried out.

Monakhov *et al.*[16] measured levels of hexokinase in normal and malignant lung, gastric, and uterine tissue. These workers concluded that hexokinase activity was increased in malignant tissue due to an increased affinity (decreased Km) of the enzyme for glucose. Novikoff hepatomas have been found to have increased activities of all key glycolytic enzymes compared to normal liver. By contrast hepatoma gluconeogenic enzyme activities are decreased and tumour glucose-6-phosphatase activity is absent.[17] These changes in glycolytic and gluconeogenic enzyme activity in malignant tissue are thought to reflect changes in the relative proportions of the low- and high-affinity isozymes of each enzyme.

3-O-methyl-D-glucose (MeG) is a D-glucose analogue that is passively transported across the blood–brain barrier (BBB) by the D-hexose carrier, but not metabolised.[18] 2-Deoxyglucose (DG) is also transported by the hexose carrier, but is then phosphorylated by hexokinase,[19] DG-6-P does not enter the glycolytic pathway and is only slowly dephosphorylated. As a consequence its rate of formation is a direct measure of hexokinase activity. A number of studies have measured the kinetics of uptake of methyl-glucose and 2-deoxyglucose into sarcoma virus transformed cells.[20–23] Their overall conclusion is that the number of D-hexose carriers is increased in transformed cells.

PET studies on the oxygen metabolism and haemodynamics of human cerebral tumours

Regional cerebral blood flow (rCBF), regional cerebral arterial oxygen extraction (rOER), and regional cerebral oxygen utilization (rCMRO$_2$), can be measured by asking subjects to inhale $C^{15}O_2$ and $^{15}O_2$ sequentially while PET scanning.[24] Regional cerebral blood volume (rCBV) can be determined using ^{11}CO or $C^{15}O$ as PET tracers.[14] These carbon monoxide tracers label haemoglobin, and so strictly measure red cell rather than blood volume. To calculate rCBV regional cerebral haematocrit must also be measured concomitantly using a plasma volume marker such as ^{11}C-methyl-albumin.[25]

Figure 7.1 (a, b) shows an enhanced CT brain scan of a patient with a cerebral metastasis from the colon, and corresponding PET images of rCBF, rOER, rCMRO$_2$ and rCBV. It can be seen that for this subject both the tumour and its surrounding oedema have low levels of blood flow, arterial oxygen extraction, and oxygen utilization compared to equivalent contralateral brain tissue. In practice, while the blood flow of cerebral tumours can be highly variable, brain tumour arterial oxygen extraction and oxygen utilization are consistently found to be low.[26] Such a finding supports Warburg's statement that respiration in malignant tumours is depressed.[15] In normal grey and white matter the rOER is 40 per cent i.e. normal

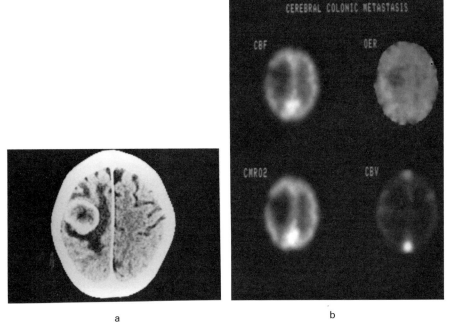

Fig. 7.1(a) CT brain scan of a patient with a cerebral metastasis from the colon, (b) Corresponding PET images of rCBF, rOER, rCMRO$_2$ and rCBV.

Table 7.2 Mean values of tumour and oedema function in patients with cerebral neoplasia

	Cerebral tumours ($n = 14$) (mean ± SD)	Oedema ($n = 11$) (mean ± SD)	Normal grey ($n = 13$) (mean ± SD)	Normal white ($n = 13$) (mean ± SD)
rCBF (ml/100 ml/min)	28 ± 28	16 ± 6	45 ± 10	27 ± 5
rOER	0.19 ± 0.12	0.44 ± 0.99	0.40 ± 0.66	0.38 ± 0.06
rCMRO$_2$ (ml O$_2$/100 ml/min)	0.9 ± 0.8	1.3 ± 0.3	3.2 ± 0.3	1.8 ± 0.2
rCBV (ml/100 ml)	4.1 ± 2.9	2.2 ± 0.8	4.1 ± 0.6	2.4 ± 0.8

brain tissue extracts 40 per cent of its arterial oxygen supply. If tissue ischaemia is present, i.e. the blood flow is too low to meet tissue oxygen demands, the rOER approaches 100 per cent. To date PET scanning has failed to detect any ischaemic regions in brain tumours in spite of the presence of necrotic tissue. The resolution of PET scanners is however at best 5 mm and so microscopic regions of ischaemia may be missed when positron tomography is used.

Regions of perifocal tumour oedema are consistently found to have low blood flow and oxygen utilization compared to equivalent contralateral brain tissue.[27] In spite of the locally raised intracranial pressure, such regions of oedema have normal 40 per cent levels of arterial oxygen extraction. This implies that the oedematous tissue is not ischaemic. Table 7.2 details mean values of regional cerebral function for normal brain tissue, cerebral tumours, and regions of perifocal tumour oedema. In normal brain tissue regional blood flow and blood volume are closely coupled, the rCBF/rCBV ratio having a value of about 10 min^{-1} for both grey and white matter. This coupling is lost in brain tumours where abnormal microvasculature is present. Brain tumour haematocrit values also vary widely compared to those of normal brain tissue. This reflects the highly variable calibre of tumour blood vessels.[28]

The effect of the presence of cerebral tumours on the metabolism of distant brain tissue has also been studied. Beaney et al.[29] showed that both the mean oxygen utilization and the blood flow of the contralateral cortical tissue of patients with hemispheric brain tumours were significantly reduced compared to the cortical function of age-matched normal controls. Following tumour excision biopsy the contralateral cortical function of the patients returned towards normal levels. Patients with acute obstructive hydrocephalus secondary to posterior fossa tumours also have a reduced cortical oxygen utilization and blood flow.[30] Unlike the patients with hemispheric tumours, the hydrocephalus patients were found to have an increased level of cortical oxygen extraction. This suggests that their raised intracranial pressure was leading to cortical ischaemia. On decompression the hydrocephalus patients all improved their cortical blood flow, but improvements in their cortical oxygen utilization occurred inconsistently.

The effects of both dexamethasone and radiotherapy on the regional cerebral oxygen metabolism and haemodynamics of patients with brain tumours has also been studied.[31, 32] Dexamethasone appears to produce a coupled decrease in regional cerebral blood flow and blood volume in tumour patients within hours of its administration, this decrease paralleling clinical improvement. It would appear that dexamethasone initially causes a vasoconstriction which may in turn lead to a reduction in intracranial pressure and blood-brain barrier permeability. Beaney et al.[32] measured the temporal lobe function of a group of patients with pituitary tumours who had received 4000–5500 rads of radiation in fractionated doses 1–10 years prior to being studied. The temporal lobe function of these patients was in no way impaired following their radiotherapy compared to that of age-matched normal controls. Radiotherapy has however been observed to cause an acute cerebral vasodilatation within days of the treatment by the same group of workers.

PET studies on glucose metabolism of human cerebral tumours

The glucose analogue ^{18}F-2-fluoro-2-deoxy-D-glucose (^{18}FDG) behaves like 2-deoxy-glucose, being transported across the blood–brain barrier by the D-hexose carrier and then being phosphorylated by hexokinase.[33] FDG-6-P is only slowly metabolized and so its rate of production reflects hexokinase activity. A number of kinetic models exist for computing regional cerebral glucose utilization (rCMRGlu) from the ^{18}FDG cerebral uptake time course.

The uptake of ^{18}FDG by gliomas has been shown to correlate with their clinical grade on the Kernohan scale,[34] aggressive tumours having a raised level of glucose utilization. Both oxygen and glucose utilization are suppressed in regions of perifocal tumour oedema.[27, 34] As might be expected, the levels of glucose utilization by brain tumours have been found retrospectively to correlate well with the eventual clinical outcome of the tumour patients.[35] As a consequence PET scanning can potentially be used to give tumour patients a clinical prognosis. A second advantage of PET scanning is that by measuring regional cerebral ^{18}FDG uptake it is possible to distinguish between recurrent tumour and regions of tissue necrosis following radiotherapy. Conventional CT brain scanning is frequently unhelpful in this situation.

The relationship between glucose and oxygen utilization by human cerebral tumours has also been investigated.[36] Using FDG, Rhodes et al. showed that the fraction of glucose extracted from arterial blood by tumours was similar to that extracted by normal brain tissue while in contrast tumour oxygen extraction was relatively depressed. These workers concluded that brain tumours preferentially utilize aerobic glycolysis rather than respiration to produce ATP. This finding is in agreement with Warburg's conclusions.[15] The effect of brain tumours on distant brain tissue function has also been studied with FDG. De La Paz et al.[37] found that the presence of hemispheric tumours led to a relative depression in the glucose utilization of both the ipsilateral cortex and of the contralateral cerebellar hemisphere. This is presumably a consequence of the disruption of pathways connecting the cortex and brainstem.

Surface-coil ^{31}P-NMR studies on brain tumour metabolism

Oberhaensli et al.[13] have studied eight patients with intrinsic brain tumours using surface coil ^{31}P-NMR spectroscopy. In six of the patients studied the ratio of phosphocreatine:ATP was lower than that of normal brain tissue. Lowest ratios were found in an oligodendroglioma and meningioma, astrocytomas having more normal ratios. The significance of these low tumour P-Cr:ATP ratios was not discussed. Taken in combination with PET findings, it is likely that these low P-Cr:ATP ratios in tumours reflect the fact that the aerobic glycolysis favoured by tumours is less efficient in generating phosophocreatine than normal respiration.

The pH of cerebral tumours

It has been suggested that the raised levels of aerobic glycolysis found in tumours should in theory lead to reduced levels of tumour pH due to increased lactic acid production.[38] Microelectrode studies, which measure interstitial tumour pH, have suggested that tumours are indeed more acidic than surrounding normal tissue.[4, 39] With the advent of PET and surface-coil ^{31}P-NMR spectroscopy, intracellular pH can now be measured non-invasively in man.

$^{11}CO_2$ and ^{11}C-dimethyl-oxazolidinedione (^{11}C-DMO) are both positron-emitting weak organic acids with a pKa of 6.12. When administered to subjects the neutral acid from of these tracers, but not the anion, passes across the intact blood–brain barrier. As a consequence the partition of these tracers between arterial plasma and brain tissue reflects the pH difference between the two compartments. Both tracers can therefore be used with PET to determine regional cerebral pH. The $^{11}CO_2$ and ^{11}C-DMO approaches yield a pH of 7.0 for normal brain tissue and show little difference between the pH of grey and white matter.[40, 41] Unlike the microelectrode studies, the PET studies with $^{11}CO_2$ and ^{11}C-DMO have found brain tumours, perifocal tumour oedema and normal brain tissue all to have approximately neutral pH, tumours being if anything slightly more alkaline than normal brain tissue.

Using surface-coil ^{31}P-NMR a pH of 7.03 has been reported for normal brain tissue in agreement with PET findings. The pH of eight gliomas and meningiomas ranged between 7.01 and 7.27; again tumours tended to be slightly more alkaline than normal brain tissue. The discrepancy between tumour pH values obtained using the microelectrode approach and those obtained using non-invasive PET and NMR approaches is difficult to explain. The close agreement between PET and ^{31}P-NMR studies suggests that if brain tumours are producing excess lactic acid via aerobic glycolysis, the lactic acid is adequately buffered by the intracellular phosphate and proteins in the malignant tissue.

Amino acid metabolism of human cerebral tumours

Amino acid metabolism is extremely complex to model as at present no metabolic analogues of amino acids have been developed which become trapped in a similar manner to ^{18}FDG. There are two carrier systems for the passive transport of amino acids across the blood–brain barrier. Following their uptake amino acids can be incorporated into protein, converted to neurotransmitters, or be metabolized and enter the Kreb's cycle. Bustany et al.[42] have developed a simplified three-compartment model to quantitate ^{11}C-methionine uptake by brain tissue using PET. They assume that ^{11}C-methionine in brain tissue is either free or incorporated into protein, and that negligible amino acid metabolism occurs. Using this model these workers have computed regional cerebral protein synthesis rates (PSR). Glioma PSRs were found to correlate with their grade of malignancy, a similar finding to that reported for glioma glucose utilization.[34]

[11]C-methionine, like [18]FDG, is a suitable PET tracer for distinguishing between tumour recurrence and tissue necrosis following radiotherapy. ^{11}C-methionine uptake is also capable of revealing deposits of brain tumours and tumour extensions that may be missed when conventional CT brain scanning or other PET tracers are employed.[6, 42] Other amino acids that have been used to image brain tumours include ^{11}C-DL-valine and ^{11}C-DL-tryptophan, their uptake being increased in brain tumours[43] compared to normal brain tissue.

Blood–brain barrier function in human cerebral tumours

Transport across the BBB can be studied using PET if tracer analogues of hexoses and amino acids are used which are not metabolized. Suitable analogues include ^{11}C-3-O-methyl-D-glucose[18] and ^{11}C-1-amino-cyclopentane carboxylic acid[44] which can be used to monitor D-glucose and neutral amino acid transport respectively. [82]Rb$^+$ is a positron-emitter which behaves both chemically and biologically in a

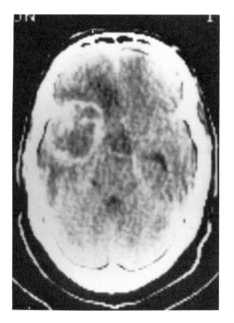
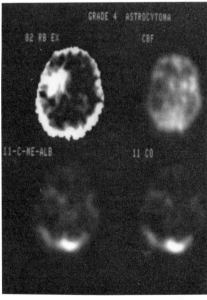

Fig. 7.2(a) CT brain scan of a patient with a grade IV astrocytoma, (b) Corresponding PET images of [82]Rb extraction, rCBF, "C-methyl-albumin uptake, and rCBV

manner similar to K^+. It has a half-life of 76 seconds[45] and can be used to study K^+ transport. ^{11}C-methyl-albumin can be used to monitor albumin leakage across the BBB.[7] In addition non-physiological tracers such as ^{68}Ga-EDTA, which has a similar molecular size to sucrose, have also been used to quantitate BBB disruption.[46] Figure 7.2 (a, b) shows a CT scan of a Grade IV astrocytoma and corresponding PET images of ^{82}Rb$^+$ extraction, rCBF, ^{11}C-methyl-albumin uptake and red cell volume. It can be seen that although the glioma has a high Rb extraction, relatively little albumin leakage into the tumour has occurred after 50 min of PET scanning.

Under fasting, resting conditions, normal brain tissue extracts about 14 per cent of arterial ^{11}C-3-O-methyl-D-glucose (^{11}C-MeG) unidirectionally. Glioma ^{11}C-MeG extraction can vary from normal levels to levels of 30 per cent.[47] Whether the increased ^{11}C-MeG extraction by tumours reflects increased transport or free diffusion of the tracer into the tumour cannot be distinguished by the PET technique. As transformed cells have been shown to have increased numbers of D-hexose carriers[20-23] it is likely that both diffusion and transport of hexoses into tumours are increased. Compared to normal controls, patients with gliomas showed reduced ^{11}C-MeG transport into contralateral cortical tissue. This is likely to reflect a depression of glucose utilization by the brain tissue of these patients.

Yen *et al.* were the first to demonstrate that cerebral tumours could be visualized using ^{82}Rb$^+$ and PET.[48] ^{82}Rb$^+$ transport across the blood-brain barrier in humans has subsequently been quantitated using both a steady-state and a dynamic approach.[49, 50] These two approaches yielded similar mean influx constants of 5.5×10^{-3} and $4.4 \times 4.4 \times 10^{-3}$ ml min^{-1} g^{-1} for ^{82}Rb$^+$ transport across the intact blood–brain barrier of contralateral brain tissue of tumour patients. Brain tumours that enhanced on CT scanning following intravenous injections of contrast medium had increased levels of ^{82}Rb extraction, but non-enhancing tumours, regions of perifocal tumour oedema, and contralateral brain tissue had similar ^{82}Rb extractions to normal brain tissue.[49]

Within 72 h of administering 100 mg doses of dexamethasone, Jarden *et al.*[50] were able to demonstrate a significant reduction in ^{82}Rb influx into tumours. The same workers found that a single dose of 200–600 rads of radiotherapy had no immediate effect on regional cerebral ^{82}Rb permeability. Increased tumour and contralateral brain extraction of Rb has been reported following higher doses of radiotherapy however when measurements were performed several days after treatment.[7] Such a finding is not surprising as radiotherapy has been shown to fragment the vasculature of Walker cell carcinomas in rats over the course of several days.[51] The Rb permeability of contralateral brain tissue of tumour patients studied 1–6 months following radiotherapy is normal[49] suggesting that any subacute blood–brain barrier disruption by radiotherapy is rapidly repaired.

Uptake of cytotoxic agents by human cerebral tumours

The kinetics of ^{11}C-BCNU into brain tumours have been studied using PET[52, 53] Initial tumour ^{11}C-BCNU uptake following intravenous injection of the tracer parallels tumour blood flow. If 20 per cent mannitol is first administered intravenously to disrupt the blood–brain barrier further, increased tumour ^{11}C-BCNU uptake results.

Highest tumour ^{11}C-BCNU concentration occurs if the tracer is administered by selective intra-arterial cannulation, rather than intravenously. In two of the 10 patients studied cold BCNU was administered intra-arterially resulting in striking regression.

Conclusions

PET studies suggest that cerebral tumours utilize aerobic glycolysis rather than respiration to produce energy for metabolism. This is in agreement with Warburg's findings in his original studies on solid tumours and suspensions of ascites cells. Surface-coil ^{31}P-NMR spectroscopy suggests that the energy derived from such aerobic glycolysis by tumours is less efficient in generating phosphocreatine. In spite of the presence of necrotic regions in cerebral tumours, PET studies, within the 0.5–1.5 cm resolution of current scanners, have found no evidence to date that such tumours are anoxic. Lack of sensitivity of brain tumours to radiotherapy is therefore unlikely to be a consequence of poor tumour oxygenation. Both PET and ^{31}P-NMR studies suggest that brain tumour pH is similar to that of normal brain tissue, i.e. close to neutrality. Cytotoxic agents should therefore ideally have a pKa value greater than 7.0 to aid free diffusion into neoplastic tissue.

Glucose and amino acid utilization by gliomas are proportional to their grade on the Kernohan scale. ^{11}C-methionine uptake by gliomas can show tumour extension using PET scanning that is not evident with conventional CT scanning. Both ^{11}C-methionine and ^{18}FDG uptake by cerebral tumours can be used to distinguish tumour recurrence from tissue necrosis following radiotherapy.

Cerebral tumours when present depress the oxygen and glucose utilization and the glucose transport of distant brain tissue. Removal of the tumour has been shown partially to reverse the depression in oxygen utilization. Treatment of brain tumour patients with dexamethasone appears to result in a generalized cerebral vasoconstriction within hours of steroid administration. This may result in a secondary fall in intracranial pressure and so explain the rapid clinical response of patients to treatment. In high doses dexamethasone therapy reduces tumour permeability to Rb^+. Radiotherapy in fractionated doses up to 5500 rads appears to produce no long-term damage to cerebral function or blood–brain barrier permeability. Acutely however, irradiation of brain tissue may result in increased blood–brain barrier permeability to Rb^+.

PET provides a means of studying the kinetics of uptake of labelled cytotoxic agents such as ^{11}C-BCNU by tumours and so optimizing their administration. In the future it should be possible to study cerebral tumour receptors using suitable PET tracers and this will hopefully aid the development of more specific anti-cancer agents.

References

1. Frei E. Combination Cancer Therapy: presidential address. *Cancer Research.* 1972; **32**, 2593–607.
2. Zubrad CG. Chemical control of cancer. *Proceedings of the National Academy of Sciences of the USA.* 1972; **69**, 1042–7.

3. Evans NTS, Naylor PFD. The effect of oxygen breathing and radiotherapy upon the tissue oxygen tension of some human tumours. *British Journal of Radiology*. 1963; **36**, 418–25.
4. Wike-Hooley JL, Van Den Berg AP, Van der Zee J, *et al*. Human tumour pH and its variation. *European Journal of Cancer and Clinical Oncology*. 1985; **21**, 785–91.
5. Patronas NJ, Di Chiro G, Brooks RA, *et al*. Work in progress: [^{18}F]Fluoro-deoxyglucose and positron emission tomography in the evaluation of radiation of necrosis of the brain. *Radiology*. 1982; **144**, 855–89.
6. Bergström M, Collins P, Ehrin E, *et al*. Discrepancies in brain tumour extent as shown by computerised tomography and positron emission tomography using [^{68}Ga]-EDTA, [^{11}C]glucose, and [^{11}C]methionine. *Journal of Computer Assisted Tomography*. 1983; **7**, 1062–6.
7. Brooks DJ, Beaney RP, Thomas DGT. The role of positron emission tomography in the study of cerebral tumours. *Seminars in Oncology*. 1986; **13**, 83–93.
8. Phelps ME, Hoffman EJ, Huang SC, et al. ECAT: A new computerised tomographic imaging system for positron-emitting radio-pharmaceuticals. *Journal of Nuclear Medicine*. 1978; **19**, 635–48.
9. Koutcher JA, Burt CT. Principles of nuclear magnetic resonance. *Journal of Nuclear Medicine*. 1984; **25**, 101–11.
10. Hoult DI, Busby SJW, Gadian DG, *et al*. Observations of tissue metabolites using ^{31}P nuclear magnetic resonance. *Nature*. 1974; **252**, 282–7.
11. Ackerman JJH, Grove TH, Wong GC, *et al*. Mapping of metabolites in whole animals by ^{31}P NMR using surface coils. *Nature*. 1980; **283**, 167–70.
12. Moon RB, Richards JH. Determination of intracellular pH by ^{31}P magnetic resonance. *Journal of Biological Chemistry*. 1973; **248**, 7276–8.
13. Oberhaensli RD, Hilton-Jones D, Bore PJ, *et al*. Biochemical investigation of human tumours *in vivo* with phosphorus-31 magnetic resonance spectroscopy. *Lancet*. 1986; **ii**, 8–11.
14. Phelps ME, Mazziota JC, Huang SC. Study of cerebral function with positron emission tomography. *Journal of Cerebral Blood Flow Metabolism*. 1982; **2**, 113–62.
15. Warburg O. On the origin of cancer cells. *Science*. 1956; **123**, 309–14.
16. Monakhov NK, Nelstadt EL, Shavlovskii NM, *et al*. Physiochemical properties and isoenzyme composition of hexokinase from normal and malignant human tissues. *Journal of the National Cancer Institute*. 1978; **61**, 27–34.
17. Weber G. Enzymology of cancer cells. *New England Journal of Medicine*. 1977; **296**, 541–50.
18. Casky TZ, Wilson JE. The fate of 3-0-^{14}CH$_3$-glucose in the rat. *Biochimica et Biophysica Acta*. 1956; **22**, 185–6.
19. Sokoloff L, Reivich M, Kennedy C, *et al*. The (^{14}C) deoxyglucose method for the measurement of local cerebral glucose utilisation: Theory, procedure, and normal values in the conscious and anaesthetised albino rat. *Journal of Neurochemistry*. 1977; **28**, 879–916.
20. Hatanaka M. Transport of sugars in tumour cell membranes. *Biochimica et Biophysica Acta*. 1974; **355**, 77–104.
21. Weber MJ. Hexose transport in normal and in rous sarcoma virus transformed cells. *Journal of Biological Chemistry*. 1973; **248**, 2978–83.
22. Hatanaka M, Augl C, Gilden RV. Evidence for a functional change in the plasma membrane of murine sarcoma virus infected mouse embryo cells. *Journal of Biological Chemistry*. 1970; **245**, 714–7.
23. Venuta S, Rubin H. Sugar transport in normal and rous sarcoma virus-transformed chick-embryo fibroblasts. *Proceedings of the National Academy of Sciences USA*. 1973; **70**, 653–7.
24. Frackowiak RSJ, Lenzi GL, Jones T, *et al*. Quantitative measurements of regional

cerebral blood flow and oxygen metabolism in man using ^{15}O and positron emission tomography. *Journal of Computer Assisted Tomography.* 1980; **4**, 727-36.
25. Lammertsma AA, Brooks DJ, Beaney RP, *et al.* In vivo measurement of regional cerebral haematocrit using positron emission tomography. *Journal of Cerebral Blood Flow Metabolism.* 1984; **4**, 317-22.
26. Ito M, Lammertsma AA, Wise RJS, *et al.* Measurement of regional cerebral blood flow and oxygen utilisation in patients with cerebral tumours using ^{15}O and positron emission tomography. *Neuroradiology.* 1982; **23**, 63-74.
27. Lammertsma AA, Wise RJS, Cox TCS, *et al.* Measurement of blood flow, oxygen utilisation, oxygen extraction ratio and fractional blood volume in human brain tumours and surrounding oedematous tissue. *British Journal of Radiology.* 1984; 58, 725-34.
28. Brooks DJ, Beaney RP, Lammertsma AA, *et al.* Studies on regional cerebral haematocrit and blood flow in patients with cerebral tumours using positron emission tomography. *Microvascular Research.* 1986; **31**, 267-76.
29. Beaney RP, Brooks DJ, Leenders KL, *et al.* Blood flow and oxygen utilisation in the contralateral cortex of patients with untreated intracranial tumours as studied by positron emission tomography. *Journal of Neurology, Neurosurgery and Psychiatry.* 1985; **48**, 310-9.
30. Brooks DJ, Beaney RP, Powell M, *et al.* Studies on cerebral oxygen metabolism, blood flow and blood volume in patients with hydrocephalus before and after surgical decompression, using positron emission tomography. *Brain.* 1986; **109**, 613-28.
31. Leenders KL, Beaney RP, Brooks DJ, *et al.* Dexamathasone treatment of brain tumour patients: effects on regional cerebral blood flow, blood volume and oxygen utilisation. *Neurology.* 1985; **35**, 1610-6.
32. Beaney RP, Brooks DJ, Gibbs JSR, *et al.* Lack of irradiation-induced ischaemic temporal lobe damage in patients with pituitary tumours. *Journal of Neuro-oncology* (in press).
33. Phelps ME, Huang SC, Hoffman EJ, *et al.* Tomographic measurement of local cerebral glucose metabolic rate in humans with (F-18) 2-fluoro-2-deoxy-D-glucose. *Annals of Neurology.* 1979; **6**, 371-88.
34. Di Chiro G, De La Paz RL, Brooks RA, *et al.* Glucose utilisation of cerebral gliomas measured by (^{18}F) fluorodeoxyglucose and positron emission tomography. *Neurology.* 1982; **32**, 1323-9.
35. Patronas NJ, Di Chiro G, Brooks RA, *et al.* [^{18}F]-Fluorodeoxyglucose and positron emission tomography in the evaluation of radiation necrosis of the brain. *Radiology.* 1982; **144**, 885-9.
36. Rhodes CG, Wise RJS, Gibbs JM, *et al.* In vivo disturbance of the oxidative metabolism of glucose in human cerebral gliomas. *Annals of Neurology.* 1983; **4**, 614-26.
37. De La Paz RL, Patroneus NJ, Brooks RA, *et al.* Positron emission tomography study of the suppression of grey matter glucose utilisation of brain tumours. *American Journal of Neuroradiology.* 1983; **4**, 826-9.
38. Griffiths JR, Stevens AN, Iles RA, *et al.* ^{31}P-NMR investigations of solid tumours in the living rat. *Bioscience Reports.* 1981; **1**, 319-25.
39. Pampus F. Die Wasserstoffionen konzentration des Hirngewebes bei raumfordernden intracraniellen Prozessen. *Acta Neurochirugica.* 1963; **11**, 305-18.
40. Brooks DJ, Beaney RP, Thomas DGT, *et al.* Studies on regional cerebral pH in patients with cerebral tumours using continuous inhalation of $^{11}CO_2$ and positron emission tomography. *Journal of Cerebral Blood Flow Metabolism.* 1986; **6**, 529-35.
41. Rottenberg DA, Gino JZ, Kearfott KJ, *et al.* In vivo measurement of brain tumour pH using [^{11}C] DMO and positron emission tomography. *Annals of Neurology.* 1985; **17**, 70-9.
42. Bustany P, Chatel M, Derlon JM, *et al.* Brain tumour protein synthesis and histological grades: A study by positron emission tomography with C-11-L-methionine. *Journal*

Neuro-oncology. 1986; **3**, 397–404.
43. Hübner KF, King P, Gibbs WD, *et al.* Clinical investigations with carbon-11 labelled amino acids using positron emission tomography in patients with neoplastic diseases. *Medical Radionuclide Imaging* IAEA (Vienna). 1981; 515–29.
44. Hayes RL, Washburn LC, Wieland BW, *et al.* Carboxyl-labelled ^{11}C-1-aminocyclopentane carboxylic acid, a potential agent for cancer detection. *Journal of Nuclear Medicine.* 1976; **17**, 748–51.
45. Yen CK, Budinger TF. Evaluation of blood–brain barrier permeability changes in rhesus monkeys and man using ^{82}Rb and positron emission tomography. *Journal of Computer Assisted Tomography.* 1981; **5**, 792–9.
46. Hawkins RA, Phelps ME, Huang SC, *et al.* A kinetic evaluation of blood–brain barrier permeability in human brain tumours with [^{68}Ga]-EDTA and positron emission tomograpy. *Journal of Cerebral Blood Flow Metabolism.* 1984; **4**, 507–15.
47. Brooks DJ, Beaney RP, Lammertsma AA, *et al.* Glucose transport across the blood–brain barrier in normal human subjects and patients with cerebral tumours studied using [^{11}C]-3-*O*-methyl-D-glucose and positron emission tomography. *Journal of Cerebral Blood Flow Metabolism.* 1986; **6**, 230–9.
48. Yen CK, Yano Y, Budinger TF, *et al.* Brain tumour evaluation using Rb-82 and positron emission tomography. *Journal of Nuclear Medicine.* 1982; **23**, 532–7.
49. Brooks DJ, Beaney RP, Lammertsma AA, *et al.* Quantitative measurement of blood–brain barrier permeability using Rb-82 and positron emission tomography. *Journal of Cerebral Blood Flow Metabolism.* 1984; **4**, 535–45.
50. Jarden JO, Dhawan V, Poltorak A, *et al.* Positron emission tomographic measurement of blood-to-brain and blood-to-tumour transport of ^{82}Rb: the effect of dexamathasone and whole-brain radiation theraphy. *Annals of Neurology.* 1985; **18**, 636–46.
51. Rubin P, Caserett G. Microcirculation of tumours: II. The supervascularised state of irradiated regressing tumours. *Clinical Radiology.* 1966; **17**, 346.
52. Yamamoto YL, Diksis M, Sako K, *et al.* Pharmacokinetic and metabolic studies in human malignant gliomas. In: Magistretti PL, ed. *Functional Radionuclide Imaging of the Brain.* New York: Raven Press, 1983: 327–335.
53. Tyler JL, Yamamoto YL, Diksic M, *et al.* Pharmacokinetics of superselective intra-arterial and intravenous [^{11}C] BCNU evaluated by PET. *Journal of Nuclear Medicine.* 1986; **27**, 775–80.

8 The epidemiology of brain tumours

Ronald O McKeran, Edward S Williams and Helen Thornton Jones

Introduction

The advent of highly sophisticated non-invasive methods of diagnosis such as CT scanning and more recently MRI, of improved anaesthetic and surgical techniques, combined with a growing tendency to consider the use of radiotherapy and chemotherapy at least in certain stages in the growth and evolution of human cerebral gliomas, has refocused attention on the possible impact of these activities on the reported incidence, characteristics and survival of these patients. Most of the earlier reports dealing with the frequency of neoplasms affecting the central nervous system were based on the clinical experience of individual clinicians, on autopsy rates or on proportionate rates of hospital admission. More recently, studies derived from tumour registry data and special case-finding surveys have yielded more accurate estimates of the morbidity, thus reducing the effect of selection bias inherent in the earlier studies. In contrast to the experience in the United States of America, the United Kingdom experience has not been frequently studied and there is no report from a Cancer Registry study currently in existence. Therefore, apart from the intrinsic interest of epidemiological studies on different populations at different periods which might suggest important genetic or environmental factors in their genesis, the question arises as to whether Cancer Registry studies in principle could allow sufficient accuracy of surveillance to determine changes in survival of brain tumour populations and thus act as a monitor of the general effect of the implementation of new treatment schedules derived from previously conducted double blind controlled studies. The results on survival in highly studied trial patients may not be the same as in the generality of patients offered the same treatment at a later date. To justify continued support to trial data and treatment schedules it would seem reasonable to attempt to obtain this data where available.

The general background

The epidemiological approach to the study of disease is concerned with the distribution and determinants of disease in populations as compared to the physician's approach, which focuses on the individual. The epidemiologist should always attempt to ensure that his observations are representative of the population under study. The categories are often crude by clinical standards. Useful data and courses of action can be defined however in the management of human disease even where a precise aetiology has not been identified.

The evidence from post-mortem studies would suggest that between 1 and 2 per cent of patients are affected with primary brain tumours.[1,2] These figures are not representative of the general population owing to the selection bias and differences in the selection of material, in post-mortem examination rates in different centres, and the criteria used for histological diagnosis. Further refinement of data collection in this area was achieved when official mortality statistics were used to obtain estimates of frequency of occurrence of brain tumours using the International Classification of Disease, Injuries and Causes of Death (WHO). An incidence of 5 per 100 000 (range 1 per 100 000 in Mexico to 7 per 100 000 in Israel) was found for all cerebral tumours in 27 countries using age-adjusted mortality rates.[3] This figure was found to be remarkably constant for death rates across North America, Europe, Australia, New Zealand and South America, and within a given country such as the USA and Denmark.[4,5] Major genetic or environmental factors might have been expected to demonstrate their effect by registering differences in these death rates between and within countries and the fact that such differences were not found indicated that, whilst there might be some regional differences, these were not sufficient to alter the effect within the total population and suggested that, unlike other types of tumours, social engineering and health education were unlikely to have much impact on the incidence of brain tumours which demonstrated a remarkably constant spontaneous occurrence across and within continents. Some caution in interpreting these figures had to be exercised however, and it was Kurtzke who fully emphasized the relationship of these figures to the number of physicians practising in a given community, the differences in mortality rates from area to area and country to country and the variation in the entry of the brain tumours in some mortality classifications.[5] The variation between centres in the development of their health programmes, availability of diagnostic facilities and clinical practice must cast further doubt on placing too much reliance on these data. As with all epidemiological studies where the search for cases has been rigorous, the figures have been higher and in general, repeated studies of the same population give rise to higher figures for incidence in successive studies. These points were underlined in the studies of Kurland and Percy et al. from Rochester, Minnesota.[6,7] They insisted upon an accurate diagnosis in the individual patient and complete ascertainment of all cases in their defined population. Their population provided an ideal opportunity to undertake epidemiological research in that it was relatively isolated from other urban centres, had a long history of availability and uptake of excellent modern medical services including those of neurology, neurosurgery, neuroradiology and neuropathology, with the required technical support of refined diagnosis in all these disciplines. For these reasons it seems highly probable that most patients with brain tumours had access to, and utilized, the available services. The implication would thus be that the reported cases are related to the defined population. In their studies which ran from 1945 to 1954 they estimated the age-adjusted prevalence rates for all cases of primary cerebral tumour (including pituitary tumours) to be 46 per 100 000 (24.7 verified cerebral tumours, 12.4 probable cases, 8.9 pituitary and 9.7 intracranial metastases).

In their second and larger study which ran from 1935 to 1968 in Rochester, they estimated 15.8 per 100 000 primary tumours of the central nervous system (cerebral tumours 12.6, pituitary tumours 1.9). The majority of these primary tumours were meningiomas (35 per cent), 28 per cent astrocytomas and 5 per cent neurinomas. These figures were considerably higher than those obtained from official mortality figures; 36 per cent were only diagnosed at post-mortem (38 per cent were found to have neurological symptoms and signs which were not appreciated to be due to a brain tumour and 62 per cent were asymptomatic at death) and 57 per cent of the cases diagnosed first at post-mortem were meningiomas and 20 per cent gliomas. This last finding altered the ratio of meningiomas to gliomas diagnosed in life from 0.7:1 to 1.2:1 when taken overall, including the cases first diagnosed at death. The age-specific incidence rates in both studies increased with age overall and in the subgroups and no sex preponderance could be demonstrated. This last point has to be compared with the ealier studies of Zulch who found a slight male preponderance (M:F 55.6:44.4 per cent).[8] Of particular relevance to the question as to whether there are any important environmental factors in the genesis of brain tumours was the finding that rural farm residents were more likely to be affected by some types of tumour compared to rural non-farm residents, but the proportion of urban to rural inhabitants of both sexes affected by any type of tumour did not differ from the general population.

Another important study from the USA was that reported by Schoenberg, Christine and Whisnant.[9] Their study from the Connecticut Tumour Registry reported on 3210 primary brain tumours diagnosed between 1934 and 1964. The registry makes considerable effort to achieve complete case ascertainment in their well-defined geographic region. This data can therefore be taken as a reliable indicator of the disease pattern in their population. Their study demonstrated for tumours of the brain and meninges an early peak, followed by a taller and sharper peak in the 55–65 year age group. They pointed out that the different types of brain tumours demonstrated sufficiently distinct epidemiological patterns to suggest that they should be regarded as different diseases and not lumped together. The Rochester data had shown an increasing incidence with increasing age and, in contrast to the Connecticut study and most other investigations, that meningiomas were more common than gliomas. These differences were studied by Schoenberg.[10] The majority of the cases first diagnosed at autopsy accounted in large part for the different age-specific incidence curves especially among the elderly in the Rochester study and for the higher percentage of meningiomas. The conclusions drawn by Schoenberg were that a substantial number of asymptomatic tumours remain undiagnosed during life in the elderly and that, as the autopsy rate increases in any given population, the age-specific incidence pattern will more clearly resemble the data reported in the Rochester study. The UK experience closely mirrors that described for the Connecticut study.[11] Gliomas again were found to be the commonest tumour (average annual incidence 3.94 per 100 000) with a lower frequency in large urban areas. Grade 3–4 astrocytomas (glioblastoma multiforme) had a peak annual incidence of 7.53 per 100 000 in the 50–59 years age group and were more common in males. The peak incidence for oligodendrogliomas was also 50–59 years, but was in the 30–39 years age group for grade 1–2 astrocytomas. Meningiomas had an average annual incidence of 1.23 per 100 000 with a peak of 2.48 per 100 000 at 60–69 years with a female predominance

There is therefore now enough evidence from a variety of sources to consider that the various histological types of brain tumours are separate disease entities with sufficiently distinct epidemiological patterns of occurrence to suggest the possibility of different aetiological factors in their causation. The point is clearly demonstrated when age-adjusted incidence rates for histological type of tumour, the anatomical site, sex distribution and average age of occurrence are considered. The hormonal influence on certain types of pituitary adenoma and meningiomas may dictate an earlier occurrence of these tumours in the female and explain apparent sex ratio differences. From an epidemiological viewpoint, childhood and adult central nervous system tumours have different biological behaviours: only haemangioblastomas have a similar incidence in both childhood and adult life. All common brain tumours demonstrate a small childhood peak and higher adult peak when age-specific incidence rates are charted. Astrocytomas demonstrate an early peak and a less rapid, flatter rise to an adult peak, whilst meningiomas increase steadily in incidence from childhood to adult life. The less common primary central nervous system tumours are more varied in their incidence profiles. The neurilemmomas demonstrate a solitary peak at age 65, haemangioblastomas a steady, slight rise from 40 to 65, followed by a decline; ependymomas have two peaks, one at 15 and another at 55, and finally medulloblastomas show a childhood segregation with much fewer cases in adult life.[12]

As with the studies on primary intracranial tumours the best estimates of the true incidence of metastatic brain disease probably come from community studies. In Kurland's study 32 per cent of intracranial tumours were secondary deposits, although this was felt to be an underestimate, with the true figure suspected to lie between 35 and 50 per cent of all brain tumours.[6] This contention was supported by the later studies of Percy *et al.* who reported a figure of 41 per cent for cerebral tumours.[7] Autopsy studies from general pathological material have supported these figures and recorded estimates of 40 per cent.[13, 14] Henson and Urich suggested that a neurosurgical department might expect 20 per cent of their patients with intracranial tumours to be due to secondary deposits.[15] These variations in reported incidence from different data sources clearly reflect wide differences in ascertainment, size of sample, diagnostic difficulties, institutional bias, geographical and historical factors.[15]

Despite the difficulties in interpreting data on survival for patients with primary cerebral neoplasms, there is evidence to suggest that there may have been a gradual improvement in survival.[12] Again the survival data suggest differences in biological behaviour with regard to survival in the different types of tumour, with haemangiomas and meningiomas demonstrating a relatively linear decline in survival with time compared with all other types of tumour which demonstrate a relatively rapid decline in the first two years after diagnosis and treatment, followed by a more rapid decline.

Genetic and environmental factors in causation

Genetic factors play a minor role in determining the occurrence of brain tumours, apart from the two rare tumours, bilateral retinoblastomas and glomus tumours, and the occasional reporting of familial gliomas.[16] Tuberose sclerosis, like the retinoblastomas and glomus tumours, is often inherited as an autosomal dominant and rarely may be associated with intracranial astrocytomas, or more rarely still a glioblastoma, ependymoma or ganglioneuroma. In the central form of neurofibromatosis characterized by multiple tumours of the cranial and spinal nerve roots (often schwannomas, particularly bilateral acoustic neuroma) other types of tumour may include multiple meningiomas, ependymomas, astrocytomas, optic nerve gliomas and astrocytic lesions of the retina, with the rarer occurrence of hamartomatous lesions and syringomyelia. The peripheral form of this condition is defined by the presence of *café au lait* spots and multiple peripheral and subcutaneous nerve sheath tumours. Von Hippel-Lindau disease, characterized by haemangioblastomas (which are often multiple and cerebellar) and retinal angiomas, may be associated with pancreatic and kidney cysts, phaeochromocytomas, ependymomas, syringomyelia and erythrocytosis. Diffuse malignant proliferation of meningeal melanocytes with large cutaneous naevi and peripheral neurofibromas characterize the rare condition of neurocutaneous melanosis. Brain tumours, lymphoreticular tumours, leukaemia, epithelial tumours and carcinoma of the stomach occur with increased frequency in females with ataxia telangiectasia. Finally, there is the group of conditions in which nervous system tumours are associated with other multiple primary tumours elsewhere in the body.

The advantages of case control studies are that they are very useful in studying rare diseases and give an immediate answer in retrospective studies. They are, however, prone to bias. It is difficult to select comparable groups with all factors taken into account. There may be a bias in measuring exposure, since the presence of an outcome, whether favourable or unfavourable, may directly affect both the exposure and the subjective recall of an exposure. Allowing for these limitations these studies do provide another source of interesting, and possibly illuminating, information in the causation of brain tumours.

Of the environmental factors that have been tentatively linked with the genesis of brain tumours, the overall impression to date would be that, as with genetic factors, they are not making a sizeable contribution to the overall incidence of brain tumours. Patients who have received X-ray therapy to the scalp have an increased incidence of brain tumours but not of any specific type, and meningiomas may be more common in women receiving medical or dental X-ray examinations. Workers in the rubber manufacturing industry may be more likely to develop brain tumours; reticulum cell sarcomas of the brain are more common in renal transplant patients receiving immunosuppressive therapy; there is a significant association between breast cancer and meningiomas in women; osteosarcomas have been described in association with bilateral familial retinoblastomas: however, no clear environmental triggers have been identified for the overwhelming majority of primary intracranial tumours in man.

Conclusion

As yet, unlike some other common tumours, no useful preventive advice can be offered to reduce the incidence of brain tumours. Whether viral or chemical induction can occur in human brain tumours with any frequency remains uncertain, despite the wealth of information from animal experiments that this is possible.

More detailed and constant surveillance of populations should enable major changes in survival to be detected as a result of double-blind randomized studies recommending different treatment schedules. In a cost-conscious age this may become more important and better supported.

References

1. Garland HG, Armitage G. Intracranial tuberculomata. *Journal of Pathology and Bacteriology*. 1933; **37**, 46–71.
2. Weil A. *Textbook of Neuropathology*, 2nd edn. London: Heinemann, 1946.
3. Goldberg ID, Kurland LT. Mortality in 33 countries from disease of the central nervous system. *World Neurology*, 1962; **3**, 444–65.
4. Kurland LT, Myrianthopoulos NC, Lessell S. Epidemiological and genetic considerations of intracranial neoplasms. In: Fields WS, Sharkey PC, eds. *The Biology and Treatment of Intracranial Tumours* Springfield: C.C. Thomas, 1962: 5.
5. Kurtzke JF. Geographic pathology of brain tumours. 1. Distribution of deaths from primary tumours. *Acta Neurologica Scandinavica*. 1969; **45**, 540–55.
6. Kurland LT. The frequency of intracranial and intraspinal neoplasms in the resident population of Rochester, Minnesota. *Journal of Neurosurgery*. 1958; **15**, 627–41.
7. Percy AK, Elveback LR, Osaki H, Kurland LT. Neoplasms of the central nervous system: epidemiological considerations. *Neurology* (Minneapolis). 1972; **22**, 40–8.
8. Zulch KJ. *Brain Tumours, their Biology and their Pathology*. 2nd edn. New York: Springer-Verlag, 1965.
9. Schoenberg BS, Christine BW, Whisnant JP. The descriptive epidemiology of primary intracranial neoplasms: The Connecticut experience. *American Journal of Epidemiology*. 1976; **104**, 5, 499–510.
10. Schoenberg BS. *Epidemiology of Primary Nervous System Tumours*. New York: Raven Press, 1978: 475–95.
11. Barker DJP, Weller RO, Garfield JS. Epidemiology of primary tumours of the brain and spinal cord: a regional survey in southern England. *Journal of Neurology, Neurosurgery and Psychiatry*. 1976; **39**, 290–6.
12. Schoenberg BS. The epidemiology of central nervous system tumours. In: Walker MD, ed. *Oncology of the Nervous System*. Boston: Martinus Nijhoff, 1983: 1.
13. Kimura Sakumo S. Zur statistik der intrakraniellen Tumoren. *Psychiatria et Neurologica Japonica* (*Seishin Shin Keigako Zassh*), 1937; **41**, 999–1013. Summary in *Zentrablatt Psychiatrice*, 1938; **89**: 83.
14. Krasting. Beitrage zur statistik and Kasuistik meta statischer Tumoren, besanders der Carcinommetastase in Zentral nerven system. *Zeitschrift fur Krebsforschung under Klinische Onkologie*. 1906; **4**, 315–79.
15. Henson and Urich. *Cancer and the Nervous System*. London: Butterworths, 1982; Ch. 2: 7–59.
16. Tijessen EC, Halprin MR, Endtz LJ. *Familial Brain Tumours, a Commented Register*. London: Martinus Nijhoff, 1982.

9 Clinical manifestations of brain tumours

David GT Thomas and Ronald O McKeran

Introduction

Malignant primary brain tumours occur with two separate peaks of incidence: childhood and in middle age. Generally the presenting symptoms of patients with malignant brain tumours are those due to focal brain dysfunction, to raised intracranial pressure or to epilepsy. These may occur singly or in combination. Examples of the first systematic descriptions in textbooks of neurology of clinical syndromes related to brain tumours appeared in the latter part of the nineteenth century[1] and are now commonplace.[2] In spite of the advent of highly sensitive and non-invasive methods of imaging the brain by computerized tomography or magnetic resonance imaging, a clinical suspicion of the presence of a brain tumour based on history and physical signs remains the essential guide that further investigation is necessary.

Focal brain damage due to malignant brain tumour may cause hemiparesis, dysphasia, hemianaesthesia or hemianopia, either as an initial symptom or as symptoms at the time when the patient presents for diagnosis in the neurosurgical unit. Mental deterioration, with changes in intellectual function and, or, changes in personality, may occur as a more general feature of impaired brain function due to tumour. Raised intracranial pressure may cause headache associated with vomiting and visual failure due to papilloedema. There is a delay between the time a patient becomes aware of an initial symptom caused by a brain tumour and the time of histological diagnosis by surgery. This, and other aspects of clinical presentation, have been studied by the authors and co-workers in a series of 653 patients with cerebral gliomas.[3] The mean delay is 1.65 years, but there is a wide range. The relative frequencies of these and other symptoms, like epilepsy, as the initial symptom or as symptoms present at the time of histological diagnosis by surgery are shown in Table 8.1. Epilepsy is a very frequent accompaniment of the development of a brain tumour and may have focal features or involve generalized convulsions. A fit occurring for the first time in life after the age of 30, i.e. epilepsy of late onset, frequently indicates structural brain disease which in many cases will be due to brain tumour. The relative frequency of signs found prior to surgery is shown in Table 8.2.

Table 9.1 Relative frequency in percentage of initial symptoms (A) and symptoms at time of diagnosis (B)[3]

	A	B
Epilepsy	38	54
Headache	35	71
Mental change	17	52
Hemiparesis	10	43
Vomiting	8	31
Dysphasia	7	27
Impaired consciousness	5	25
Visual failure	4	18
Hemianaesthesia	3	14
Hemianopia	2	8
Cranial nerve palsy	2	1

Table 9.2 Relative frequency in percentage of signs at time of diagnosis[3]

Hemiparesis	62
Cranial nerve palsy	54
Mental deterioration	53
Papilloedema	52
Hemianaesthesia	35
Hemianopia	33
Dysphasia	28
Visual failure	21

Symptoms of focal neurological deficit and raised intracranial pressure

The nature of a focal deficit, for example lateralized or localized motor deficit, or the site of focal epileptic manifestations may be helpful in indicating the probable site of the brain tumour. Headache is a non-specific symptom, but the headache associated with malignant brain tumour is usually of moderately severe intensity, generally worse in the early morning on waking and gradually lessening through the day. Sometimes the most helpful diagnostic feature is that the headache is different in character and duration from previous ones experienced by the patient. Sometimes it is localized to the site, or side, of the tumour, but more frequently this is not the case. Vomiting associated with raised intracranial pressure due to brain tumour is also often worse in the early morning. Visual failure, due to raised intracranial pressure and papilloedema, may be tolerated for so long by the patient that there may be virtual blindness at the time of presentation. Usually visual failure is less severe than this and is detected on physical examination by finding impaired visual acuity associated with the presence of papilloedema, together with exudates and haemorrhages and sometimes optic atrophy. Field defects, due to involvement of the optic radiation, may be detected on perimetry. Diplopia may be present due to partial sixth or third nerve palsies related to incipient brain herniation at the tentorium. These two cranial nerves are those most often involved when brain tumours present with cranial nerve palsy. On rare occasions acute brain herniation with abrupt coma may be the first presenting manifestation of a malignant brain tumour. Where such attacks are not fatal the patient will generally be brought to hospital and investigated urgently.

Brain tumour syndromes

Malignant brain tumours occurring at particular sites within the brain can give rise to typical patterns of symptoms and signs. There is a wide variation in the abruptness of onset of symptoms due to brain tumour, as well as in the length of time between the initial symptom and diagnosis and treatment as noted above. Both these aspects vary with the histological grade and the site of tumour.

Cerebral hemisphere tumours

Frontal lobe

Changes in personality with intellectual failure and emotional lability coupled with facetiousness are often the first symptoms of tumours affecting the anterior and basal frontal lobes. In the left (dominant) hemisphere, dysphasia accompanies the spastic hemiparesis which develops in the contralateral limbs when such tumours involve the posterior frontal lobe. Relatively large tumours involving the superficial cortical structures may give rise to weakness affecting a small anatomical distribution, appropriate to the motor function of the relevant cortex. Thus, tumours of the superior and medial part of the frontal lobe will cause severe weakness of the foot and leg. Tumours occurring deeper in the white matter, where fibres projecting from the pyramidal tract converge, may cause a relatively more extensive pattern of weakness and a small tumour at a critical site can cause a hemiplegia. Where brain posterior to the central sulcus is affected by tumour spreading from the frontal lobe, sentation will also be impaired. Epilepsy, either as focal motor manifestations in the contralateral face and limbs or as generalized convulsions, often occurs. Focal (Jacksonian) motor epilepsies are due to tumours in the motor region of the posterior frontal lobe. Such attacks may affect the hand, face, or foot, for example and spread causing more general clonic and/or adversive movements. Early physical signs of frontal tumours are the presence of abnormal grasp reflexes, abnormal plantar response and slight facial weakness or hemiparesis, frequently associated with papilloedema. Frequency and urgency of micturition may also occur.

Corpus callosum

Gliomas which involve the corpus callosum and typically affect both frontal lobes cause a progressively severe dementia associated with incontinence and bilateral pyramidal signs generally most marked in the lower limbs. When the more posterior part of the corpus callosum is affected, a much less common site than the butterfly tumour found in the anterior corpus callosum, pressure on the superior colliculi may cause impairment of upward gaze.

Parietal lobe

Involvement of the sensory cortex leads to neglect of the contralateral side of the body, commonly associated with visual inattention. Tumours of the dominant parietal lobe cause receptive dysphasia, while those in the right parietal lobe generally impair left–right discrimination and orientation of the body image. When the more anterior part of the parietal lobe is affected, in the post-central gyrus, joint sensation, vibration, and light touch sensation will be particularly disturbed. Testing of two-point discrimination and stereognosis will elicit clinical signs of these deficits, and commonly there will also be signs of associated frontal motor cortex disturbance by the tumour, with weakness of upper motor neurone pattern. More posterior and deeper parietal tumours disturb the optic radiation and give rise to a lower quadrantanopia. In addition to dysphasia and dyslexia, both dysgraphia and dyscalculia may also arise. Sensory inattention, and sensory extinction[4] may occur, whereby when both sides of the body are stimulated the sensation coming to the affected parietal lobe is ignored. Tumours of the parietal lobe may also give rise to agnosia or apraxia. Epilepsy is also a frequent manifestation of parietal tumours. Sometimes this takes the form of focal sensory features of paraesthesia perceived in a limb or the face.

Occipital lobe

Tumours in this site, which are relatively uncommon, cause a homonymous hemianopia. Presentation in such cases is often late, after the patient has developed other symptoms and/or signs due to raised intracranial pressure.

Temporal lobe

Tumours of the temporal lobe cause hemiparesis, homonymous hemianopia and, in the dominant hemisphere, dysphasia. Epilepsy of the temporal lobe type, generally associated with olfactory or gustatory hallucinations, feelings of fear or pleasure, repetitive pyschomotor movements or absences is relatively frequent in tumours affecting the temporal lobe. However, temporal lobe tumours may be relatively "silent" until the continued growth of the tumour leads to symptoms of raised intracranial pressure. Sometimes the initial effect of the temporal lobe tumour on the optic radiation is simply to cause a superior quadrantanopia which may become apparent on formal field testing. Medial temporal tumours may present with impairment of memory and a change to a more irritable personality. Sometimes the hallucinations may be auditory or visual in character and there may be a feeling of *déjà vu*. Salivation and chewing movements of the mouth together with flushing and automatic behaviour may occur during temporal lobe seizures.

Third ventricle region tumours

Pineal region, thalamus, lateral ventricle, third ventricle, hypothalamus and optic chiasm

Germinoma and teratomas of the pineal region grow at the posterior end of the third ventricle. Gliomas can also occur in the posterior third ventricle and may mimic pineal tumours. The local effect of pressure on the quadrigeminal plate usually causes palsy of upward gaze, ptosis and dilatation of the pupils. Gliomas which grow in the thalamus and basal ganglia generally cause contralateral sensory and motor neurological deficits and may progress to cause the symptoms of raised intracranial pressure, particularly if hydrocephalus also supervenes.

Colloid cysts and craniopharyngiomas tend to affect the anterior part of the third ventricle. The local effect of pressure from posterior third ventricle tumours on the quadrigemical plate usually causes failure of upward gaze, ptosis and dilatation of the pupils. Any of the tumours at this site, which is critical for circulation of CSF, may cause hydrocephalus which can be acute, presenting with excruciating headache and drop attacks, or chronic, presenting with remittent or progressive dementia and chronic signs of raised pressure.

Gliomas which grow in the thalamus, or in the basal ganglia generally cause contralateral sensory and motor neurological deficits and may progress to cause symptoms of raised intracranial pressure, particularly if hydrocephalus also supervenes. If the internal capsule is affected by such tumours the resulting neurological deficits may be very dense. Involuntary movements are only a very rare manifestation of tumours in the basal ganglia. Tumours which grow into the lateral ventricle include glioma, meningioma, choroid plexus papilloma and epidermoids. Symptoms of such lesions tend to be rather non-specific motor or sensory deficits, sometimes associated with hemianopia. Gliomas may also occur in the hypothalamus or optic chiasm, particularly in children. Such tumours in the floor of the ventricle can cause failure of growth, voracious appetite and failure of temperature control. They may also cause impaired sexual development or, sometimes, precocious puberty. They may also cause diabetes insipidus, visual failure and disturbance in sleep patterns as well as raised intracranial pressure due to associated hydrocephalus.

Brain stem

Intrinsic malignant tumours affecting the brain stem cause a constellation of lower cranial nerve palsies associated with symptoms due to involvement of the sensory and motor tracts passing through the brain stem. Frequently the pattern is of gradual progressive deterioration, but sometimes the course may be step-wise and it may fluctuate. Change in facial sensation (trigeminal (V) nerve), diplopia, (abducens (VI) nerve), facial weakness, (facial (VII) nerve), deafness, (acoustic (VIII) nerve), or difficulty in swallowing and speaking (glossopharyngeal (IX), vagus (X), hypoglossal (XII) nerves) singly or in combination may be the presenting symptoms of cranial nerve dysfunction. Sensory impairment or ataxia, frequently combined with weakness and clumsiness of the limbs, may also be associated with these symptoms. However, raised intracranial pressure and hydrocephalus are unusual with tumours at this site. Typically children and young adults are affected by brain stem tumours.

Cerebellum and fourth ventricle

Brain tumours which affect the cerebellar hemispheres commonly cause ataxia of the ipsilateral limbs, associated with nystagmus. Often there are associated signs of hydrocephalus with raised intracranial pressure and papilloedema with or without, optic atrophy. Tumours of the cerebellar vermis and fourth ventricle cause truncal ataxia, often associated with vomiting, headache and neck stiffness which are due, in part, to hydrocephalus with associated raised intracranial pressure and, in part, to local pressure within the posterior fossa.

Epilepsy in relation to malignant brain tumours

Epilepsy may develop due to many forms of structural brain disease. The nature of fits due to brain tumours is the same as those due to other causes. However, a temporary paresis, Todd's palsy, may occur and persist for a few hours afterwards. Failure to recover function, or a progressive deterioration after consecutive episodes, are indications of progressive organic brain damage due to a tumour. A change in the character of epileptic manifestations, resistance to drug therapy and the recurrence of *status epilepticus* as well as associated signs of focal neurological deficit or raised intracranial pressure are further indications that an underlying brain tumour may be responsible. The likelihood of developing epilepsy due to an intracranial tumour is related both to the site and nature of the neoplasm. Tumours affecting the sensori-motor cortex are most likely to lead to epileptic manifestations, while those affecting the occipital cortex are least likely to do so. Tumours adjacent to the cortex are more likely to cause epilepsy than those deep within white matter. Oligodendrogliomas and low-grade astrocytomas are relatively more likely to cause epilepsy than high-grade gliomas. The onset of epilepsy is generally a dramatic event for the patient, most frequently noted as the first manifestation of his illness (Table 8.1) and the symptom which prompts the seeking of specialist advice and investigation. Long periods of time, frequently several years, may pass between the first fit and the onset of other symptoms. In general epilepsy is a favourable prognostic sign.

Differential diagnosis

The differential diagnosis of brain tumour remains that of other space-occupying lesions including benign tumours, e.g. meningioma, chronic subdural haematoma, brain abscess and other inflammatory masses such as tuberculoma. Cerebrovascular accident with infarction or with haemorrhage and haematoma may also cause similar syndromes. Degenerative neurological diseases such as the presenile dementias and multiple sclerosis may also enter into the differential diagnosis.

Conclusion

A carefully taken clinical history, and a thorough physical examination, remain the starting points in the detection of patients with brain tumours. The widespread introduction of imaging techniques, in the form of computerized axial tomography and magnetic resonance imaging, which are not only relatively non-invasive but are also reliable and sensitive, has revolutionized the clinical management of such patients. In neurological centres which are equipped with these modern neuroradiological facilities there should be little delay in obtaining confirmation of the presence of an intracranial lesion. With the improvements in conventional neurosurgical methods, as well as with the introduction of image-directed stereotactic biopsy, histological diagnosis and, where appropriate, surgical excision should generally be achievable at an earlier stage in the disease than in the past. This places an increased responsibility on all clinicians to be alert to early clinical symptoms and signs of intracranial tumours in their patients so that modern methods of investigation and treatment may be applied quickly.

References

1. Gowers WR. *A Manual of Diseases of the Nervous System.* Vol. 2. London: J and A Churchill, 1888.
2. Thomas DGT. Brain tumours. In: Harrison MJG, ed. *Contemporary Neurology.* London Butterworths, 1984: 511–30.
3. McKeran RO, Thomas DGT. The clinical study of gliomas. In: Thomas DGT, Graham DI, eds. *Brain Tumours: Scientific Basis, Clinical Investigation and Current Therapy* 1980: 194–230.
4. Critchley McD. The phenomenon of tactile inattention with special reference to parietal lesions. *Brain.* 1949; **44**, 538–61.

10 Advances in surgery for malignant brain tumour

R Bradford and DGT Thomas

Introduction

Surgical treatment of malignant glioma began over one hundred years ago on 25 November 1884. Sir Rickman Godlee, under the direction of Dr Hughes Bennett, removed a right parietal glioma from a 25-year-old labourer suffering from Jacksonian epilepsy.[1] This early attempt at glioma surgery preceded radiological localization and relied on the concept of cerebral function localization introduced by Ferrier and Jackson.

The introduction of air ventriculography by Dandy in 1918 and arteriography by Moniz in 1927 mark the beginning of the modern era of neurosurgery.[2] These techniques allowed some attempt at preoperative diagnosis regarding tumour type as well as demonstrating their intracranial location. Over the ensuing years the principles of brain tumour surgery have been established. Although surgery cannot be regarded as curative for malignant glioma, it is a most useful component of adjuvant therapy. Shapiro has outlined five objectives for the surgical treatment of malignant glioma.[3] First, it enables the histologist to establish a pathological diagnosis. Second, the bulk of the tumour is removed. Third, distressing symptoms are relieved. Fourth, tumour volume reduction permits time for adjuvant therapy. Finally, removal of tumour bulk will induce those cells that are not in cycle to resume an active phase of growth and thus increase their susceptibility to radio- or chemotherapy.

The development of computerized tomography (CT) and magnetic resonance imaging (MRI) has allowed direct visualization of lesions within the central nervous system. Moreover data obtained from these imaging techniques when integrated with stereotactic technology allow the neurosurgeon to locate precisely areas within a tumour as well as its imaged boundary within three-dimensional space. These developments have made a considerable advance in the diagnosis and surgical treatment of malignant glioma and will form the subject of this chapter.

Pathological diagnosis of malignant glioma

Despite the two major advances in neuroimaging (CT and MRI) in the last 20 years a diagnosis of malignant glioma remains dependent on the histological examination of pathological tissue. The undoubted poor prognosis for the patient harbouring what appears radiologically to be a malignant glioma is no excuse for the failure of the neurosurgeon to make a tissue diagnosis. The fear of diagnostic error must continue to be one of the main justifications for surgical biopsy. Conventional stereotaxis, prior to CT scanning, relied on intracranial landmarks defined by plain skull radiographs, ventriculography and angiography. This has proved adequate for functional neurosurgery where targets are estimated from known parameters, most frequently estimates of normal anatomical variation derived from standard stereotactic atlases. The application of stereotactic technique to brain tumour surgery prior to the CT era was, however, severely limited due to the distortion of normal brain anatomy by the intracranial mass and the consequent difficulty of locating it in stereotactic space. Prior to CT, stereotaxis, the biopsy of intracranial mass lesions had, been performed freehand either via a burr hole or open craniotomy. Freehand biopsy is associated with two problems which appear to be inversely proportional to each other, i.e. the failure to achieve a diagnosis and morbidity/mortality. An early comparison of biopsy versus resection by Hitchcock and Sato showed that there was a 27 per cent mortality associated with burr hole biopsy in contrast to 4 per cent mortality with definitive removal of tumour volume.[4] Improvements in preoperative management, particularly with the introduction of steroids, reduced mortality to approximately 5 per cent.[5] A tissue diagnosis was, however, only made in 88 per cent of patients. Increasing the yield of positive tissue diagnoses to 95 per cent necessitates multiple freehand biopsies and results in an increase in neurological morbidity.[6] Brain biopsy with CT stereotactic techniques has reduced mortality to less than 1 per cent and achieved a diagnostic accuracy as high as 96 per cent.[7]

CT-directed stereotactic biopsy

The potential benefits of integrating stereotactic technique with CT data were quickly realized. Several existing stereotactic frames were modified for CT compatibility and several new systems designed *de novo*.[8-11]

The "BRW" stereotactic system was developed by Brown, Roberts and Wells[12-15] and is manufactured by Trent Wells Inc, Southgate, California and distributed by Radionics Inc, Burlington, Massachusetts, USA and RDG Electro Medical Equipment, Croydon, Surrey, UK. This is an "arc-type" apparatus[16] in which the target point is in the centre of an arc or series of arcs (Fig. 9.1). The BRW system was designed *de novo* as a CT-guided apparatus using computer graphics techniques.[17] The design included the following aims: firstly ease of transformation of the two-dimensional coordinates of a CT image to a three-dimensional point in stereotactic space and secondly to provide an infinite number of trajectories to any three-dimensionally defined point in space. These design objectives have been met and

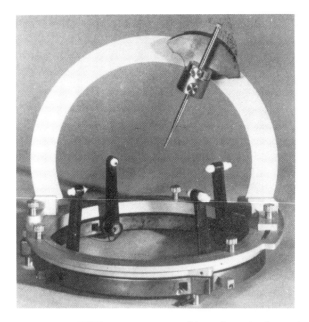

Fig. 10.1 The BRW arc system positioned on the base ring.

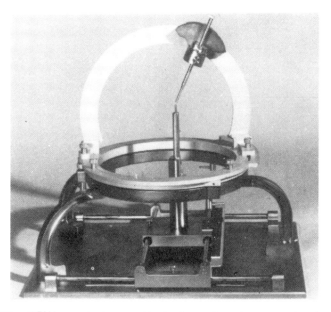

Fig. 10.2 The BRW surgical arc attached to the phantom simulator allows determination of the X, Y and Z coordinates of the chosen skull entry point.

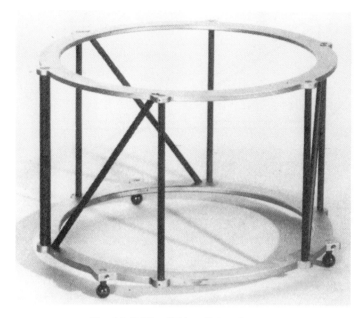

Fig. 10.3 The CT localizing frame.

have resulted in an extremely flexible and easy-to-use instrument which is one of the most commonly used CT-directed systems.[18]

In general we have preferred to perform our stereotactic procedures under general anaesthetic. The base ring (reference plane) is attached to the patient's head by four conically pointed metal screws mounted on adjustable carbon-fibre arms. The desired entry point in the skull is then defined by clamping the arc system to the base ring and bringing a blunt probe into contact with the scalp. The X, Y and Z coordinates of this entry point are then determined by attaching the surgical arc to a phantom simulator which consists of a base ring and a moveable pointed tip (Fig. 10.2). The patient is then transferred to the CT scanner where a localizing frame is attached to the base ring (Fig. 10.3). The localizing frame enables the two- to three-dimensional transformation of the CT-selected plane to be accomplished. The localizing frame consists of three sets of three rods arranged in an "N" shape. The height above the reference plane of any point on the diagonal rod is determined by the ratio of the variable distance between one of the vertical rods and the diagonal rod and the fixed distance between the two vertical rods (Fig. 10.4). This method of localization has been termed the "picket fence".[18] The combination of the three sets of picket fences defines three points in space in the image plane thereby fixing its position relative to the reference plane. The X, Y and Z coordinates of any other point in that plane can then be calculated (Fig. 10.5). By using the picket fence method of localization, the exact position and angle of the base ring is not critical provided it lies on the skull below the level of the lesion. The X and Y coordinates

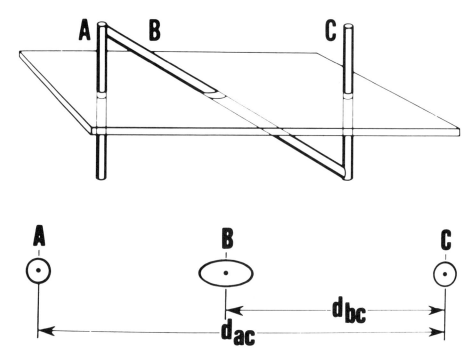

Fig. 10.4 The height above the reference plane of any point on the diagonal rod is determined by d_{bc}/d_{ac} (from Heilburn[18]).

for all nine localizing rods (fiducials) and target points can be obtained directly from the CT scanner console and calculation of target points in three-dimensional space can be performed on a portable computer (Epson HX-20). The calculations also produce four frame settings and a depth which, when set by the surgeon, produce a trajectory between the entry point and the target.

The ability of the BRW arc guidance system to connect any skull entry point with any intracranial target is achieved by using two categories of movement. The first relates to the perpendicular arc which is perpendicular to the base ring and can rotate through 360° (Fig. 10.1). In addition it has a fixed fulcrum which permits a 40° swing from the base ring. The combination of these two movements creates an infinite number of vertical two-dimensional planes, one of which will contain the chosen entry point and target. On the arc is a radial slide which supports the probe holder (Fig. 10.1). The radial slide is capable of 200° of movement along the arc and additionally the probe holder can rotate 110° about its fixation point on the slide. This second combination of movements allows the calculation of a unique trajectory between any two points within the chosen vertical plane. The combination of the four frame settings and depth establish a trajectory and distance between any chosen points within the sphere created by the arc.

Although it is perfectly feasible to perform tumour biopsies through a twist drill opening,[18] we have preferred to use a burr hole. This allows direct inspection of the

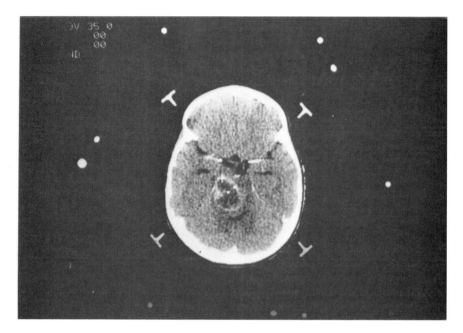

Fig. 10.5 The picket fence method of localization fixes the image plane relative to the reference plane and allows the determination of any other point in that plane. Here three targets within and on the enhancing rim of the tumour have been chosen.

cortex and surface vessels can therefore be avoided. Also, multiple targets, which will require varying trajectories, can be reached through the same skull entry point. Biopsies are taken with a Sidan-type side-cutting needle which produces a core of tissue of approximately 5 × 2 mm. Generally four biopsies from each quadrant of the target are taken and histological examination performed by immediate smear and paraffin sections. The problems of making a neuropathological diagnosis on small tissue samples are to some extent offset by the ease and safety with which multiple tissue samples can be obtained with precision from various specific areas of interest seen on the CT scan.

It has been our practice to obtain tissue samples from the contrast-enhanced edge as well as the body of the tumour. In over 40 per cent of the gliomas we have biopsied, there has been a clear histological difference between the tumour centre and its edge as defined by CT. Indeed, in 46 per cent of biopsies of malignant glioma the enhancing edge has been tumour-free,[19] suggesting that in certain selected cases radical local treatment may be warranted for tumour control.

It has also been possible to obtain cell cultures from stereotactic biopsy samples of cerebral glioma using the explant coverslip overlay technique.[20] This opens up the possibility of using cultured biopsy samples for detailed *in vitro* studies of intratumoural variability. Tissue culture studies may ultimately provide fundamental information on the biological variability of human gliomas.

MRI-directed stereotactic biopsy

Cerebral abnormalities visualized with MRI were first published in 1980 by Hawkes et al.[21] Since then the value of MR imaging of the brain has become well recognized. Production of an image by MR is considerably more complex than with CT and it is related to the MR signal of specific nuclei, the strength of external magnetic fields, and the T_1 and T_2 relaxation times of tissues being imaged.[22] MRI has, however, a number of advantages over CT. Bone artefact is not a problem with MRI of the posterior fossa,[23] and a high level of contrast is seen between grey and white matter.[24] Direct coronal and sagittal images can be produced without recourse to computer reconstructions. In addition, it has recently become apparent that MRI may reveal cerebral lesions which are not clearly visualized by CT.[25]

As with CT, the imaging technology awaited modifications of existing stereotactic coordinate frames in order that tissue from targets visualized on the MR image could be obtained with the precision and accuracy of stereotactic technique. Leksell et al. described a stereotactic system suitable for use with MRI as well as the use of conventional MRI to confirm the location functional lesions produced under CT guidance.[26, 27]

The first use of MRI-directed stereotactic tumour biopsy in clinical practice was reported by Thomas et al.[28] Subseqently, Lunsford reported three cases in which he had performed CT- and MRI-directed biopsy using a modification of the Leksell frame.[7] We have subsequently reported MRI-directed biopsies in five patients whose intracerebral lesions were not clearly shown by CT.[29, 30] Unlike Lunsford's series we have reserved MRI-directed biopsy for a small subset of patients who require stereotactic biopsy of lesions which are not shown at all or are not clearly delineated on CT scanning. In these cases MRI has revealed the lesion or given more detail with regard to selecting target sites for biopsy (Figs 10.6(a) and (b)).

The stereotactic frame used for biopsy under MRI control was a prototype modification of the BRW CT-directed stereotactic system. Basically frames must be free of ferromagnetic components to make them suitable for use in strong magnetic fields and closed conducting loops must be eliminated to avoid artefact from eddy currents. For MRI compatibility the aluminium alloy base ring of the BRW frame was replaced by one constructed of non-metallic paxolin and carbon-fibre. The ferromagnetic stainless steel skull fixation pins were replaced with titanium. In the prototype, the localizing frame consisted of 12 carbon-fibre tubes containing a solution of gadolinium-DTPA or weak copper sulphate with a T_1 of approximately 200 ms enabling them to be seen on MR images when appropriately windowed. Target and fiducial coordinates can be obtained directly from the MR visual display unit. The use of 12 fiducials in the localizing frame necessitates the use of a separate computer program to calculate the X, Y and Z coordinates of the target. Once obtained these data can be fed into the standard BRW software used for CT-directed biopsy in order to obtain the settings for the BRW arc system.

At present there is little information regarding the accuracy of MRI for stereotactic surgery. MRI has been shown to produce spatial distortion, particularly in the coronal and saggital planes.[31] Two studies have been performed using the MRI modification of the Leksell frame.[7, 32] Wyper et al., using an agar filled phantom into which aluminium pellets were inserted stereotactically to act as targets, found MRI produced an accuracy of better than 2 mm.[31] Lunsford et al. performed intraoperative CT in three cases immediately following MRI-directed biopsy and

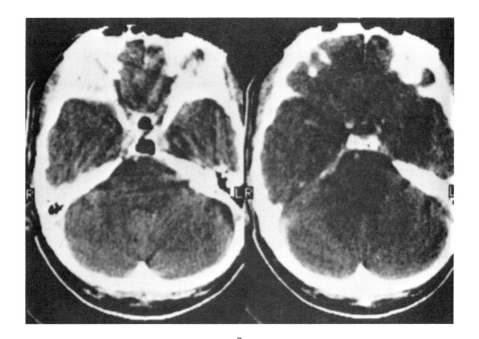

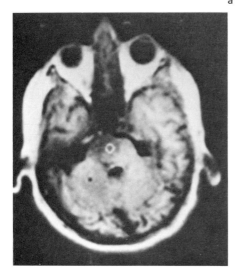

Fig. 10.6 (a) CT scan of a patient with a progressive brain stem syndrome; (b) MRI of the same patient reveals the pontine lesion. The cursor shows the proposed target for biopsy.

claimed an accuracy for Leksell system of 1 mm.[7] In our own studies using the modified BRW frame and defined targets within a phantom, we have found some discrepancy in the calculated coordinates derived from either CT or MRI.[39] If CT is used as the standard then MRI appears to be less accurate. We feel, however, that the accuracy is adequate for obtaining tissue samples from cerebral mass lesions but further studies on the linearity of MRI are needed before its use in functional neurosurgery is considered. Future modifications to the localizing frame which will allow stereotactic biopsy of targets defined in the coronal and saggital planes may improve the accuracy in the Z axis.

In our series of stereotactic biopsies we have found MRI-directed biopsy to be a useful adjunct to CT in the management of difficult cases. It is technically feasible to perform MRI-directed biopsy in cases where CT controlled biopsy would not be possible and in the majority of cases obtain a pathological diagnosis. Undoubtedly MRI is a major advance in brain imaging but it is still not possible to reach an accurate diagnosis without histological examination of tissue samples. Stereotactic biopsy represents an extension of the scope of MRI and promises to have valuable clinical and research applications particularly in the definition of tumour boundaries with different pulse sequences.

Stereotactic biopsy of brain stem lesions

Advanced generation CT scanners and MR imagers have enabled the detection of small lesions deep within the brain and brain stem. The management of these intrinsic brain stem lesions, however, remains controversial. The surgical inaccessibility of these lesions has produced empirical therapists who assume the poor prognosis of the patient and because of the dangers do not advocate biopsy.[32]

Open biopsy or decompression of mass lesions of the brain stem via the subtemporal,[33] the retromastoid,[34] or the suboccipital[35] route represent major surgical procedures. Although recent series of patients subjected to open biopsy demonstrate low incidences of morbidity and mortality, a high rate of non-diagnostic tissue was obtained particularly if a clearly exophytic or surface lesion was not visualized.[33] A stereotactic approach to brain stem lesions can, potentially, provide a high yield of positive histological diagnosis with a low incidence of morbidity. That this is the case is evident from two recently published series.[36, 37] We have performed a number of stereotactic biopsies of intrinsic brain stem lesions under either CT or MRI control with a high diagnostic rate and minimal morbidity.[38] In non-neoplastic cases where it was possible to aspirate haematoma, considerable neurological improvement occurred in the early postoperative period.

Stereotactic trajectories to the brain stem include the transfrontal, transtentorial and transcerebellar. The latter route has been advocated for the lateral pons or cerebellar peduncle. We have performed our brain stem biopsies through a transfrontal approach. The flexibility of the BRW system, described earlier, allows precise placement of the burr hole parasagittally on or just behind the coronal suture ipsilateral to the selected targets. The trajectory is entirely transparenchymal and avoids the posterior clinoid processes and the free edge of the tentorium. The transfrontal trajectory permits a route to all divisions of the brain stem while avoiding the risk of haemorrhage from the pial surface of the cerebellum or mesencephalon. The trajectory also allows tissue sampling at various depths along the brain stem axis. This is an advantage since most neoplastic lesions are not confined to one division but infiltrate along the brain stem axis.

It is too early at present to assess the impact of stereotactic biopsy on the management of the patient with a brain stem lesion. Reported series have at present merely assessed the technical feasibility and the diagnostic accuracy. It seems likely that the prognosis for patients with brain stem tumours depends on the tumour grade.[39] Reported trials of therapy for these lesions have not required a histological diagnosis and therefore valid conclusions are difficult to reach.[40] Since CT or MRI-directed biopsy of brain stem lesions is potentially the safest and most reliable method for the diagnosis of lesions within the mesencephalon and pons, this procedure should be considered for all patients entering any controlled therapy studies. Only then can statistically meaningful research into novel therapies be performed.

Computer-interactive stereotactic tumour excision

Several therapeutic approaches to intracranial lesions in which volume has been determined by CT scanning have been described. Shalit *et at.* have described total resection of intracranial gliomas using intraoperative CT scanning.[41] Unfortunately, few neurosurgeons have the luxury of a dedicated CT scanner situated within the operating theatre. Combined CT-directed stereotactic techniques have been used to guide the neurosurgeon to tumours located in sensitive areas of the brain where major tumour resection has been performed.[18,42] This method, while providing accurate localization of the tumour, does not make use of the tumour boundaries defined by CT. The problem of distinction between the primary glial neoplasm and oedematous but intact brain perenchyma remains unresolved. In the early 1980s, Kelly and co-workers began development of a computer-interactive stereotactic system which allows the precise three-dimensional data obtainable from the CT scan to be placed into a stereotactic coordinate system. The second model of this stereotactic system, which consists of custom-built hardware and software, was installed in Maida Vale Hospital, London, in 1984 and has been used for total resection of centrally located and deeply seated intra-axial malignant gliomas. Computer-assisted stereotactic tumour resections are performed in three stages, which Kelly *et al.* have termed data acquisition, surgical planning and the computer-interactive operative procedure.[43]

The data acquisition stage resembles any other CT-directed stereotactic procedure. A CT-compatible stereotactic head-holder,[44] which consists of a round metal base with four vertical molybdenum supports, is fixed to the patient's head by four carbon-fibre pins inserted into twist drill holes in the outer table of the skull. The patient then undergoes CT scanning with a localizer system attached to the head holder. This localizer is of the picket-fence variety discussed above and produces nine artefacts on each CT slice.

During the planning procedure a three-dimensional software reconstruction package is used which transposes lesions appearing on serial CT slices into three-dimensional stereotactic space. On each CT slice which demonstrates the lesion the nine fiducial markers are digitized by an intensity sweep program which automatically marks the coordinates of their centre. The enhancing edge of the tumour is then digitized using the cross-hair cursor and trackball systems of the display console (Fig. 10.7). The X and Y coordinates of each digitized point are connected by the computer program and stored as a continual outline within the three-dimensional image matrix related to the stereotactic coordinate system. The tumour is digitized

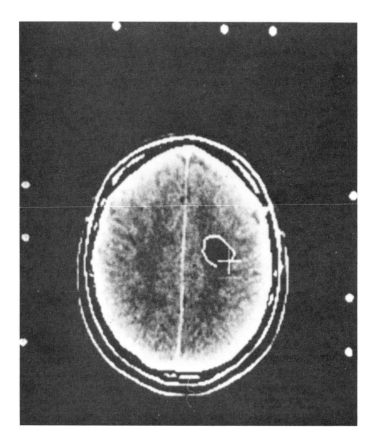

Fig. 10.7 Digitization of the tumour edge.

on each slice that it appears. On one CT slice on which the cross-sectional area of the tumour is largest a single point within the tumour is chosen as a target point and digitized. The entire image is then reconstructed around this point in the image matrix. The three-dimensional image of the tumour is created by a program which interpolates intermediate slices at 1 mm intervals.[45,46] Cross-sections of the "digitized" and prepared image may then be sliced orthogonal to any safe surgical trajectory and reformatted slices can be displayed on an operating theatre video monitor. The program allows entry of any surgical trajectory based on the angulations of the arc-quadrant stereotactic table. The surgical trajectory should, ideally, cross non-essential brain in the direction of the major white matter fibres. The computer also calculates the mechanical adjustments on the stereotactic frame that will position the selected target point at the focal point of the arc-quadrant system.

The surgical procedure is performed using the custom built Kelly–Goerss computer-interactive arc-quadrant stereotactic instrument (Fig. 10.8).[45] The patient is fixed to the table by means of the stereotactic head-holder which is moved in the X, Y or Z directions by means of motorized slides. These three degrees of freedom

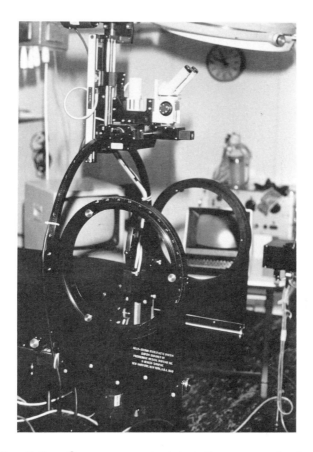

Fig. 10.8 The Kelly – Goerss computer-interactive arc-quadrant stereotactic instrument.

enable the head to be moved such that the predetermined target point within the tumour is at the centre of the sphere generated by the arc and quadrant. A standard craniotomy is then performed and arc and quadrant angles specified which allow a safe trajectory to the tumour. Subcortical tumours are approached through a cortical incision and a self-retaining cylindrical stereotactic retractor inserted. As the tumour is approached the surgeon calls up the superficial tumour slices on the operating theatre graphics display. These are cut orthogonal to the surgical viewing angle. Attached to the stereotactic arc are an operating microscope and a helium–argon laser which acts as an aiming device. The distance of the focal points of the microscope and the laser from the focal point of the stereotactic frame is measured by optical encoders and displayed on a digital readout. By means of a remote joystick which is manipulated by the surgeon or his assistant and optical encoders the X, Y position of the aiming laser beam is transmitted to the computer which sets the position of the laser beam in the surgical field and displays its position on the graphics terminal in the form of a cursor. Thus, if the graphics terminal cursor is moved

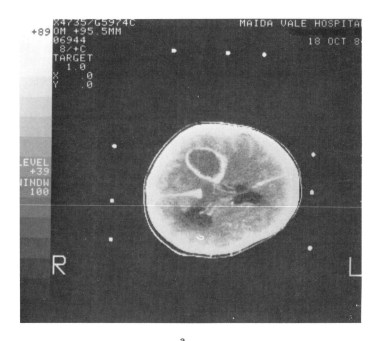

Fig. 10.9 (a) and (b) Pre- and postoperative scans of a patient whose malignant glioma was resected by stereotactic craniotomy using the Kelly – Goerss instrument.

(by means of the joystick) around the orthogonally sliced graphics representation of the tumour boundary this, will be translated into movement of the laser beam which in turn will trace the tumour contour on the surface of the brain. The tumour can then be removed slice by slice using the ultrasonic aspirator from the most superficial to deep. The position of the laser beam and the surgical excision is monitored through the operating microscope. The Kelly–Goerss system allows complete excision of tumour defined by the CT enhancing edge.

We have now performed a number of stereotactic craniotomies for subcortical gliomas situated in eloquent areas of the brain with minimal morbidity. Postoperative CT scans show that complete excision has been achieved (Fig. 10.9(a) and (b)). At present it is too early to assess the effects of this technique on the survival of patients harbouring malignant glioma. Kelly *et al.* have published their results using this method and have found that the long-term survival figures are no better than those treated by more conventional surgical methods.[43] It is now possible, however, to remove tumours from previously inaccessible areas of the brain using this technology, and offer such patients some prolongation of survival. Further hope of a "cure" for patients harbouring a malignant glioma must await developments in adjuvant therapy.

Conclusions

Modern technology has not altered the principles of surgery for malignant glioma. Advances in neuroradiology have, however, allowed the application of stereotactic techniques and have facilitated biopsy and surgical resection of deep-seated tumours. Integration of the operating microscope, which offers magnification and illumination, together with the increased precision of tools such as the laser and ultrasonic aspirator will ensure the increasing importance of stereotactic microsurgery in the management of malignant glioma.

References

1. Davis CH, Bradford R. A surgical history of Maida Vale Hospital. In: Walker MD, Thomas DGT, eds. *Biology of Brain Tumours*. Boston: Martinus Nijhoff, 1986: 245–9.
2. Garfield J. Surgery of cerebral gliomas. In: *Brain Tumours: Thomas DGT, Graham DI, eds. Scientific Basis, Clinical Investigation and Current Therapy*. London: Butterworths, 1980: 301–21.
3. Shapiro WR. Treatment of neuroectodermal brain tumours. *Annals of Neurology*. 1982; **12**, 231–7.
4. Hitchcock E, Sato F. Treatment of malignant gliomata. *Journal of Neurosurgery*. 1964; **21**, 497–505.
5. Marshall LF, Jennett B, Langfitt TW. Needle biopsy for the diagnosis of malignant glioma. *Journal of the American Medical Association*. 1974; **228**, 1417–8.
6. Shetter AG, Bertuccini TV, Pittman HW. Closed needle biopsy in the diagnosis of intracranial mass lesions. *Surgical Neurology*. 1977; **8**, 341–5.
7. Lunsford LD, Martinez J, Latchaw RE. Stereotaxic surgery with a magnetic resonance- and computerized tomography-compatible system. *Journal of Neurosurgery*. 1986; **64**, 872–8.
8. Koslow M, Abele MG, Griffith RC, *et al*. Stereotactic surgical system controlled by computed tomography. *Neurosurgery*. 1981; **8**, 72–82.

9. Perry JH, Rosenbaum AE, Lunsford LD, et al. Computed tomography/guided stereotactic surgery: conception and development of a new stereotactic methodology. Neurosurgery. 1980; **7**, 376-81.
10. Mundinger F, Birg W, Klar M. Computer-assisted stereotactic brain operations by means including computerized axial tomography. Applied Neurophysiology. 1978; **41**, 169-82.
11. Penn RD, Whisler WW, Smith CA, et al. Stereotactic surgery with image processing of computerized tomographic scans. Neurosurgery. 1978; **3**, 157-63.
12. Brown RA. A stereotactic head frame for use with CT body scanners. Investigative Radiology. 1979; **14**, 300-4.
13. Brown RA. A computerized tomography–computer graphics approach to stereotaxic localization. Journal of Neurosurgery. 1979; **50**, 715-20.
14. Roberts TS, Brown R. Technical and clinical aspects of CT-directed stereotaxis. Applied Neurophysiology. 1980; **43**, 170-1.
15. Brown RA, Roberts TS, Osborn AG. Stereotaxic frame and computer software for CT-directed neurosurgical localization. Investigative Radiology. 1980; **15**, 308-12.
16. Gildenberg PL. Functional neurosurgery. In: Schmidek HH, Sweet WH, eds. Operative Neurosurgical Techniques: Indications, Methods and Results. Vol. 2. New York: Grune and Stratton, 1982; 993-1043.
17. Thomas DGT, Anderson RE, du Boulay GH. CT-guided stereotactic neurosurgery: experience in 24 cases with a new stereotactic system. Journal of Neurology, Neurosurgery and Psychiatry. 1984; **47**, 9-16.
18. Heilbrun MP. Computed tomography-guided stereotactic systems. Clinical Neurosurgery. 1984; **31**, 564-81.
19. Thomas DGT, Powell MP, Bradford R, et al. Correlation of CT-directed target site with histology and cell culture in cerebral glioma. Applied Neurophysiology. 1985; **48**, 460-2.
20. Thomas DGT, Darling JL, Watkins BA, et al. A simple method for the growth of cell cultures from small biopsies of brain tumours taken during CT-directed stereotactic procedures. Acta Neurochirugica. 1984; 33 suppl, 243-5.
21. Hawkes RC, Holland GN, Moore WS, et al. Nuclear magnetic resonance (NMR) tomography of the brain: A preliminary clinical assessment with demonstration of pathology. Journal of Computer Assisted Tomography. 1980; **4**, 577-86.
22. Wehrli FW, MacFall JR, Newton TH. Parameters determining the appearance of NMR images. In: Newton TH, Potts DG, eds. Advanced Imaging Techniques. Modern Neuroradiology. Vol. 2. San Anselmo: Clavadel Press, 81-117.
23. Young IR, Burl M, Clarke GJ, et al. Posterior fossa: Magnetic resonance properties. American Journal of Roentgenology. 1981; **137**, 895-901.
24. Doyle FH, Gore JC, Pennock JM, et al. Imaging of the brain by nuclear magnetic resonance. Lancet. 1981; **ii**, 53-7.
25. Bydder GM, Steiner RE, Young IR et al. Clinical NMR imaging of the brain: 140 cases, American Journal of Radiology. 1982; **139**, 215-36.
26. Leksell L, Leksell D, Schwebel J. Stereotaxis and nuclear magnetic resonance. Journal of Neurology, Neurosurgery and Psychiatry. 1985; **48**, 14-18.
27. Leksell L, Herner T, Leksell D, et al. Visualisation of stereotactic radiolesions by nuclear magnetic resonance. Journal of Neurology, Neurosurgery and Psychiatry. 1985; **48**, 19-20.
28. Thomas, DGT, Davis, CH, Ingram, S., et al. (1986). Stereotaxic biopsy of the brain under MR imaging control. American Journal of Neurology 161.
29. Thomas DGT, Bradford R, Bydder G. Magnetic resonance directed stereotactic brain biopsy. Journal of Neurology, Neurosurgery, and Psychiatry. 1987; **50**, 645.
30. Bradford R, Bydder GM, Thomas DGT. MRI-directed stereotactic biopsy of cerebral lesions. Acta Neurochirurgica. Suppl. 1987: **39**; 25-27.

31. Wyper DJ, Turner JW, Patterson J, *et al*. Accuracy of stereotaxic localisation using MRI and CT. *Journal of Neurology, Neurosurgery and Psychiatry*. 1986; **49**, 1445–8.
32. Lassman LP. Tumours of the pons and medulla oblongata. In: Vicken PJ, Bruyn GW, eds. *Tumours of the Brain and Skull, Part II. Handbook of Clinical Neurology*. Vol. 17. Amsterdam: North Holland, 1974; 693–706.
33. Lassiter KRL, Alexander E Jr, Davis CH Jr, *et al*. Surgical treatment of brain stem gliomas. *Journal of Neurosurgery*. 1971; **34**, 719–25.
34. O'Laoire SA, Crockard HA, Thomas DGT, *et al*. Brain stem haematoma: A report of six surgically treated cases. *Journal of Neurosurgery*. 1982; **56**, 222–7.
35. Pool JL. Gliomas in the region of the brain stem. *Journal of Neurosurgery*. 1968; **29**, 164–9.
36. Coffey RJ, Lunsford LD. Stereotactic surgery for mass lesions of the midbrain and pons. *Neurosurgery*. 1985; **17**, 12–18.
37. Hood TW, Gebarski, SS, McKeevar PE, *et al*. Stereotaxic biopsy of intrinsic lesions of brain stem. *Journal of Neurosurgery*. 1986: **65**: 172–6.
38. Bradford R, Davis CH, Thomas DGT. Stereotaxic biopsy of intrinsic brain stem lesions. *Journal of Neurology, Neurosurgery and Psychiatry*. 1987. **50**; 1097.
39. Littman P, Jarrett P, Bilanuik LT, *et al*. Pediatric brain stem gliomas. *Cancer*. 1980; **45**, 2787–92.
40. Levin VA, Edwards MS, Wara WM, *et al*. 5-Fluorouracil and 1-(2-chloroethyl)-3-cyclohexyl-1-nitrosourea (CCNU) followed by hydroxyurea, misonidazole and irradiation for brain stem gliomas: a pilot study of the Brain Tumour Research Center and the Children Cancer Group. *Neurosurgery*. 1984; **14**, 679–81.
41. Shalit MN, Israeli Y, Matz S, *et al*. Intraoperative computerized axial tomography. *Surgical Neurology*. 1979; **11**, 382–4.
42. Moser RP. Tumours, tools and technology: the role of the neurosurgeon. *Progress in Experimental Tumour Research*. 1985; **29**, 256–68.
43. Kelly PJ, Kall BA, Goerss S, *et al*. Computer-assisted stereotaxic laser resection of intra-axial brain neoplasms. *Journal of Neurosurgery*. 1986; **64**, 427–39.
44. Goerss S, Kelly PJ, Kall B, *et al*. A computed tomographic stereotactic adaptation system. *Neurosurgery*. 1982; **10**, 375–9.
45. Kall BA, Kelly PJ, Goerss SJ. Interactive stereotactic surgical system for the removal of intracranial tumours utilizing the CO_2 laser and CT-derived data base. EEE *Transactions on Biomedical Engineering*. 1985; **32**, 112–6.
46. Kelly PJ, Kall B, Goerss S. Transposition of volumetric information derived from computed tomography scanning into stereotactic space. *Surgical Neurology*. 1984; **21**, 465–71.

11 Brain and spinal cord tumours in children

Jeffrey S Tobias and Richard D Hayward

Introduction

Brain tumours represent just under one-fifth of all childhood malignancy, and tumours of the central nervous system (CNS) are numerically the most common solid tumours of childhood. Taken together, tumours are the commonest natural cause of death in children, being second only to trauma in children under 14 years of age. Overall, the five-year survival of children with brain tumours is approximately 40 per cent.

Very little is known of the aetiology of childhood brain tumours. Although many chromosomal abnormalities such as Down's and Klinefelter's syndromes are known to predispose to various childhood malignancies including leukaemia, Wilms' tumour and retinoblastoma, brain tumours have not been associated in this way. However, there is an increased incidence of childhood neural tumours in certain neurological–cutaneous disorders, including von Recklinghausen's syndrome and tuberous sclerosis (both autosomal dominant disorders), in which gliomas, generally of low grade, can be a feature. In addition, the von Hippel–Lindau syndrome is associated with an increased incidence of haemangioblastoma,[1] although this tumour is rare in children. Apart from these inherited chromosomal and congenital disorders, there is some evidence of a familial risk for childhood brain tumours. One study identified 38 families from more than 5000 patients in whom a cancer had been diagnosed in two or more children.[2] Siblings of children with brain tumours have an excess mortality from sarcomas and gliomas.

Although there are wide demographic differences in the incidence of children's cancers, the incidence of tumours of the CNS is generally constant and in both the United Kingdom and the United States accounts for about 20 per cent of the total. Like other childhood tumours, there is a peak age incidence of 2–8 years.

Pathological classification of childhood brain tumours

All of the adult brain tumours can occur in childhood, and the classification given in Chapter 5 accurately describes the childhood group. However, there are some important differences.

1. The frequency of the various tumours is quite different in children. In one large index series of brain tumours seen in a single centre within the United Kingdom over the past 20 years, the predominant tumours were medulloblastoma, low-grade glioma and ependymoma (Table 11.1). Medulloblastoma, the commonest of childhood brain tumours, is exceedingly unusual above the age of 25 years.
2. Cerebral metastases from solid primary tumours outside the CNS are extremely rare in children.
3. Most childhood CNS tumours are composed of cells which are of neuro-ectodermal origin. They range in their malignancy from the primitive neuro-ectodermal tumour (which includes medulloblastoma when the growth arises in the cerebellar vermis) to the highly differentiated (grade I) astrocytomas which may be difficult to distinguish histologically from a hamartoma. Despite the active myelination taking place in young children, oligodendrogliomas are relatively uncommon.[3]

Within the group of cerebral gliomas, the degree of differentiation differs

Table 11.1 Incidence of intracranial tumours at all ages and in children under 15 years of age[a]

Tumour	All ages (%)	Children (%)
Glioma	45	70
Astrocytoma	15	30
Glioblastoma	15	5
Oligodendroglioma	8	1
Medulloblastoma	4	20
Ependymoma	4	10
Meningioma	15	1
Neurinoma	6	<0.5
Pituitary adenoma	6	1
Metastases	5–20	<0.5
Craniopharyngioma	3	10
Choroid plexus papilloma	0.5	3
Pinealoma	1	2
Haemangioma	3	1
Epidermoid	2	0.5
Dermoids-teratoma	<0.5	3
Sarcoma	2	4
Optic glioma	1	4

[a]The figures are approximate and are based on reports collected from the literature (from ref. 5).

markedly between children and adults. In children, most gliomas are of low grade (Kernohan I and II) whereas in adults high grade lesions (Kernohan grades III and IV) are commoner. True glioblastoma multiforme is very rare in children. These differences have implications not only from the point of view of surgical resectability but also for prognosis.

4. There are also important differences in site. The anatomical areas most frequently involved in childhood CNS tumours lie within the posterior fossa, the frequency of medulloblastoma in childhood making an important difference in this respect. In addition, gliomas of the brain stem are much more common in children than in adults, in whom the overwhelming majority of gliomas arise within the cerebral hemispheres, a site rather more unusual in children.

5. Malignant CNS tumours in childhood have a tendencey to metastasize by seeding throughout the subarachnoid space. Whether this is because of any biological difference in these tumours due to the patients' ages, or whether the usually longer survival times following treatment of malignant childhood tumours allow a greater chance for metastases to become clinically manifest, remains unknown. In any event, it has now been recognized that myelography should be performed as part of the routine investigation of all children diagnosed as having malignant CNS tumours, because the presence of occult spinal metastases may necessitate a change in management, as well as affecting the ultimate prognosis. It is because of this tendency for subarachnoid seeding that whole neuraxis irradiation has now become such an important part of the treatment of these children.

6. The spectrum of tumours seen in the pituitary region is very different in childhood. Pituitary adenomas are most uncommon, and the commonest tumours are craniopharyngiomas, followed by gliomas of the optic chiasm (see below).

7. Against these pathological and anatomical differences should be set the differences that exist in the nature of the child's nervous system. During the first two years of life, and particularly during the first six months, the brain is involved in a continuing growth spurt. Its increase in size is due both to progressive myelination, and also to arborization of neuronal dendrites. This means that although the infant brain is more plastic in its response to surgical and accidental trauma, the effects of hypoxia, radiotherapy and chemotherapy on these vital developmental processes may produce long-term interference with intellectual, motor and hormonal functions.[4]

Table 11.2 Tumours of the posterior fossa (collected series, modified from ref. 27)

Tumour	Boston (%)	Vienna (%)	Tokyo (%)	Melbourne (%)	London (%)
Astrocytoma	32	33	35	36	24
Medulloblastoma	30	33	36	29	52
Ependymoma	8	8	9	18	10
Brain stem glioma	18	13	—	16	10
Total	418	350	225	260	119

Tumours of the posterior fossa

This site is dealt with first because these tumours together represent the largest single group in childhood.[5] The relative incidence is shown in Table 11.2; astrocytoma, medulloblastoma and brain stem glioma are the commonest tumours, though there appear to be genuine geographic variations. The age-related incidence for one large series is shown in Fig. 11.1.

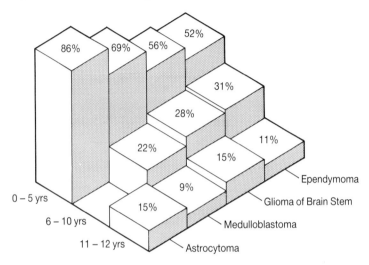

Fig. 11.1 Age-related incidence of childhood brain tumour. (Reprinted with permission from: Jones PG, Campbell PG, eds. *Tumours in Infancy in Childhood*, Oxford: Blackwell Scientific Publications, 1976.)

Clinical presentation

The symptoms and signs of a childhood posterior fossa tumours result from a combination of those due to local brain dysfunction coupled with those relating to the raised intracranial pressure resulting from the hydrocephalus that is so frequently present. Despite the size of these tumours when they are eventually diagnosed,[6] the child's illness has often been comparatively brief, presumably reflecting the ability of the young brain to adapt even when increasing pressures are placed upon it. As the tumours grow most commonly in the cerebellar vermis or cerebellar hemispheres, most children present with ataxia, particularly affecting their gait. Any disturbance of the brain stem can lead to diplopia while the presence of a bulbar palsy, dysarthria and facial weakness of lower motor neurone type suggest that the tumour may lie within the brain stem itself.

Enlargement of the tumour may be sufficient to compress the corticospinal tracts as they run through the brain stem, eventually producing a contralateral hemiparesis.

168 *Brain and spinal cord tumours in children*

Evidence for raised intracranial pressure include an enlarged head circumference (especially in young children), drowsiness, papilloedema and vomiting, the last being particularly prominent when the floor of the fourth ventricle is involved.

Investigations

A lumbar puncture has absolutely no place in the investigation of a child in whom a diagnosis of intracerebral tumour is being considered. It is unlikely to produce useful diagnostic information and in the presence of raised intracranial pressure it can be positively dangerous. Plain X-rays of the skull may reveal spreading or widening of the sutures or a copper-beaten appearance as signs of raised pressure, but most

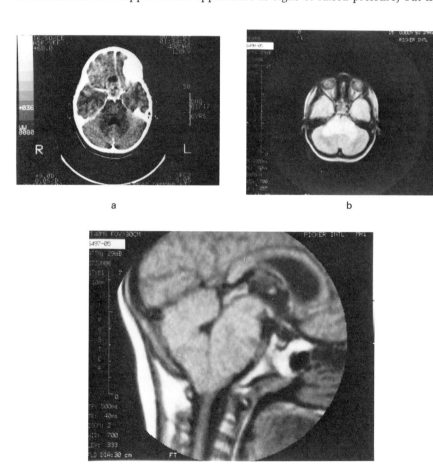

Fig. 11.2 (a) CT scan appearances in brain stem glioma, showing typical hypodense area but with few other features. (b) MRI Scanning shows the lesion with greater clarity. (c) Sagittal view from the same case, showing extensive swelling involving the whole of the brain stem.

children nowadays are diagnosed on the basis of computed tomographic (CT) scans. These not only demonstrate the size of the ventricles but in most cases give an excellent image of the size, site and extent of the tumour itself. Enhancement of the tumour is often usefully shown by intravenous injection of iodine-containing contrast material. Magnetic resonance imaging (MRI) is now becoming more available. It has a definite role in the detection of intrinsic brain stem glioma which may be poorly demonstrated by CT scanning, even with contrast (Fig. 11.2).

Surgical management

As in any other branch of surgery, the indications for an operation include the necessity of making a histological diagnosis, the relief of symptoms, and if possible the cure of the patient. Since the advent of stereotactic biopsy techniques, it is now becoming less common to leave tumours, even those lying within the brain stem, unbiopsied. All tumours within the cerebellar hemispheres and vermis should be surgically resected, with an attempt made to achieve complete surgical excision. The aim is to remove as much tumour bulk as possible and thus relieve local pressure on the brain. At the same time, if obstruction to the flow of CSF through the posterior fossa has resulted in hydrocephalus, then tumour removal will hopefully allow the intracranial pressure to return to normal levels without the need for the insertion of a shunt system. More details concerning the role of surgery are given in the sections below. Neurosurgeons vary in their treatment of the hydrocephalus, and some will always proceed to a shunt insertion before contemplating a direct procedure on the tumour itself. Our own policy is to treat the hydrocephalus first only in the minority of cases where the intracranial pressure is high enough to present an immediate danger to the child. In all other cases we hope that the removal of the bulk of the tumour will relieve the obstruction to the CSF flow; if this does not occur, then a shunt system can be inserted at a later date.

Astrocytoma

Many of these predominantly low-grade tumours are completely resectable and have a good prognosis following complete surgical removal without additional treatment. This is particularly likely in the relatively common juvenile fibrillary astrocytomas which lack the nuclear variability more common in the adult type of tumour.

As a group, the cerebellar astrocytomas have a relatively good prognosis, and the majority of these children are alive and well, presumably cured, between 10 and 20 years after surgical treatment.[5,7] In children in whom resection is not complete, usually because of tumour extension into the brain stem or where a local recurrence is either inoperable or cannot be totally removed, external-beam treatment is undoubtedly the treatment of choice, using laterally placed wedged or open fields to a total tumour dose of 45–50 Gy (4500–5000 rad) given over 4.5 to 5.5 weeks. However, following an incomplete removal of the very slow growing grade I astrocytoma, many clinicians prefer to adopt a policy of careful follow-up using frequent CT scanning, particularly if the child is under the age of two years and therefore most vulnerable to the harmful effects of radiotherapy.

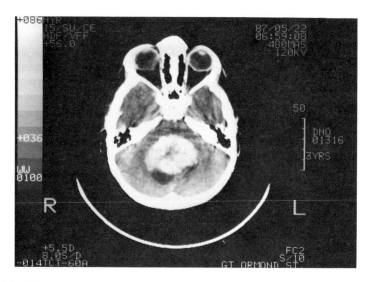

Fig. 11.3 CT scan appearance of modulloblastoma showing typical enhancing midline lesion. This was completely resectable at surgery.

Medulloblastoma (Fig. 11.3)

Although reportedly less common throughout the world than the cerebellar astrocytoma, medulloblastoma is the commonest childhood brain tumour in the United Kingdom.[5] Treatment by surgery alone is almost always unsuccessful, and radical postoperative radiotherapy is essential even where a naked-eye "complete" surgical removal has been achieved. During the past 25 years, medulloblastoma has been shown to be amongst the most radiosensitive of tumours, and routine postsurgical irradiation has improved the cure at experienced referral centres to over 40 per cent.[8]

It is generally accepted that dissemination of tumour by direct spread within the cerebrospinal fluid is particularly common in medulloblastoma and may even be recognized at operation, with tumour visible as nodules or sheets of malignant cells over the surface of the cerebellum. Spinal seeding, with metastases within the spinal theca is common (Fig. 11.4), though often clinically undetectable unless routine myelography is performed in all cases. Spinal deposits are clearly more common than previously thought[9] and our routine investigations now include postoperative myelography in every patient.

Radiotherapy technique (Fig. 11.5) The whole craniospinal axis should be irradiated as soon after surgery as possible. Treatment planning must be meticulous, taking care to treat areas such as the base of the brain, retro-orbital area, and brain stem, which might easily be missed. These sites can be undertreated if adult surface anatomical boundaries are used without regard to the anatomy of the developing brain. A variety of techniques are in use, and at University College Hospital we have adopted the following guidelines.

Tumours of the posterior fossa 171

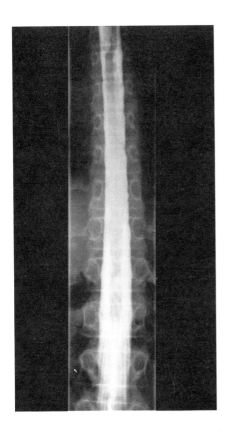

Fig. 11.4 Myelographic findings in a child with spinal seedlings from medulloblastoma. The child was treated using boost irradiation to these areas and is alive and well two years later.

1. Irradiation of the whole brain, using large lateral opposed fields, including the mid-brain and upper cervical vertebrae as far as the lower limit of C2, to a midline dose of 30 Gy (3000 rad) in 3 weeks;
2. Boosting of the posterior fossa and mid-brain as far anteriorly as the anterior clinoid process, to 40 Gy (4000 rad), treating at the same rate;
3. At the same time that the posterior fossa boost is commenced, spinal irradiation is started, using a direct posterior field to treat the whole spine from the lower border of the cerebral fields to the termination of the subarachnoid space (usually at about the level of S2) so that the entire spinal cord and the cauda equina are treated. Radiotherapy details are outside the scope of this chapter but in general, a single field is used wherever possible, to avoid potentially dangerous areas of under- or overtreatment. In taller children this is not always possible and in these cases, the junctional level is varied throughout treatment to minimize these risks. A dose of at least 30 Gy min (3000 rad) is given (as an applied dose) to the chosen length of the spine over 5 weeks;
4. For the final part of treatment, a posterior fossa boost is given, taking the initial site of the tumour and its immediate surrounding area to a final dose of 50–55 Gy (5000–5500 rad) in 7–8 weeks; with a mid-brain dose of 45 Gy (4500 rad) in 5–6 weeks, a dose to the cerebral hemispheres and anterior part of brain of 35 Gy

172 *Brain and spinal cord tumours in children*

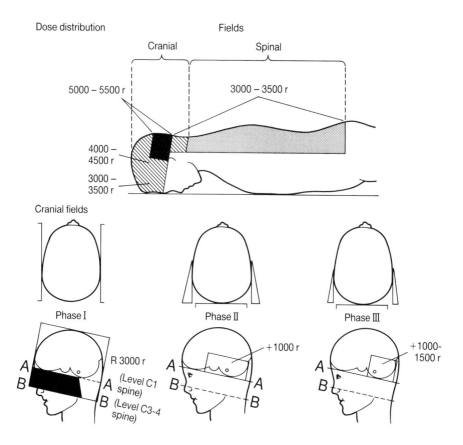

Fig. 11.5 Technique for whole craniospinal irradiation, as described by Bloom HJG (Reprinted with permission from: Voute PA, Banett A, Bloom HJG, Lemerle J, Neidhardt MK, eds.) *Cancer in Children – Clinical Management.* Berlin: Springer Verlag, 1986.

(3500 rad) in 4 weeks, and a final spinal dose of 30 Gy (3000 rad) minimum, given over 5 weeks. The whole treatment usually takes 8 weeks to complete;

5. If spinal seedlings have been identified by myelography (with or without clinical signs), we attempt additional treatment to the site of the metastases, though this may be difficult where there is extensive disease, since neutropenia from suppression of the vertebral bone marrow may develop during spinal irradiation even without boosting. Nonetheless it is generally possible to give a boost to a limited area, of an additional 10 Gy (1000 rad), at a rate of 1.8–2.0 Gy daily, given if possible during the early part of treatment, and before the start of the irradiation of the whole spine, so as to complete the entire treatment within the 8-week period.

Despite the demands of this vigorous postoperative whole CNS treatment, most children withstand the radiotherapy without overwhelming difficulty or undue delay because of toxicity. Nausea is not uncommon but can usually be managed conservatively; many children require a modest dose of dexamethasome (2–8 mg daily, in divided doses, by mouth) or an antiemetic such as prochlorperazine or metoclopramide. Although the total leucocyte count may fall during the period of spinal irradiation, it is not generally necessary to discontinue treatment because the fall is chiefly due to lymphopenia rather than neutropenia. We do not usually interrupt what could be curative treatment unless the total white blood cell count falls below $2 \times 10^9/1$. It is sometimes possible to give at least part of the treatment as an outpatient, though many children are unwell during the immediate postoperative and early radiation period.

Irradiation complications have become an increasingly important consideration in this group of children, since many will survive into adult life without recurrence of the tumour. These unavoidable effects result from direct radiation damage either to the hypothalamic–pituitary axis, to other parts of the brain, to the growing spine, or to organs also affected by the spinal irradiation – most notably the thyroid gland and ovaries which may lie within the scattered beam.

The most important and common problem is growth failure, due either to a direct effect on vertebral growth, a reduction of growth hormone secretion, or a combination of both.[10] In our own series from Great Ormond Street/University College Hospitals and the Royal Marsden Hospital, which comprises a follow-up group of 122 children treated between 6 months and 15 years previously, clinical evidence of growth delay was seen in well over 75 per cent of all surviving children.[11] It was particularly noted in the modulloblastoma group, who had all undergone spinal irradiation. With free availability of synthetically produced growth hormone, it has now become essential that all children with brain tumours treated with radiotherapy should be closely followed in a growth clinic, so that early growth failure can be readily detected, and corrected as far as possible.

Hypothyroidism has also been reported,[7, 12] and is presumably due to the exit dose from the posterior spinal field acting on the thyroid gland itself, since most children have elevated TSH levels. This biochemical abnormality, the most common evidence of direct thyroid radiation damage, is much more frequently encountered than clinical hypothyroidism.

Primary ovarian failure is less commonly a problem, and almost always results from direct irradiation damage to the developing ovary from the spinal field. FSH levels are usually elevated, so the pituitary gonadotrophin-releasing cells are apparently little affected by the high radiation dose they invariably receive.

Intellectual impairment has been reported but evidence for its development is controversial. Over three-quarters of surviving children with medulloblastoma lead independent and active lives, and at least one study has shown that intellectual achievement in these children is not reduced below normal.[13] However, in another study where children who had been irradiated for medulloblastoma were compared with a group of children who had been treated surgically (but without irradiation) for cerebellar astrocytoma, a significant reduction in intellectual ability was noted in the irradiated group.[14]

Carcinogenesis is also important, though fortunately uncommon. The latent period is usually over 10 years, and thyroid and skin cancers (often multiple) are probably the commonest.

In the context of a high probability of cure,[15] there seems no doubt that the possible hazards of treatment have to be accepted. One of the dilemmas of current research in the management of medulloblastoma is the difficulty of designing new clinical trials which are likely to increase the cure rate still further, without causing an inevitable increase in the long-term toxicity of treatment.

Chemotherapy in medulloblastoma Despite the undoubted radiosensitivity of this tumour, both local recurrence and dissemination of disease (chiefly via the cerebrospinal fluid) remain relatively common, and in such cases the prognosis becomes very poor indeed. It has been clear for many years that a variety of cytotoxic agents have activity in this condition,[5] including vinca alkaloids such as vincristine, nitrosoureas including BCNU, CCNU, and antimetabolites such as methotrexate and others. Cis-platinum, more recently introduced, clearly has activity,[16] though its side-effects of severe nausea, vomiting, renal dysfunction and ototoxicity make it a more difficult agent to use, particularly in the very young.

Responses are usually short-lived, and combination chemotherapy, which is generally preferred to treatment with single agents, may be difficult to deliver in full dosage if relapse follows soon after completion of the craniospinal irradiation because of the large area of bone marrow which has been irradiated. Methotrexate, one of the more active agents, may be hazardous if given within 6 months of radiotherapy as it can cause a severe leucoencephalopathy.

Because of the partial effectiveness of such chemotherapy, an international collaborative study was set up by the International Society of Paediatric Oncology (SIOP), which attempted to investigate the effect of combination chemotherapy as an adjuvant to surgery and radiotherapy given to the whole CNS as described above. Half of the children were randomized to receive chemotherapy which included vincristine (1 mg/m^2 weekly until the end of the radiotherapy, then at less frequent intervals for one year) together with CCNU (100 mg/m^2 starting after the end of the radiotherapy and given every six weeks for one year). The chemotherapy group did marginally better, with a trend towards an improved overall survival but without any statistically significant advantage in the group taken as a whole.[5, 17] There was however a subgroup of patients who did significantly better with the addition of chemotherapy. This included children of less than two years of age (57 per cent actuarial five-year survival *vs.* 31 per cent with radiotherapy alone) and also children who had undergone partial rather than total surgical excision or in whom there was brain stem involvement. In children with all these risk factors, the survival was very significantly improved (53 *vs.* 25 per cent). Although these highly suggestive results warrant independant confirmation, it would be difficult to mount such a large study again, and the current SIOP study for medulloblastoma includes more intensive chemotherapy with additional agents. It is worth pointing out that long-term treatment-related damage, for example to the thyroid gland, appears to be more in children who have undergone chemotherapy as well as irradiation.[12]

Medulloblastoma may, on occasion, metastasize more widely than within the CNS, most notably to bone (Fig. 11.6). In such circumstances, palliative treatment with radiotherapy and/or chemotherapy is often of value, though the overall outlook is very poor. Occasionally, a very late ($>$ 5 years) recurrence may occur, either at the primary site within the posterior fossa, or elsewhere within the CNS, and the clinician must then exercise great judgement in deciding whether or not to re-treat with radiotherapy, and to what dose. Radiation tolerance of the brain is further discussed in Chapter 12.

Tumours of the posterior fossa 175

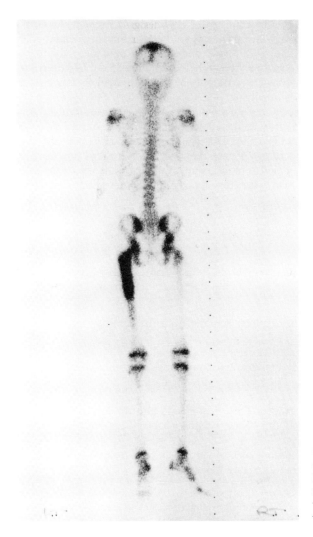

Fig. 11.6 Isotope bone scan in a child with medulloblastoma who developed bone metastases three years after initial treatment.

Ependymoma of the fourth ventricle

These less common tumours share some important characteristics with medulloblastomas, particularly the tendency to seed into other parts of the CNS via the subarachnoid space, a feature which is much commoner in posterior fossa (infratentorial) ependymoma than in ependymomas at other sites. In addition, ependymoma is relatively radiosensitive so that once again, full craniospinal irradiation is an essential part of treatment. Although some ependymomas may appear to be histologically of low grade, this is no guarantee of a "benign" behaviour, and most radiotherapists would now agree that an infratentorial ependymoma of any grade should be treated in this way. Treatment details are as described above, and identical dose and fractionation schedules are generally used.

Much less is known of the chemosensitivity of ependymoma, though there have been recent encouraging reports.[16] No large-scale studies of adjuvant chemotherapy have been reported though the SIOP have undertaken a similar study to the medulloblastoma trial described above.[18] Nonetheless it is clear that in children with recurrent disease, useful responses are sometimes observed, though these are rarely complete and further relapse is inevitable.

The prognosis for infratentorial ependymoma has clearly improved with routine craniospinal irradiation. The dose delivered is critical and the overall five-year survival is approximately 50 per cent.[5] At 10 years, the survival rate (from the same series) for infratentorial tumours was 43 per cent; for supratentorial tumours, the survival rate was 26 per cent. Prior to radiotherapy, overall results were very poor, though it has been known for many years that ependymoma, even when arising from the more adverse infratentorial site, can sometimes run a slow course over many years.

Brain stem glioma

Despite recent technical advances, the brain stem remains a relatively inaccessible surgical site, and radiotherapy is therefore the mainstay of treatment. These tumours may be classified as follows.

1. Extensions of cerebellar hemisphere tumours into the brain stem, which are usually of low grade.
2. Diffuse gliomas of the pons. These are the commonest brain stem tumours of childhood. They are usually malignant although on CT scanning they appear to be either of low attenuation or isodense with surrounding brain tissue, despite contrast enhancement (Fig. 11.2).
3. Rarely, focal low-grade tumours. They may extend into the fourth ventricle or cerebellopontine angle, and thus cause hydrocephalus. They may also have a prominent cystic component.
4. Occasionally a brain-stem tumour seems to represent the upward extension of an intrinsic tumour of the spinal cord (see below).

Many of these children are extremely unwell when first seen, with multiple cranial nerve palsies, usually affecting the lower cranial nerves, so that a bulbar palsy, often resulting in recurrent aspiration of food, is particularly common and distressing. Compression of the corticospinal tracts running through the brain stem may produce a hemiplegia. Hydrocephalus usually occurs only when the tumour has expanded into the CSF pathways – either into the fourth ventricle or cerebellopontine angle (Fig. 11.7). Because of the malignant nature of many of these tumours and their location in such an eloquent area of the CNS, surgery has proved generally disappointing[19] except in cases where low-grade tumours extend upwards from the spinal cord or where there is a prominent cystic or exophytic component. Apart from these instances, surgery is reserved for the treatment of hydrocephalus and for biopsy (using stereotactic techniques) when histological confirmation is required prior to radiothererapy.

Despite these unpromising features, brain stem gliomas can be rewarding to treat since some tumours may display a surprising degree of radiosensitivity, and cure is by no means unknown. In one series, 23 per cent of cases survived for more than 5

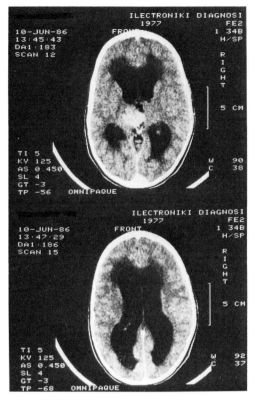

Fig. 11.7 Gross hydrocephalus from ventricular outflow obstruction from a brain stem glioma. Following treatment, this child is alive and well at 15 months.

years.[20] Routine use of MRI imaging has provided much more information on the anatomy and local invasiveness of these tumours, at a site where CT scanning is often disappointingly uninformative.[21] Biopsy and autopsy material confirm that these lesions can be a mixture of low-, intermediate, and high-grade gliomas, and as pointed out by Bloom,[5] they should not be grouped together with tumours of the mid-brain, fourth ventricle or hypothalamus since the true brain stem glioma carries a very different prognosis.

Treatment consists of local irradiation, usually with small lateral fields to encompass the tumour with a generous margin. CT and, if possible, MRI scanning are essential for adequate determination of the tumour volume; MRI scanning in the sagittal plane is invaluable and may demonstrate inferior extension into the medulla or cervical cord which would otherwise go undetected. Whole craniospinal irradiation is not recommended since dissemination is extremely unusual. Doses of 50 Gy tumour midline dose over 5 weeks (daily fractionation) to 55 Gy over 7 weeks have generally been used, and it seems clear that doses below 40 Gy are inadequate.[22] In children with tumours that enhanced on CT scanning and who have had a good clinical response, the average survival is over five years. Long-term cures have been reported[5] and may even occur in patients who presented with extreme hydrocephalus (Fig. 11.7). However, a satisfactory initial response to radiotherapy in patients with malignant pontine gliomas, though not unusual, does not necessarily indicate a favourable outcome, and most children die rapidly, often within six months from diagnosis. The use of adjuvant chemotherapy has so far proved disappointing.[23]

Tumours of the pituitary region

This is a very heterogeneous group, comprising four main sites. These are:

1. pituitary stalk
2. optic chiasm
3. hypothalamus
4. pituitary gland (not discussed in this chapter).

Craniopharyngioma

This is the commonest developmental brain tumour in children, accounting for 5 to 10 per cent of all reported childhood tumours. It is thought to arise from remnants of Rathke's pouch, itself a diverticulum of the primitive stomodaeum, and can contain both cystic and solid areas. Heavy calcification of the solid portion is usually present, presumably a reflection of the slow growth of the tumour, often over many years. It is this hardness of the solid part of the tumour together with its tendency to adhere to adjacent structures such as the optic chiasm, hypothalamus and internal carotid arteries that may make surgical excision extremely difficult.

These tumours often present with growth failure or other endocrinopathies. High-resolution CT scanning has been invaluable in demonstrating small tumours which would otherwise have been undetectable.

Surgical resection has in the past carried a high mortality (up to 40 per cent[5]) yet local recurrence was common after surgery alone, and long-term survival figures ranged from 20 to 50 per cent. Although using modern surgical and anaesthetic techniques, complete removal is the ideal form of treatment for these tumours, neurosurgeons vary in their assessment of the proportion of cases in which this can safely be achieved.[24, 25] However there now appears to be a general consensus that postoperative radiotherapy will either prevent or at least retard the growth of any residual tumour fragments, whether they be cystic or solid. Adequate local excision (complete wherever possible) with postoperative irradiation for those with incomplete removal has become established as the most successful form of treatment for these children. This has led to a much reduced postoperative mortality since the surgeon no longer has to strive for a radical local excision. Although the tumour is clearly radiosensitive, high doses are required, of the order of 50 Gy over 6 weeks (daily fractionation), normally delivered using a three-field technique similar to that used for adult pituitary tumours. As with brain stem tumours, it is clear that lower doses lead to inferior survival,[26] though lower doses may of course be a reflection of a worse overall clinical state leading to early discontinuation of therapy. A five-year survival rate of approximately 80 per cent has regularly been documented in several series of patients treated by surgical excision and routine postoperative irradiation,[5, 26] though late recurrences probably reduce the true long-term survival rate to 75 per cent. Although some radiotherapists advocate the use of intracystic radiocolloid, there is no evidence that this approach is superior to external-beam irradiation. Accumulation of cyst fluid is however a common clinical problem, often requiring repeated aspiration during therapy. In our experience, however, external-beam irradiation is often effective in achieving long-term control of this complication.

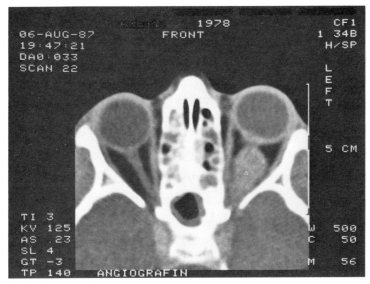

a

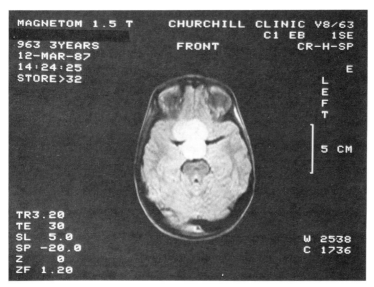

b

Fig. 11.8 (a) Large optic nerve glioma confined to the left optic nerve involvement of the chiasm. (b) Optic nerve glioma arising from the chiasm itself.

Optic nerve and chiasmal tumours

These tumours tend to occur in early childhood, and account for about a third of all anterior third ventricular tumours, an area in which occur approximately 5 per cent of all intracranial childhood tumours. There is no doubt that children with von Recklinghausen's disease are at high risk from this condition. In one series, almost half of all children with optic nerve glioma showed some of the features of the syndrome.[27] The tumour may arise in the chiasm or anywhere along the optic nerve (Fig. 11.8), and usually presents with visual impairment and proptosis if the orbital component is large, together with hydrocephalus when a chiasmatic tumour is large enough to obstruct the third ventricle.

The typical CT scan appearance[28] shows a suprasellar hyperdense mass often with extensions anteriorly along the optic nerves and posteriorly along the optic tracts. There may even be a suggestion of intracranial metastases (Fig. 11.9). Occasionally

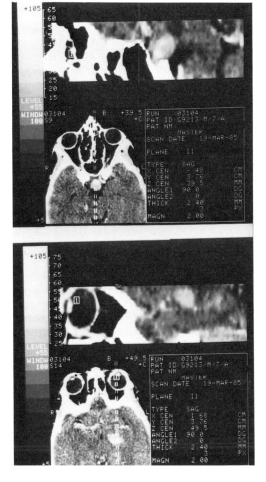

Fig. 11.9 Optic nerve glioma extending posteriorly along optic radiation. This appearance is sometimes mistaken for intracerebral metastasis.

the CT scan abnormality is much more subtle even though the visual fields can be grossly restricted. The tumour may be bilateral, involving the chiasm and both optic nerves, with risk of total blindness from compression of optic nerve fibres or their vascular supply. Opinions vary markedly as to the malignant potential of the tumours. Jones and Campbell, for example, claim that up to 25 per cent may undergo spontaneous arrest of growth,[27] with many of their cases showing histological appearances of only a very low grade of activity. Others have suggested that these tumours, particularly those confined to a single optic nerve, are in fact congenital, self-limiting lesions similar to hamartomas.[29] Nonetheless there is no doubt that the chiasmatic tumours can indeed extend well beyond their primary site, and infiltrate the base of the brain or other vital structures. Unfortunately, involvement at a single site such as a single optic nerve is less common than bilateral or chiasmal involvement. Where biopsy material is available, the most common appearance is of a low-grade glioma, generally a pilocytic astrocytoma. The slow clinical evolution is consistent with that of low-grade gliomas at other sites both in chilhood and adult life.

An interesting feature of the optic chiasm glioma is the frequency of endocrine abnormalities, particulary precocious puberty, which in one series occured in over a fifth of all cases,[30] and may be manifest as increased libido even in the absence of clinical or biochemical features. Although the cause of this abnormality is not entirely clear, it is assumed to result from hypothalamic involvement by tumour, with stimulation of gonadotrophins.

Although some surgeons will try to reduce the bulk of a large chiasmatic tumour, complete excision is impossible, and, in most cases, surgery is limited either to biopsy (preferably stereotactic) or excision of a single optic nerve when an obviously enlarging tumour seems entirely confined to that site and it seems justifiable to sacrifice residual vision in one eye before the chiasm is invaded and while a long-term cure is still possible. In most cases, radiotherapy is the mainstay of treatment, and several series now confirm that this approach confers an excellent prognosis, often with both visual improvement and reduction in proptosis.[31] Radiotherapy should be given at a moderately high dose; we normally employ a total dose of 50 Gy over 5 weeks using daily fractionation, generally delivered by parallel opposed radiation fields.

Our own view would be, that despite the low-grade nature of the tumour, treatment is essential since the disease carries an overall mortality of approximately 25 per cent,[30] not to mention the problems of advancing blindness, and with an even worse prognosis in children with chiasmal involvement. Long-term follow-up is important since associated endocrinopathies may need careful assessment and management, particularly in older children who seem to be most at risk from precocious puberty. Because some children may present with a progressive deterioration at under two years of age, there has been increasing interest in the use of chemotherapy as the primary method of treatment.[32]

Tumours of the hypothalamus

These are more uncommon than tumours seen at other sites within or adjacent to the anterior part of the third ventricle. They usually present with raised intracranial pressure as a result of obstruction to ventricular outflow, coupled with the behavioural and endocrine problems that might be expected from involvement of this sensitive area of the brain. The differential diagnosis is usually from a chiasmatic glioma or, occasionally, a craniopharyngioma. Because of the deep-seated nature of these tumours, biopsy is not usually attempted although with the advent of stereotactic techniques, this may well change in the future. Of histologically proven cases, the commonest diagnosis is a low-grade glioma. Apart from the question of whether or not to biopsy, the only surgical consideration is to decide whether a shunt insertion might be useful, in order to reduce the intracranial pressure by relieving the hydrocephalus. Treatment with radiotherapy produces disappointing results, with only 20 per cent of children surviving five years, at best.

Tumours of the pineal region

These unusual tumours are best considered together with the paediatric brain tumours since they are less commonly encountered in adults. There is an important pathological distinction to be drawn between, on the one hand, the pineal germ cell tumours (both pure germinoma and the less common teratoma), and on the other, the group of non-germ-cell pineal tumours. The latter group includes both the primitive neuroectodermal pinealoblastoma and the more mature pineocytoma. Tumours of the glial series, both benign and malignant, may also occur in this area.

Tumours of the pineal region, like any intracerebral tumours, may present with a constellation of focal neurological symptoms and signs, with or without evidence of raised intracranial pressure. Compression downwards upon the upper part of the brain stem (midbrain) causes a distinctive ocular abnormality with restriction of upward gaze, pupillary abnormalities and often a divergent squint (Parinaud's syndrome).[33] Raised intracranial pressure, with headache, vomiting and papilloedema is usually due to hydrocephalus.

Excision of pineal region tumours using a supercerebellar approach is now performed by many neurosurgeons, but because the commonest tumour is a germinoma which is best treated by radiotherapy (with or without chemotherapy), it is obviously important to establish the pathological diagnosis, if possible, before embarking upon such a major procedure. The diagnosis can often be made in the following ways.

1. By the CT and MRI appearances.
2. By the presence in blood or CSF (usually obtained during a shunt procedure) of the specific tumour markers α-fetoprotein (AFP) and/or human chorionic gonadotrophin (HCG). These may be raised in teratomatous germinomas but never in non-germ cell tumours of the pineal. AFP, produced by yolk-sac elements, always indicates a teratoma though hCG may be modestly raised even in cases of "pure" (i.e. non-teratomatous) germinoma.
3. Surgically, by obtaining a stereotactic biopsy.
4. By assessing the tumour response to a modest dose of local irradiation (see below).

Whichever type of treatment is selected, it may still be necessary to insert a ventriculoperitoneal shunt in order to relieve hydrocephalus, especially if the intracranial pressure is sufficiently high to produce impairment of consciousness.

Both main varieties of germ cell tumour are generally regarded as radiosensitive, though, as with adult germ cell tumours, it is the pure germinoma (seminoma) which is more reliably responsive. There is no doubt that both of these tumours have a propensity for subarachnoid and ventricular seeding, and in one series of pineal and suprasellar germinoma distant spread was present in almost 40 per cent of cases.[34] For this reason, all patients with this diagnosis should have a post-operative myelogram followed by whole CNS irradiation. This has now become our standard practice. We use a radiotherapy technique with boosting to the primary site, generally to a final dose of 45–55 Gy. Where the primary tumour has been shown to be a teratoma, either on histological grounds or because of high levels of AFP or hCG in the blood or CSF, the dose to the primary site should if possible be raised to not less than 55 Gy (over 5.5–6 weeks with daily fractionation), because of the lower radiosensitivity of this tumour compared with the true (pure) germinoma. An alternative approach is to use chemotherapy as primary treatment (see below).

For pinealoblastoma, a primitive neuroectodermal tumour (dealt with more fully on p. 188) with a similarly high rate of seeding within the CSF, the radiotherapeutic technique is identical, once again aiming to treat the whole CNS and raise the final dose to the primary site to not less than 50 Gy. If the tumour has been histologically verified as the more benign pineocytoma, then local irradiation, without whole CNS treatment, is sufficient. In unbiopsied cases, or where AFP and hCG are undetectable in the blood, the most useful means of attempting a diagnostic distinction between the radiosensitive group of tumours and the rest may be to give a short two-week course of local irradiation to the primary site, and repeat the CT scan. The sensitive tumours will often show unequivocal volume reduction even at this early stage. Since this then implies that the tumour is likely to be a germinoma or pineloblastoma with a high risk of spinal seeding, treatment should then be extended to include the whole CNS (see above). In non-responsive cases, local treatment should be continued to the full dose (50–55 Gy over 5–6.5 weeks) to the primary site alone, but in these circumstances it may be best to proceed to a formal operative removal before considering further irradiation. In the same way, tumours whose preliminary biopsy has shown them to be unlikely to respond to radiotherapy (low-grade astrocytomas, well-differentiated teratomas, dermoid cysts etc.) should be treated in the first instance by an attempt at surgical excision.

As with germ cell tumours arising at other sites, primary intracranial germ cell tumours are undoubtedly chemosensitive,[16, 35] often to a remarkable degree (Fig. 11.10). Chemotherapy has assumed an increasing role in the management of these tumours (see below) and is clearly indicated in children with recurrences after primary treatment. Long-term survival is still possible, even where the tumour has metastasized.

It may also be appropriate to use chemotherapy as primary treatment in pineal germ cell tumours,[35] though no large series has yet been reported. The advantages of such an approach are considerable. First, it is clear that successful treatment with chemotherapy may be associated with less profound late damage, particularly growth failure (see p. 173). Secondly, tumours in the teratomatuous group are generally felt to be less radiosensitive than the pure germinomas so that irradiation of these tumours as definitive primary therapy is less certain to produce a cure. Thirdly, whole CNS irradiation in children who later require chemotherapy because of recurrence of the tumour clearly makes such treatment more hazardous because of reduced marrow reserve. At present our own policy in a child with a large pineal teratoma (either biopsy-proven or diagnosed by serum marker analysis) would be to

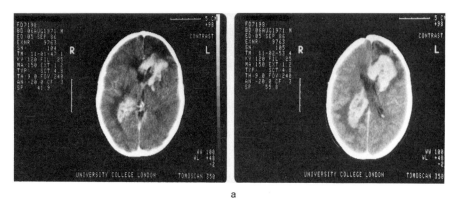

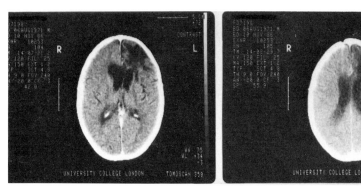

Fig. 11.10 (a) Large primary intracranial germinoma recurrent after craniotomy, showing extensive intracerebral involvement. (b) Dramatic response after two courses of chemotherapy with BEP (see text). Both films with intravenous contrast.

employ chemotherapy in the first instance and to follow progress with serial CT scanning and repeat marker estimation. We normally use a combination of bleomycin, etoposide and cisplatin (BEP), using an in-dwelling Hickman line to obviate multiple venepunctures. The combination is well tolerated and highly effective at producing remission, though most of the evidence has accumulated through treatment of metastatic teratoma outside the CNS.[36] Our experience (for example see Fig. 11.10) clearly suggests that these drugs, given intravenously, enter the CNS and can produce remarkable tumour reduction. It is certainly possible in these cases to follow the chemotherapy with whole-CNS irradiation though it is not yet clear in cases where the CT or MRI scan is completely normal following chemotherapy whether such treatment is necesarry.

Cerebral hemisphere tumours

These tumours are less common than tumours of the posterior fossa, and account for less than a quarter of all childhood intracranial tumours. They occur at all periods

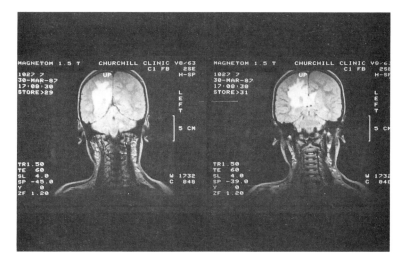

a

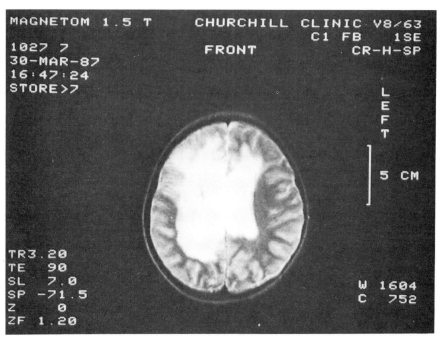

b

Fig. 11.11 (a) Large low-grade cerebral hemisphere tumour (coronal view, MRI scan). (b) Extensive and bilateral intracerebral involvement in the same case.

throughout childhood, with a slight male preponderance. The commonest sites are the parietal and frontal lobes; the temporal and occipital lobes are affected much less commonly. They can present as tumours of unusually large size (Fig. 11.11) and occasionally, multiple tumours are encountered (Fig. 11.12). Pathologically, astrocytomas are most common, usually of moderate or low-grade, malignant varieties tending to merge with the primitive neuroectodermal tumours (see below). Glioblastoma multiforme is much less common than in adults. Ependymoma is commoner in children than in adults, but oligodendrogliomas are very rare. A further type of tumour, the choroid plexus papilloma, is almost never found beyond the first decade of life, and is a rare tumour even in childhood. About 10 per cent are histologically malignant and are best described as choroid plexus carcinomas.

Little is known of the aetiology of these hemisphere tumours, though children with tuberous sclerosis have a high incidence of astrocytoma which is often of the giant-cell variety, and typically develops in the anterior end of the third ventricle with obstruction of the foramina of Munro.

As with adults, the clinical presentation usually results from the effects of raised

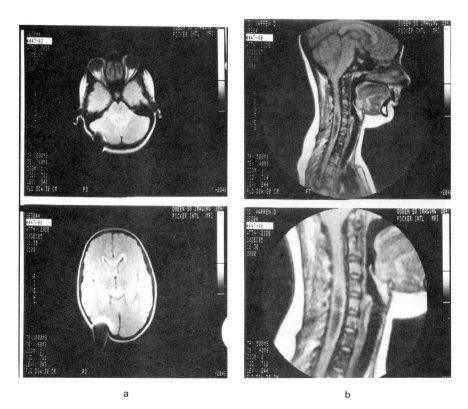

Fig. 11.12 Multiple intracranial glioma. (a) Tumour present in cerebellopontine angle and adjacent to ventricles. (b) The same patient had a spinal glioma with syrinx formation in the cervical spine (MRI views).

intracranial pressure, notably headache and nausea with vomiting, coupled with a focal deficit whose nature depends on the site of the lesion. Epilepsy, sometimes of many years duration, may be an important part of the clinical history in patients with a low-grade glioma that infiltrates a cerebral hemisphere.

Surgery, with a view to establishing the histological diagnosis and removing as much of the tumour as possible, has always been the initial treatment of choice for all of the cerebral hemisphere tumours of childhood. However the presence of a small and poorly demarcated lesion deep within the dominant hemisphere, particularly in a patient with only minimal neurological problems has often led to a request for primary treatment with irradiation, without histological verification. Hopefully with the increasing acceptance of stereotactic biopsy techniques these cases will become a rarity.

For low-grade tumours, surgical resection should always be attempted, although where the tumours are diffusely infiltrating or involving eloquent areas such as the speech centre or the motor cortex, this may not always be possible. As with adults, tumours involving the anterior part of the frontal or temporal lobes, especially in the non-dominant hemisphere, are ideally situated for surgical resection. Although it is not clear whether postoperative irradiation is essential when an apparently complete resection has been achieved, there is little doubt that for unresectable tumours, radiotherapy has an important role. Overall, the postoperative survival rate is certainly higher with radiotherapy than with surgery alone.[37] Routine pre- and postoperative CT scanning (and more recently MRI scanning) have made it much easier for the radiotherapist to deliver high local doses to the tumour (or tumour bed), and local postoperative irradiation no longer needs to include such generous portions of normal brain which are clearly well outside the radiologically abnormal area. If surgical resection is incomplete, the radiation dose should be at least 50 Gy over 5 weeks (daily fractionation) though some authorities advocate a lower dose where total naked eye excision has been carried out. For recurrent tumours, a number of groups have investigated treatment with chemotherapy, and responses have been claimed to a number of agents, including cisplatin, vincristine, nitrosoureas and procarbazine,[5] though these responses are rarely durable.

For the less common high-grade lesions, the proportion of truly resectable tumours is clearly lower and the prognosis correspondingly worse. However, once again there is good evidence that postoperative irradiation is of value, particularly in grade III astrocytomas. Unfortunately, as with adults, local recurrence at the primary site reduces the overall survival rate to a disappointing 10 per cent at two years.

Adjuvant chemotherapy is of interest in this high-risk group. In one recent study, treatment with a combination of CCNU, procarbazine and prednisone in addition to surgery and radiotherapy resulted in a disease-free survival rate of 44 per cent at 2.5 years compared with 21 per cent in a similar group of children treated without chemotherapy.[23] This may suggest a more profound effect with cytotoxic agents in children with cerebral glioma than in the case with adults, and this encouraging study needs further amplification.

Ependymoma is discussed on page 175, though about 40 per cent of childhood ependymomas are supratentorial. Their presentation and surgical management are similar to those described for other cerebral hemisphere tumours. With regard to postoperative treatment, the major question facing the radiotherapist is whether or not to irradiate the whole CNS, as for infratentorial ependymoma, or to limit the treatment to the primary site with a generous margin. In our experience, it is wiser to irradiate the whole CNS since there seems to be a clear-cut tendency to subarachnoid seeding even though this is admittedly less common than with infratentorial tumours. Whole CNS irradiation is undoubtedly required in the unusual variant of ependymoblastoma, a highly malignant lesion that generally occurs in early childhood and carries a high risk of spinal seeding.

For recurrent cases, chemotherapy has again been claimed to be of value,[16] but responses are generally short-lived. In the SIOP study of adjuvant chemotherapy for childhood ependymoma, no firm evidence of improved long-term survival has yet been noted.[5]

Primitive neuroectodermal tumours of the cerebrum

The category primitive neuroectodermal tumour (PNET) was coined by Hart and Earle[38] to describe tumours occurring in the cerebral hemispheres which resemble medulloblastoma histologically but arise in an area distant from the characteristic site of origin of the medulloblastoma. The term cerebral neuroblastoma has also been used, but seems less appropriate since we cannot be certain that it is similar in behaviour and treatment response to other neuroblastomas. They can arise at any supratentorial site (Fig. 11.13) and are often extremely large and radiologically bizarre. They are highly malignant, generally running a rapid course and with an

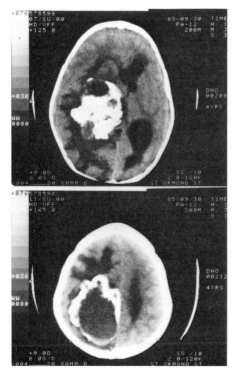

Fig. 11.13 Large supratentorial primitive neuroectodermal tumour, with areas of cystic formation and gross hydrocephalus.

average survival time of only 18 months despite the short-lived responses to radiotherapy which frequently seem to occur. Recurrence may be local or elsewhere within the CNS. In the 14 cases described by Gaffney et al.[39] and treated with radiotherapy, five were alive at two years, with three alive at five years. No survivors were seen in the group with undifferentiated histology. Treatment along the principles outlined for medulloblastoma seems indicated, with whole-CNS irradiation as a routine part of management for every case.

Cerebral tumours in children under one year of age

Thanks to advances in diagnostic and surgical techniques, paediatric neurologists and neurosurgeons are increasingly presented with very young children harbouring cerebral tumours. The plasticity of their immature brains coupled with their open skull sutures means that they are more likely to present with raised intracranial pressure and an increased head circumstances so that the initial clinical diagnosis is usually one of hydrocephalus, until a CT scan reveals the true situation. Apart from the occasional choroid plexus papilloma most of these tumours are highly malignant and very large at the time of presentation.[40, 41]

No satisfactory regimen for their management has yet been devised. Surgery to remove the bulk of the tumour rarely achieves a complete excision, and the operative hazards are great because of the child's small blood volume relative to the size of the tumour. Postoperative irradiation may slow the growth of the tumour but invariably at this young age it must affect the development of the brain by interfering with both cerebral myelination and dendritic arborization. Current interest centres on the use of chemotherapy but here too there are problems, both of delivery of the cytotoxic agent and also of tumour sensitivity to the drugs presently available.

Tumours of the spinal cord

Intramedullary spinal cord tumours are rare, and when they occur in childhood are more likely to be astrocytomas than ependymomas. They usually present with a combination of mechanical spinal problems (local pain, restriction of movement and deformity) and evidence of spinal cord compression – a spastic weakness of the legs (and the arms too if the lesion is high enough) and interference with micturition.

The diagnosis is usually made at myelography (with or without CT scanning) but where available, MRI scanning is now the imaging procedure of choice as it demonstrates not only the anatomy of the tumour but is also capable of differentiating the solid from the cystic components (Figs 11.12(b) and 14).

Most of these tumours are low-grade, partly cystic astrocytomas with a relatively benign behaviour, similar to that of cerebellar hemisphere tumours. At one time surgical resection was rarely attempted, but since the advent of the operating microscope, the Cavitron ultrasonic aspirator and the surgical laser, more paediatric neurosurgeons are operating with a view to achieving a complete removal of the solid part of the tumour.[42, 43]

It remains to be seen how many genuine cures are being achieved in this way, expecially since the tumours are often so slow in their growth rate. In general, it still

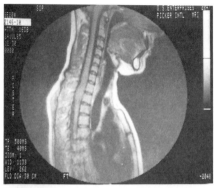

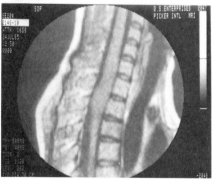

Fig. 11.14 MRI views showing swelling of cervical and upper thoracic spinal cord. Biopsy suggestive of low-grade glioma. No syrinx present in this example (compare Fig. 11.12(b)).

seems advisable to recommend postoperative irradiation in cases where there is evidence of residual tumour even after radical surgery.

References

1. Christoferson LA, Gustafson MB, Petersen AG. Von Hippel–Lindau's Disease *Journal of the American Medical Association*. 1961; **178**, 280.
2. Li FP Tucker MA, Fraumeni JF. Childhood cancer in sibs. *Journal of Pediatrics*. 1976; **88**, 419.
3. Packer RJ, Sutton LN, Rorke LB, et al. Oligodendroglioma of the posterior fossa in childhood. *Cancer*. 1985; **56**, 195.
4. Davis PC, Hoffman JC, Pearl GS, Braun JF. CT evaluation of effects of cranial radiation therapy in childhood. *American Journal of Roentgenology*. 1986; **147**, 587.
5. Bloom HJG. Tumours of the central nervous system. In: Voûte PA, Barrett A, Bloom HJG, Lemerle J, Neidhardt MK, eds. *Cancer in Children – Clinical Management*. 2nd edn. Berlin: Springer-Verlag, 1986.
6. Flores LE, Williams DL, Bell BA, O'Brien M, Ragab AH. Delay in the diagnosis of pediatric brain tumors. *American Journal of Diseases of Childhood*. 1986; **140**, 684.
7. Gjerris F, Klinken L. Long-term prognosis in children with benign cerebellar astrocytoma. *Journal of Neurosurgery*. 1978; **49**, 179.
8. Al-Mefty O, Jinkins JR, El-Senoussi M, El-Shaker M, Fox, JL. Medulloblastomas: a

review of modern management with a report on 75 cases. *Surgical Neurology.* 1985; **24**, 606.
9. Deutsch M, Reigel DH. The value of myelography in the management of childhood medulloblastoma. *Cancer.* 1980; **45**, 2194.
10. Shalet SM, Beardwell CG, Morris Jones PN, Pearson D. Pituitary function after treatment of intracranial tumours in children. *Lancet.* 1975; **ii**, 104.
11. Livesey EA, Brook CGD, Whitton AC, Britton JA, Tobias JS, Bloom HJG. Growth failure following irradiation in children with brain tumours. *Proceedings of the British Oncology Association.* Oxford, 1987; **2**.
12. Livesey EA, Brook CGD, Whitton AC, Tobias JS, Bloom HJG. Endocrine disorders following treatment of brain tumours in childhood. *Proceedings of the British Oncology Association.* Oxford, 1987; **2**.
13. Danoff BF, Cowchock FS, Marquette C, Mulgrew L, Kramer S. Assessment of the long-term effects of primary radiation therapy for brain tumours in children. *Cancer.* 1982; **49**, 1580.
14. Raimondi AJ, Tomita T. The disadvantage of whole-CNS postoperative radiation therapy for medulloblastoma. In: Paoletti P, Walker MD, Butti G, *et al. Multidisciplinary Aspects of Brain Tumor Therapy.* Amsterdam: North-Holland, 1979: 209–18.
15. Berry MP, Jenkin RDT, Keen CW, Nair BD, Simpson WJ. Radiation treatment for medulloblastoma. A 21 year review. *Journal of Neurosurgery.* 1981; **55**, 43.
16. Kahn AB, D'Souza BJ, Wharam MD, Champion LAA, Sinks LF, Woo SY, McCullough DC, Leventhal BG. Cisplatin therapy in recurrent childhood brain tumours. *Cancer Treatment Reports.* 1982; **66**, 2013–20.
17. Bloom HJG, Thornton-Jones H. Adjuvant chemotherapy for medulloblastoma: The multicentre controlled trial of the International Society of Paediatric Oncology (SIOP). *Proceedings of 13th International Congress of Chemotherapy.* Vienna, 1983.
18. Bloom HJG. Intracranial tumours: Response and resistance to therapeutic endeavours, 1970–1980. *International Journal of Radiation Oncology and Biological Physics.* 1982; **8**, 1083–13.
19. Epstein F, McLeary EL. Intrinsic brainstem tumours of childhood: surgical indications. *Journal of Neurosurgery.* 1986; **64**, 11.
20. Freeman CR, Suissa S. Brain stem tumours in children: results of a survey of 62 patients treated with radiotherapy. *International Journal of Radiation Oncology and Biological Physics.* 1986; **12**, 1823.
21. Peterman SB, Steiner RE, Bydder GM, Thomas DJ, Tobias JS, Young IR. Nuclear magnetic resonance imaging (NMR, MRI) of brain stem tumours. *Neuroradiology.* 1985; **27**, 202.
22. Whyte TR, Colby MY, Layton DD. Radiation therapy of brain-stem tumours. *Radiology.* 1969; **93**, 413–21.
23. Allen JC, Bloom HJG, Ertel I, Evans A, Hammond D, Jones H, Levin V, Jenkin D, Sposto R. Brain tumours in children: current cooperative and institutional chemotherapy trials in newly diagnosed and recurrent disease. *Seminars in Oncology.* 1986; **13**, 110.
24. Hoffman HJ, Chuang S, Ehrlich R, Buncic R, Netley C, Hendrick EB, Humphries RP. The microsurgical removal of craniopharyngiomas in childhood. *Concepts of Pediattic Neurosurgery.* 1985; **6**, 52–62.
25. Baskin DS, Wilson CB. Surgical management of craniopharyngiomas: a review of 74 cases. *Journal of Neurosurgery.* 1986; **65**, 22.
26. Hoogenhout J, Otten BJ, Kazem I, Stoelinga GBA, Walder AHD. Surgery and radiation therapy in the management of craniopharyngiomas. *International Journal of Radiation Oncology, and Biological Physics.* 1984; **10**, 2293–7.
27. Hooper R, Campbell PE, Colebatch JH. Intracranial and spinal tumours. In:

Jones PG, Campbell PE, eds. *Tumours of Infancy and Childhood.* Oxford: Blackwell Scientific Publications, 1976: 231-94.
28. Fletcher WA, Imes RK, Imes RK, Hoyt WF. Chiasmal gliomas: appearance and long-term changes demonstrated by computerised tomography. *Journal of Neurosurgery.* 1986; **65**, 154.
29. Hoyte WF, Baghdassarian SA. Optic glioma in childhood. *British Journal of Ophthalmology.* 1969; **53**,793-8.
30. Horwich A, Bloom HJG. Optic gliomas: Radiation therapy and prognosis. *International Journal of Radiation Oncology and Biological Physics* 1985; **11**, 1067-79.
31. Kanamori M, Shibuya M, Yoshida J. Long term follow-up of patients with optic glioma. *Child's Nervous System.* 1985; **1**, 272.
32. Rosenstock JG, Packer RJ, Bilanuik L, *et al.* Chiasmatic optic glioma treated with chemotherapy; a preliminary report. *Neurosurgery* 1985; **63**, 862.
33. Baloh RW, Furman JM, Yee RD, Dorsal midbrain syndrome: clinical and oculographic findings. *Neurology.* 1985; **35**, 54.
34. Dayan AD, Marshall AHE, Miller AA, Pick FJ, Rankin NE. Atypical teratomas of the pineal and hypothalamus. *Journal of Pathology and Bacteriology.* 1966; **92**, 1-28.
35. Rustin GJS, Newlands ES, Bagshawe KD, Begent RHJ, Crawford SM. Successful management of metastatic and primary germ cell tumors in the brain. *Cancer.* 1986; **57**, 2108-13.
36. Peckham MJ, Horwich A, Blackmore C, Hendry WF. Etoposide and cisplatin with or without bleomycin as first-line chemotherapy for patients with small-volume metastases of testicular nonseminoma. *Cancer Treatment Reports.* 1985; **69**, 483.
37. Leibel SA, Sheline GE, Wara WM, Boldrey EB, Neilson SL. The role of radiation therapy in the treatment of astrocytomas. *Cancer.* 1975; **35**, 1551-7.
38. Hart MN, Earle, KM. Primitive neuroectodermal tumours of the brain in children. *Cancer.* 1973; **32**, 890.
39. Gaffney CC, Sloane JP, Bradley NJ, Bloom HJG. Primitive neuroectodermal tumours of the cerebrum: pathlogy and treatment. *Journal of Neuro-oncology.* 1985; **3**, 23.
40. Tomita T, McLone DG. Brain tumours during the first twenty-four months of life. *Neurosurgery.* 1985; **17**, 913.
41 Jooma R, Hayward RD, Grant DN. Intracranial neoplasms during the first year of life: analysis of one hundred consecutive cases. *Neurosurgery.* 1984; **14**, 31.
42. Epstein F, Epstein N. Surgical treatment of spinal cord astrocytomas of childhood. A series of 19 patients. *Journal of Neurosurgery.* 1982; **57**, 685.
43. Reimer R, Onofrio BM. Astrocytomas of the spinal cord in children and adolescents. *Journal of Neurosurgery.* 1985; **63**, 669.

12 Radiotherapy in the treatment of cerebral astrocytomas

Steven A Leibel and Glenn E Sheline

Introduction

The majority of intracranial astrocytic gliomas are malignant or high-grade tumors. Because of their aggressive behaviour and poor prognosis, the treatment of malignant gliomas represents a substantial therapeutic challenge. Prospective studies in patients with anaplastic astrocytomas and glioblastoma multiforme have demonstrated the efficacy of radiation therapy in the management of these tumors. It is clear, however, that new approaches to the treatment of malignant gliomas need to be explored if survival is to be improved to a clinically significant degree. Unlike the malignant gliomas, there has been an absence of prospective studies for low-grade astrocytomas. The rationale for radiation therapy in these lesions is based solely on retrospective reviews of patients treated in single institutions over long periods of time.

This chapter details the rationale and the results of radiation therapy in the treatment of patients with the diagnoses of astrocytoma, anaplastic astrocytoma, and glioblastoma multiforme. As the selection of radiation dose is restricted by the tolerance of the normal brain, this chapter begins with a review of the adverse effects of therapeutic irradiation that may result from the irradiation of primary brain tumours.

Tolerance of the brain to therapeutic irradiation

The ability to deliver therapeutic doses of radiation to brain tumours is limited by the tolerance of the normal brain. Adverse effects may develop either during or following therapeutic irradiation. The various forms of injury that my occur vary in pathogenesis and can be classified into three groups according to their time of presentation: (1) acute reactions which occur during the course of treatment; (2) early delayed reactions presenting a few weeks to 2–3 months after irradiation; and (3) late delayed reactions which develop several months to years after treatment.[1,2] There are a number of factors which influence the occurrence and severity of these reactions including the individual radiation fraction size, total radiation dose, and the volume of tissue irradiated. The risk of injury may be influenced also by the age of the patient at the time of treatment, the presence of pre-existing brain injury by tumour or surgery, as well as infection and underlying vascular disease, and by chemotherapy.[3]

Acute reactions

Acute reactions occur during the course of radiation therapy and are distinguished by symptoms suggesting increased intracranial pressure or an intensification of pre-existing neurological symptoms or signs. The aetiology of the acute syndrome is thought to be radiation-induced oedema.[2] However, this has been difficult to demonstrate on computerized tomographic (CT) scans obtained during the course of treatment.[4] Clinical practice has established that daily doses of 1.8–2 Gy to all or a part of the brain are well tolerated and that, with such fractionation, total doses of 60–80 Gy can be administered without clinically significant *acute* adverse effects.[3,5] The acute tolerance of individual dose fractions up to 6 Gy is acceptable provided that total doses are appropriately reduced coincident with the increase in fraction size.[6] Acute complications have been reported with fraction sizes larger than 6 Gy.[7,8] Higher daily dose fractions should, therefore, be applied with discretion. Acute reactions, when they occur, are usually mild and transient. Occasionally corticosteroids occasionally may be necessary for the alleviation of symptoms.

Early delayed reactions

Early delayed reactions develop within a few weeks to a few months after the delivery of cranial irradiation. This reaction is heralded by transient somnolence or a temporary exacerbation of pre-existing signs and symptoms. Following treatment for intracranial neoplasms, this syndrome may go unrecognized or be ascribed to the recently treated tumour.[3] The early delayed reaction is thought to be the result of a temporary inhibition of myelin synthesis due to the effects of radiation on oligodendroglial cells.[3,9,10] X-ray evidence of transient demyelination may be exhibited by CT scan during the period of deterioration.[11] Although the syndrome usually is self-limited and mild, in rare instances the severity of the reaction may require intensive medical support. Corticosteroids may be useful in ameliorating signs and symptoms. The early delayed reaction may be seen after treatment of either benign or malignant neoplasms. Boldrey and Sheline[12] described eight patients who developed temporary neurological deterioration appearing within 10 weeks after radiation therapy for low-grade gliomas, meningiomas, and pituitary adenomas. These reactions could not be attributed to tumour progression and the symptoms resolved spontaneously within 6 weeks. Hoffman *et al*.[9] reported 51 patients with malignant gliomas who received 50 Gy (1.7–1.8 Gy/fraction) to the whole brain and a 10 Gy boost to a reduced field with concomitant 1,3-bis(2-chloroethyl)-1-nitrosourea (BCNU) given at eight-week intervals. Clinical and radiographic changes suggesting tumour progression occurred in 49 per cent (25/51) of the patients within 18 weeks of treatment. However, improvement occurred over the ensuing 16 weeks in 28 per cent (7/25) of these patients without a modification in therapy.

The importance of recognizing the early delayed syndrome is that it is generally transitory and that the appearance of new symptoms at this time is not necessarily an indication of treatment failure or the need for a change in therapy.[3]

Late delayed reactions

Late delayed injury may develop several months or years following treatment. These reactions range from asymptomatic narrowing of large vessels[13] to loss of function,[3] necrosis,[2] and secondary neoplasia.[14] Radiation necrosis constitutes the major hazard of exposure of the brain to therapeutic irradiation. This process tends to be progressive and irreversible and potentially is fatal. The clinical presentation of radiation injury depends on the site and volume of the brain irradiated. Late delayed brain injury occurs primarily in the white matter.[15] The breakdown of white matter with release of necrotic cellular material may result in oedema and mass effect.[10] Late radiation-induced injury has been attributed to vascular (small and medium arterioles) injury[16,17] or to a direct effect on glial cells.[18] It is probable that multiple mechanisms are involved, and the importance of each depends on the radiation dose and latent interval.[3] While demyelination appears to be important in the early delayed reaction, the effect on the vasculature becomes increasingly more important over time.[2]

Although there is considerable literature on radiation-induced brain necrosis, there is little information on the incidence of late radiation injury as a function of dose and fractionation. Time – dose relationships have been derived largely from case reports gathered from the literature. Sheline et al.[2] suggested that threshold doses for necrosis with conventionally fractionated (1.8–2.0 Gy/fraction/day) radiation therapy are approximately 35 Gy for 10 fractions, 60 Gy for 35 fractions, and 76 Gy for 60 fractions. Sheline et al. defined the lower limits of tolerance by an isoeffect line with a slope of 0.44. An equivalent single dose quantity termed "neuret" was derived. The formula:

$$\text{neuret} = D \times N^{-0.41} \times T^{\times 0.03}$$

(where D is the total dose, N is the fractions, and T is the total time in days) was based on the slope of the isoeffect line of 0.44 and the presumption that the exponent of T is -0.03. These exponents imply that the tolerance of the CNS is predominantly dependent on the number of radiation dose fractions or, conversely, dose per fraction and minimally dependent on the overall time. While this formula appears to be appropriate over the commonly used fraction numbers and treatment times, the formula may not be applicable to very small or very large numbers of fractions or to very short or prolonged overall treatment times. For example, Ang et al.[19] concluded that for rat spinal cord a reduction in individual fraction size from 2 Gy to 1.3 Gy did not result in a further increase in tolerance.

An accurate assessment of the incidence of cerebral necrosis as a function of dose has been difficult to establish because autopsies are performed infrequently and most studies do not report the number of exposed patients who have survived a sufficient length of time to develop the injury. Marks et al.[20] however, reported a series of 139 consecutive patients who received irradiation for primary brain tumours with at least 45 Gy in daily dose fractions of 1.8–2.0 Gy. Their review disclosed seven incidences of brain necrosis. Utilizing the equivalent dose formula:

$$(ED) = D \times N^{-0.377} \times T^{-0.058}$$

there were no instances of necrosis in 51 patients with an ED of less than 1250. Two of 60 patients developed necrosis with ED between 1251 and 1330. The incidence of necrosis in the ED range of 1331–1460 was five of 28 patients. These ED values can be recalculated into total dose assuming a daily dose of 1.8 Gy given five times per week. Recalculating the data in this fashion demonstrates that for total doses of 57.6 Gy or less, there were no cases of necrosis in 51 patients. Between 57.6 and 64.8 Gy, there were two instances of necrosis in 60 patients. In the 28 patients who received 64.8–75.6 Gy, there were five cases of necrosis or an incidence of 18 per cent.[6] These data suggest that the dose–response curve is quite steep; a similary steep dose response curve has been found for radiation injury of the dog brain.[15]

Surgical resection of favourably situated focal radiation-induced lesions may result in considerable improvement or complete recovery from the secondary effects of brain injury. Surgical procedures involving less than total resection of the necrotic tissue (i.e. biopsy) provide little benefit. Corticosteroids may result in temporary improvement or stability of neurological deficit when surgery is not possible.[10]

Children, especially under the age of 2–3 years, are thought to be more susceptible to injury than adults due to incomplete development and myelination of the central nervous system.[2, 21] Patients with underlying vascular disease such as that due to diabetes mellitus, Cushing's disease, acromegaly, or collagen vascular disease may have an increased propensity to radiation injury.[22-24] Underlying CNS infection also may predispose the patient to radiation neurotoxicity.[25]

The extent to which chemotherapeutic agents influence the production of radiation necrosis is poorly documented. However, there is evidence suggesting that some of these agents amplify the risk of injury. The most dramatic example occurs in children with acute lymphoblastic leukaemia (ALL) treated with aggressive chemotherapy administered intravenously and intrathecally with prophylactic brain irradiation. Brain injury has occured in these children with doses as low as 24 Gy in 1.5–2 Gy daily increments which without chemotherapy would be well below normal tolerance levels.[3] Two delayed syndromes, necrotizing leucoencephalopathy and mineralizing microangiopathy have been recognized in these children.[26]

There is less information in adults who have received combined therapy for primary brain tumors. Pratt et al.[27] reported a case of fatal cerebral necrosis after administration of 30 Gy in 10 fractions with multiagent chemotherapy, a dose that one would expect to be well tolerated. Burger et al.[28] reported four cases of radiation necrosis in 24 brains examined at post-mortem following 60 Gy in 6–6.5 to weeks for malignant gliomas. Of the four patients, three had had multiple courses of chemotherapy which included procarbazine, BCNU, and dibromodulcitol. There was a predilection for necrosis to occur in the white matter adjacent to the persistent neoplasm suggesting that the tumour may have played a role in causing the injury.

Foo et al.[29] reviewed 37 patients treated for malignant gliomas treated with radiation therapy and chemotherapy (BCNU or 1-(2-chlorethyl)-3-cyclohexyl-1-nitrosourea MeCCNU) who survived at least two years. Forty-five per cent developed severe cerebral atrophy, in a median of 46 months with a concomitant fall in Karnofsky Performance score of 20 or more. Whereas 17 per cent treated with moderate dose whole-brain irradiation (43 Gy at 1.8–2 Gy per fraction) developed severe cerebral atrophy, 39 per cent with higher dose whole brain irradiation (60 Gy at 1.8–2 Gy per fraction) developed severe cerebral atrophy. Both 17 per cent at 43 Gy and 39 per cent at 60 Gy are well above the incidence expected from irradiation alone. Eight-five per cent of the patients with severe cerebral atrophy developed CNS complications including intracerebral haemorrhage, stroke, transient ischaemia attack, subdural haematoma, and necrosis. It was concluded that, following such combined therapy for malignant gliomas, long-term survivors suffer from a high incidence of cerebral atrophy, dementia, cerebrovascular disease, and necrosis. Prospective studies are needed to establish the true incidence of injury when radiation therapy is combined with chemotherapy and the cause or relationship to the various agents used.

It is often difficult to confirm the clinical diagnosis of radiation necrosis in patients with intracranial neoplasms who deteriorate neurologically after receiving a substantial dose of cranial irradiation. Radiation-induced sequelae can be mistaken for tumour recurrence as both conditions may present similar but inconstant and nonspecific clinical and radiographic findings.[30] The lesions may present with loss of volume due to atrophy, a glial reaction appearing as a localized mass lesion with peripheral or central contrast enhancement or as a low density, enhancing or mineralized area on CT scan.[6, 30, 31] Magnetic resonance imaging (MRI) changes following cranial irradiation include ventricular enlargement and/or deposition of haemosiderin in the basal ganglia, and discrete or multiple confluent areas of high signal intensity in the white matter on T_2 weighted images.[32-34] New diagnostic methods to differentiate recurrent tumour from necrosis are being investigated; these include positron emission tomography[35] and quantitative CT scanning.[36] While CT or MRI findings may suggest radiation-induced changes if the injury occurs near or at the tumour site, only a biopsy can confirm the diagnosis.

There have been numerous reports of a decreased level of intellectual function in children after radiation therapy for brain tumours and ALL. While it is clear that some patients will exhibit a decreased level of intellectual function, it is often difficult to determine the specific cause of the impairment. The tumour, its location, presence of increased intracranial pressure and surgical treatment may contribute to the development of injury.[37] Children undergoing radiation to the supratentorial region appear to be more susceptible to intellectual dysfunction than those who receive radiotherapy to the infratentorial region.[38] Studies have suggested that mental retardation is more common in patients with tumours involving the hypothalamic or thalamic regions,[39] or the brain stem.[40] Children undergoing treatment when older than 3 years seem to be less susceptible to injury than those less than 3 years.[39] Most patients have been treated within a narrow dose range, and hence little information relating radiation dose to the development of intellectual deficit is available. Prophylactic CNS irradiation together with chemotherapy for ALL induces a small but significant reduction in IQ scores accompanied by perceptual and learning disabilities.[37-43] The decrements in IQ score that have been observed in patients receiving brain irradiation for ALL or for a primary brain tumour generally reflect a reduction in the performance score, although in some series a decrease in verbal scores also has been reported.[37, 38, 41, 44-47] Both early and late neuropsychological deterioration have been recognized in long-term surviving patients with small-cell carcinoma of the lung receiving prophylactic cranial irradiation with doses of approximately 30 Gy in 10 fractions.[48-50] As in the case of ALL, these patients received a variety of chemotherapeutic agents which may have enhanced the effect of radiation on the CNS.

It is probable that high-dose ($\geq$ 60 Gy conventionally fractionated) radiation in some degree of intellectual impairment in adults but little quantitative information exists. Such impairment seems accentuated by concurrent or subsequent multiagent chemotherapy, and it is also more evident in patients who have had whole-brain irradiation. Hochberg and Slotnick[45] studied 13 patients with high-grade astrocytomas after the combination of surgery, external-beam irradiation (45 Gy to the whole brain with 15 Gy boost) and lomustine (CCNU). The 13 patients selected for this study had survived at least one year after treatment and had failed to return to pretreatment work levels; thus, they represented a small fraction of the total group and were preselected for having functional problems. Testing revealed difficulties solving or coping with newly learned tasks requiring attention. The relative roles of tumour, treatment, and failure to return to work are unclear. Previously acquired ability, overlearned information, and judgement were not impaired. Maire et al.[51] reported on adult patients with primary intracranial tumours and showed that during the first four months following partial or whole brain irradiation (3/4 of these patients also received chemotherapy) full scale IQ coefficients were normal. Between five and 30 months there was intellectual deterioration which subsequently disappeared. Full scale IQ scores fell after 30 months but recovery was seen in four or five patients less than 30 years of age and in two patients between 30 and 50 years of age who returned to work early after treatment. They recommended early neuropyschological testing with psychological assistance when necessary and an early return to normal activity.

Prospective serial studies of both children and adults with brain tumours with proper controls are needed to assess and distinguish the effect of the tumour and its treatment, the effect of the host and the effect of environmental factors. By carefully monitoring the neuropsychological effects of the disease and treatment, the precise mechanisms of impairment can be established and corrective measures instituted.

Classification of astrocytic gliomas

The use of different pathological classification systems makes the reported data on the treatment and prognosis of the astrocytic gliomas difficult to interpret. Some of these difficulties are discussed in Chapter 5. One system, favoured by the current authors, represents a modification of the classification of Bailey and Cushing[52] and is based on the presumed histogenesis of the tumour. This system and variations thereof have been presented by Rubinstein,[53] Russell and Rubinstein,[54] and Burger and Vogel.[55] It categorizes the astrocytic gliomas into astrocytoma, anaplastic or malignant astrocytoma, and glioblastoma multiforme. Another widely used method of classification, orginally proposed by Kernohan et al. in 1949,[56] is based on grading of the degree of malignancy. This system assumes that astrocytomas and glioblastoma multiforme represent different degrees of astrocytic anaplasia and dedifferentiation. In the Kernohan–Sayer system astrocytomas are graded from I to IV, in ascending order of malignancy, as determined by the extent of pleomorphism, hyperchromasia, and mitotic activity.[57] Subjectivity of the grading procedure and the lack of explicit criteria for the separation of tumours in this scheme makes reproducibility between pathologists difficult to achieve.[53, 54, 58] Some authors have used the term "glioblastoma multiforme" to be synonymous with Kernohan grade IV astrocytomas, while others (as advocated by Kernohan and Sayer)[57] have combined grade III and IV under this term. In practice the grading system, as generally applied, has correlated poorly with prognosis. In the original publication of the grading

Table 12.1 Malignant gliomas: comparison of the prognosis by tumour grade with classification based histological characteristics

	Survival	
	Median (months)	18 months
Grade III	10.3	—
Grade IV	8.9	—
Astrocytoma with atypical or anaplastic foci	27.4*	64%*
Glioblastoma multiforme	8.4*	15%*

* Difference in survival rate ($p < 0.00001$)
— = data not available.
Data from Tables 3 and 4 of ref. 58.

system by Svien et al.[59] the three-year survival rates for grade II and III were similar. Patients with grade I tumours, however, had a significantly longer median survival than those with grade IV tumours. The system has not been prognostically useful in separating grade I from II or III from IV. Laws et al.[60] found no significant difference in survival for patients with grade I and II lesions. Fazekas reported a higher five-year survival rate for grade II than grade I, namely, 53 vs. 20 per cent respectively.[61] In a prospective randomized trial conducted by the Radiation Therapy Oncology Group (RTOG) and the Eastern Cooperative Oncology Group (ECOG) the difference in survival between grade III and IV lesions was not significant. The median survival for grade III astrocytomas was 10.3 months while the median survival for patients with grade IV astrocytomas was 8.9 months. When the pathology material was reviewed and histologically grouped as astrocytoma with anaplastic foci or as glioblastoma multiforme (based on the presence of one or more foci of coagulation necrosis involving neoplastic astrocytes) there were marked differences in both the median survival time and the 18-month survival rate[58, 62] (Table 12.1). These findings are consistent with the prognostic differences between anaplastic astrocytoma (or malignant astrocytoma) and glioblastoma multiforme reported in several retrospective studies.[63]

While the Kernohan grading system appears to be of little use, histological features are of considerable prognostic importance. The University of California, San Francisco (UCSF) experience shows a clear separation of survival curves for incompletely resected astrocytomas with decreasing survival in the following order: juvenile pilocytic astrocytoma, astrocytoma, anaplastic astrocytoma, and glioblastoma multiforme. Preliminary UCSF data suggest that the anaplastic astrocytomas can be separated histologically into two different prognostic categories which are referred to as "moderately" anaplastic and "highly" anaplastic astrocytoma. The survival curves for the highly anaplastic astrocytoma and gemistocytic astrocytoma are almost superimposable and lie between those for moderately anaplastic astrocytoma and glioblastoma multiforme.[64]

Astrocytoma

The lack of prospective randomized studies has led to considerable controversy regarding the use of radiotherapy for the treatment of the more differentiated or "low-grade" astrocytomas. The interpretation of retrospective reports is difficult because of the absence of adequate consideration for factors of prognostic significance such as selection factors, patient characteristics, tumour location, extent of surgery and radiation therapy techniques. Recent studies that have been limited to the era of CT scanning are difficult to compare with earlier studies because patients in the former have been diagnosed and treated earlier in the course of their disease and the length of their follow up is more limited. It is now well-recognized that factors such as the age of patients performance status, histology, location of lesion and extent of resection are of major prognostic significance and must be taken into consideration, if comparison of various treatment groups is to be meaningful. The lack of suitable control groups and the use of different classification systems has also contributed to problems of interpretation.[65]

Reported survival rates following surgery alone (either complete or incomplete) and surgery combined with postoperative irradiation and low-grade astrocytomas are shown in Table 12.2.[60, 61, 66–69] In order to evaluate the data summarized in this table a number of factors should be considered. One of the most important, if not the single most important, prognostic factor, is age; younger patients have a better prognosis than older ones. Laws *et al.* reported a five-year survival rate of 83 per cent for patients less than 20 years of age, 35 per cent for ages 24–49 years, and 12 per cent for those older than 50 years.[60] They also found that the functional status of the patient plays a significant role. With no postoperative performance deficit, no alteration of consciousness, and no personality change overall, survival rates range from 38–42 per cent. These rates decreased to 9–16 per cent when one of these features was present. Laws *et al.* identified a "good-risk" group of patient as being those with a 15-year survival of 87 per cent; the good-risk patients were those with totally resected supratentorial astrocytomas, age less than 20 years, surgery in 1950 or later, absence of personality change, absence of alteration of consciousness, and only minimal or no postoperative neurological deficit.[60] The appearance of the tumour on CT scan may also be of prognostic importance. Piepmeier[70] found the mean survival of patients with tumours which showed CT enhancement with contrast media was 3.92 years compared with 7.94 years for non-enhancing lesions ($p = 0.008$). This finding was independent of the age of the patient. The tumour grading system has been of variable prognostic value. The influence of tumour grade on survival is summarized in Table 11.3.[60, 61, 66, 68, 71]

It is generally agreed that postoperative irradiation is not indicated when complete surgical resection has been achieved. At the University of California, San Francisco (UCSF) the five-year survival was 100 per cent with complete resection. Eleven of the 14 lesions amenable to complete resection occurred in the cerebellum; nine of these 11 patients were less than 20 years of age.[66] Thus, at least for cystic cerebellar astrocytomas in children where the tumour is confined to a resectable mural nodule, the control rate for surgical resection alone approaches 100 per cent and radiation is not recommended. Similarly, in a series of 12 patients with complete resection of juvenile pilocytic astrocytomas at UCSF, the five- and 10-year survival rates were 100 per cent.[72]

Retrospective studies have suggested that postoperative radiotherapy is of value for incompletely resected astrocytomas. Reported five-year survival rates range from 13 to 19 per cent following incomplete resection alone and 41 to 46 per cent for incomplete resection and radiation therapy (Table 12.2). Laws *et al.* in a review of

Astrocytoma 201

Table 12.2 Low-grade astrocytomas: survival rates following treatment

Author and year	Reference	Site	No. of cases	Treatment	Percentage survival		
					5-year	10-year	15-year
Complete resection							
Leibel et al., 1975	66	IC	14	S	100	100	88
Fazekas, 1977	61	IC	22	S, S+RT	90	25	—
Laws et al., 1984	60	CH	57	S, S+RT	61	—	59
Incomplete resection							
Leibel et al., 1975	66	IC	37	S	19	11	4
			71	S+RT	46	35	35
Fazekas, 1977	61	IC	14	S	13	—	—
			32	S+RT	41	28	—
Extent of resection unknown							
Marsa et al., 1975 Scanlon and Taylor, 1979	67	CH	40	S+RT	41	22	—
	68	IC	134	S+RT	64	—	—
Laws et al., 1984	60	CH	252	0–<40 Gy	34	—	—
			74	>40 Gy	49	—	—
*Dewit et al., 1984	69	IC	35	S+RT	87	70	—

* All under age 15, 30/35 infratentional lesions.
— = no data available.
IC = all intracranial sites.
CH = cerebral hemispheric lesions only.

Table 12.3 Low-grade astrocytomas: influence of tumour grade on prognosis

Author and year	Reference	Site	No. of patients	Treatment	Five-year survival	
					Grade 1 (%)	Grade 2 (%)
Leibel et al., 1975	66	IC	37	*S	25	0
			71	*S+RT	58	25
Fazekas, 1977	61	IC	68	†S, †S+RT	20	53
Laws et al., 1984	60	CH	461	†S, †S+RT	44	34
Bloom, 1982	71	CH	120	‡S+RT	33	21
Scanlon and Taylor, 1979	68	IC	134	‡S+RT	76	58

* All incomplete resection.
† Includes patients with subtotal and total resections.
‡ Extent of resected not known some may have been complete.
IC = all intracranial sites.
CH = cerebral hemispheric lesions.
S = surgery.
RT = radiotherapy.

the Mayo Clinic experience with cerebral hemisphere low-grade astrocytomas, concluded by multivariate regression analysis that "radiation therapy was of clear benefit primarily in older patients with incompletely removed tumours".[60] Fazekas analysed the results of 68 patients with grade I and II intracranial astrocytomas.[61] Prognostically, the non-irradiated patients represented a more favourable group than did the radiated group because it contained a greater percentage of patients 16 years or age or less (74 *vs.* 22 per cent) and gross excision was more frequent (39 *vs.* 29 per cent). Nonetheless, the five-year survival rate for patients who had received radiation therapy (54 per cent) was better than for those not receiving it (32 per cent). For patients with incomplete excision, the five-year survival rate was 41 per cent with radiotherapy and 13 per cent without, even though the irradiated patients appeared to have been a less favourable group.

Leibel *et al.* reviewed the records of 122 consecutive patients with astrocytoma treated at the UCSF.[66] Of the 108 patients with incompletely resected tumours, 71 received postoperative radiotherapy whereas the other 37 did not. The extent of resection was similar in the groups who did or did not receive radiotherapy. Twenty-two per cent of the patients treated with surgery only and 30 per cent of the patients with surgery plus radiotherapy were less than 20 years of age. The available information did not permit a comparative evaluation of functional performance status of patients in the two groups; however, as far as could be ascertained, the groups were similar in this respect. The usual dose was 50–55 Gy given in 1.8 Gy fractions, five fractions per week. The overall five-year recurrence-free survival rate for incompletely resection alone was 19 per cent compared with 46 per cent for incomplete resection and radiotherapy. The 10-year survival rates were 11 and 35 per cent, respectively. For adults, the five-year survival rate was 10 per cent for surgery alone *vs.* 32 per cent when radiotherapy was added. At all time intervals from three to 20 years, the survival of patients with incomplete resection and postoperative radiation therapy was superior to that of those who had incomplete resection alone. When the grading system was applied retrospectively, the five-year survival was 58 per cent for grade I astrocytoma and 25 per cent for grade II lesions in patients who received postoperative irradiation compared with survival rates of 25 per cent for grade I and zero for grade II in the non-irradiated patients (Table 12.3).

The 10- and 20-year rates of freedom from progression for 19 patients with incompletely resected juvenile pilocytic astrocytomas receiving postoperative irradiation at UCSF were 74 per cent and 41 per cent, respectively. All recurrences were at the primary site. Unfortunately, a control group of incompletely resected, non-irradiated patients was not available for comparison. While some investigators have recommended observation only for incompletely resected juvenile pilocytic astrocytomas, it would appear that despite their "benign" nature, the risk of recurrence following incomplete resection may be high, even when postoperative irradiation is administered.[72]

With currently available data it is difficult to take a categorical position regarding the use of postoperative radiation therapy for low-grade astrocytomas. Nevertheless, therapy decisions must be made and they must be based on the evidence that is available. Except for selected patients, including those with completely resected juvenile pilocytic astrocytomas of the cerebellum and the "good-risk" group of Laws *et al.*, the so-call low-grade tumours are highly lethal and should bot be considered as "bening" lesions.[65] At five years the survival rate for all low-grade astrocytoma patients at the Mayo Clinic was about one-third of that calculated for a comparable normal population; by 15 years, it was down to one-fifth of that expected (16 vs. 90 per cent).[60] It is evident that complacency with the diagnosis of "low-grade" should not lead to inadequate therapy. Present evidence favours the position that postoperative radiation therapy is beneficial for those patients with incompletely resected astrocytomas. Although these astrocytomas are generally lethal, they tend to be slowly progressive. Thus the therapy should be relatively conservative so that it does not of itself lessen life expectancy or produce excessive morbidity or loss of function.[70]

With conventionally fractionated radiation therapy (1.8–2.0 Gy per fraction) doses of 50–55 Gy are advocated. The close is reduced for children under 2–3 years of age. It is expected that this will control some tumours or at least significantly delay their recurrence with a minimum risk of radiation injury. Generous but limited radiation fields, rather than whole brain fields, are used at UCSF. The fields encompass the tumour as demonstrated on CT scan with a 2–3 cm margin and at least 1 cm beyond the T_2 weighted MR image, whichever volume is larger.

Very young children (less than two or three years of age) and infants pose a special problem in that an adequate radiation dose is likely to lead to unacceptable late sequelae. Therefore, in such patients the initiation of radiotherapy is delayed as long as possible. Chemotherapy may be of value in delaying the necessity for irradiation but its efficacy is unproven. Unless there is evidence that immediate irradiation is necessary, close clinical observation together with repeated high quality CT and or MRI scans are used to gauge disease progression. Radiotherapy is withheld until there is evidence of clinically and functionally significant tumour growth.[65]

Properly designed prospective and controlled studies are needed to determine which patients and which tumours should be irradiated as part of the primary treatment. Such studies are now being formulated in the United States both by the Brain Tumour Cooperative Group and the Northern California Oncology Group. It seems clear, however, that for patients with incompletely resected tumours improved therapeutic strategies are needed.

Anaplastic astrocytoma and glioblastoma multiforme

Retrospective reviews of historical material have generally indicated that as a rule there are no five-year survivors among patients with anaplastic astrocytoma treated with surgery alone compared with around 20 per cent for those treated with surgery and postoperative irradiation. For glioblastoma multiforme, these retrospective reviews have suggested that postoperative irradiation extends survival time but does not yield five-year survivors even with radiation therapy.[63] The value of radiation therapy, at least for glioblastoma multiforme, has been proven in two prospective clinical trials. In 1969, the United States Brain Tumour Study Group (BTSG) began a prospective randomized trial for patients with malignant gliomas. In that study (study 6901) patients with malignant gliomas were randomized postoperatively to one of four treatment options including: (1) supportive therapy only; (2) BCNU, 30 mg/m^2 intravenously on three successive days, repeated every 6–8 weeks; (3) whole brain radiotherapy, 1.7–2.0 Gy/week, to a total of 50–60 Gy; and (4) BCNU plus radiotherapy. Two hundred and twenty-two patients constituted the "valid study group" of whom 90 per cent were classified as having glioblastoma multiforme, 9 per cent anaplastic astrocytoma, and 1 per cent other histologies. The median survival times in weeks were: supportive care, 14; BCNU 19; radiotherapy 36; and BCNU plus radiotherapy, 35. The difference in survival time between radiotherapy and either supportive care or BCNU alone was significant ($p = 0.001$).[73] Similar results were obtained in the prospective randomized trial conducted by the Scandinavian Glioblastoma Study Group.[74]

The results of the clinical trials of the BTSG are summarized in Table 12.4.[73, 75-79] Although the addition of BCNU to radiotherapy did not significantly improve the median survival compared with radiotherapy alone in either study 6901[73] or the subsequent BTSG study 7201,[76] there was a greater surviving fraction of patients at the end of 18 months in the groups receiving combined radiotherapy and chemotherapy. Furthermore, when the data from the two studies were combined, it appeared that the addition of BCNU to radiotherapy provided an increase of approximately 10 per cent in 18-month survival as compared with that produced by radiotherapy alone.[77] Thus the addition of BCNU to radiotherapy appears to result in a modest improvement in survival time and in the number of patients alive at 18 months; however, the latter represents only a small fraction of the total group. Other chemotherapeutic agents studied by the BTSG, including procarbazine, MeCCNU and streptozotocin, were similar in efficacy to BCNU.[76-78] Chemotherapeutic combinations studied in BTSG protocol 8001, including BCNU together with procarbazine and BCNU plus hydroxyurea alternating with procarbazine and teniposide (VM 26), were not superior to BCNU alone.[79] High-dose corticosteroids had no chemotherapeutic activity.[77]

The RTOG and ECOG[62, 80] conducted a joint trial between 1974 and 1979 in which 626 patients with malignant gliomas (including both anaplastic astrocytomas and glioblastoma multiforme) were randomized to one of the following treatment options: (1) 60 Gy delivered over 6–7 weeks administered to the whole brain; (2) 60 Gy given to the whole brain with a boost of 10 Gy in one week directed to the tumour volume; (3) 60 Gy given to the whole brain with BCNU; and (4) 60 Gy to the whole brain with MeCCNU and imidazole-4-(or 5)-carboxamide, 5-(or 4)-(3, 3 dimethyl-1-trizene) (DTIC). The radiation dose of 70 Gy yielded essentially the same survival time as did the lower dose of 60 Gy. For patients less than 40 years of age, the addition of the 10 Gy boost increased the median survival to 47 months compared with 21 months for 60 Gy. However, the difference appeared to be due to a disproportionate and very small (six) number of patients with anaplastic astrocytomas in the high-dose group. The survival of patients receiving either radiation and BCNU or radiotherapy with DTIC and MeCCNU was better than those for radiation alone; the latter combination, however, was more toxic. When the data were considered according to age of patients, the only significant difference occurred in the 40–60 year age range where patients treated with BCNU and radiotherapy had a significantly ($p < 0.01$) improved survival compared with patients who received irradiation alone; with BCNU the two-year survival increased from 8 to 23 per cent. Forty- to 60-year-old patients who received MeCCNU plus DTIC and radiotherapy also did better ($p = 0.04$) than the similar age group treated with radiation alone. For patients less than 40 years of age, the addition of BCNU increased the median survival from 21.3 to 29.9 months and the number of long-term (three-year)

Table 12.4 Malignant gliomas: summary of results of brain tumour study group phase III trials of postoperative therapy*

Treatment	Reference no.	No. of patients	Median survival (weeks)	18-month survival (%)	Comments
Trial 6901	73	222			RT and RT + BCNU significantly better than support
Support			14	0	
BCNU			19	4	
RT			36	4	
RT + BCNU			35	19	
Trial 7201	76	358			RT, RT + BCNU, and RT + MeCCNU significantly better than MeCCNU
MeCCNU			24	10	
RT			36	15	
RT + MeCCNU			42	23	
RT + BCNU			51	27	
Trial 7501	77	527			RT + BCNU and RT + procarbazine significantly better than RT + Medrol
RT + medrol			40	15	
RT + procarbazine			47	29	
RT + BCNU			50	24	
RT + BCNU + Medrol			41	23	
Trial 7702	78	557			No significant difference among the four arms
RT + BCNU			44	16	
Hyperfractionated RT + BCNU			45	25	
RT + misonidazole + BCNU			40	16	
RT + streptozotocin			43	25	

RT = radiotherapy.
Medrol = methylprednisolone.
* Table from ref. 75 (reprinted with permission).

survivors from 28 per cent to 44 per cent, but the patient numbers were too small for the differences to reach statistical significance. The addition of chemotherapy did not improve survival in patients older than 60 years.[80]

Levin *et al.* reported a randomized clinical trial of the Northern California Oncology Group (NCOG) in which radiation therapy plus BCNU was compared with radiation therapy plus BCNU and hydroxyurea. Radiation therapy was conventionally fractionated (1.7–2.0 Gy per day). The whole brain received 50 Gy and the tumour volume an additional 10 Gy boost. The median time to tumour progression for patients with glioblastoma multiforme was 41 weeks for those receiving hydroxyurea and BCNU compared with 31 weeks for those receiving BCNU alone ($p = 0.03$). The median time for progression for non-glioblastoma multiforme malignant gliomas (72 weeks) was not improved by the addition of hydroxyurea (50 weeks).[81]

Several important prognostic variables have been identified in the cooperative group trials. Most notably these include patient age, extent of surgical resection, performance status, and histological diagnosis. Age represents a very important prognostic factor. In the RTOG–ECOG study, for patients less than 40, 40–60, or greater than 60 years of age, the 18-month survival rates were 64, 20 and 8 per cent, respectively.[62] The combined BTSG studies also identified an age effect. Patients aged less than 45, 45–54, 55–64, or 65 years or older had relative death rates of 1, 1.75, 2.5, and 3.5, respectively. Age remained a significant prognostic factor even with adjustment for duration of symptoms, performance status, and histological tumour type as well as other identifiable prognostic variables.[82]

Another important variable was functional performance status. More intact and functional patients survive longer than those with poor status regardless of other factors. In the RTOG–ECOG studies patients with a Karnofsky Performance score of 70–100 had a median survival of 12 months, and 34 per cent survived 18 months; whereas with a score of 40–60, the median survival was 6 months and 13 per cent survived 18 months.[62] Review of the BTSG trial showed that for Karnofsky scores of 90–100, 70–80, 50–60, and 10–40, the relative death rates were 1, 1.4, 2, and 2.9, respectively.[82]

The third independent variable of significance is histological diagnosis. The RTOG–ECOG data showing better survival for anaplastic astrocytoma than for glioblastoma multiforme are presented in Table 12.1.[62, 80] In the BTSG trial, the death rate for patients with glioblastoma multiforme was 1.5 to 2 times higher than that for other malignant gliomas.[82] Nelson *et al.* also found that the extent of tumour resection was a significant independent prognostic factor in patients with anaplastic astrocytomas.[83] The median survival of patients with partial or total excision was 46.8 months compared with 15.2 months for patients who had a biopsy only. The three-year actuarial survival rates were 60.1 and 33.3 per cent, respectively.

Thus, although other factors such as history of seizures, duration of symptoms, and the occurrence of neurological abnormalities may correlate to some extent with prognosis, it is clear that age, extent of surgery, performance status and histological category are strong prognostic variables. When comparing results within or between randomized studies, it is important either to ensure that the subsets being compared are in fact comparable or that, utilizing information about prognostic factors, an adjustment for differences in composition of the subsets has been made. This is, of course, even more important when using data from non-randomized and from retrospective studies.

Two important issues in the treatment of malignant gliomas with radiation therapy include the tissue volume to be irradiated and the radiation dose. There has been considerable discussion regarding the volume of brain that should be included in the radiation treatment portal. Glioblastomas generally are diffusely infiltrating neoplasms which can extend into the subarachnoid space, may occasionally be multicentric and even may metastasize. Some of the uncertainty regarding the appropriate treatment volume results from studies attempting to correlate clinical and radiographic tumour extent with findings at autopsy.[84-86] These studies usually revealed that the tumour was more extensive than determined clinically. Often the patients studied in these series had died relatively soon after establishment of their diagnosis, and hence were a group with particularly poor prognosis. Thus, autopsy findings tend to be biased towards very advanced aggressive tumours. Futhermore, extent at autopsy represents the end-stage of disease and can be expected in the majority of patients to be greater than that at time of diagnosis and treatment. Concannon *et al.* in 1960, compared postmortem tumour volumes with previously planned radiation treatment volumes that were based on the then available contrast X-ray examinations.[84] In only two of the 21 patients studied was the tumour plus a surrounding 1 cm margin of brain tissue included in the planned treatment volume. A portion of the tumour was definitely missed in eight patients and in 11 others tumour coverage was questionable. If the high-dose treatment volume had been increased from a volume of approximately 8 × 8 × 10 cm to 9 × 10 × 12 cm the number of geographic misses would have been reduced from over 33 per cent to 20 per cent and those with questionable coverage from 33 per cent to 10 per cent of the patients. Based on this analysis Concannon *et al.* recommended that large fields be used in the treatment of patients with malignant gliomas.[84] Kramer concluded that failure from radiation therapy could be due to inadequate tumour coverage and recommended that the entire intracranial contents be irradiated for glioblastomas (astrocytic gliomas grade III and IV).[85] Salazar *et al.* reported an improved survival in patients treated to the whole brain compared with those who had limited fields.[87] As a result of such recommendations and because of difficulties in defining tumour volume many of the major randomized clinical trials (including those of the BTSG and RTOG-ECOG) have utilized whole brain irradiation. However, the earlier studies cited above were performed prior to the availability of CT and MRI scans, which provide much improved information on the definition of the target volume.

Hochberg and Pruitt[88] compared CT scans performed within two months before death with postmortem findings and found the gross and microscopic margins of the tumour in 29 of 35 patients to be within 2 cm of that predicted from the CT scans. Only one of 35 autopsied patients showed microscopic infiltration more than 2 cm beyond the tumour margin as indicated by the CT scan. The major source of error was subependymal spread which occurred in 15 per cent of cases. Multicentricity occurred in 4 to 6 per cent of the patients and in each case was identified by pretreatment CT scan. Ninety per cent of 42 patients with glioblastoma studied by serial CT scan showed tumour recurrence within a 2 cm margin of the primary site.

Kelly *et al.* studied 40 previously untreated patients with intracranial gliomas with CT and MRI based stereotaxic serial biopsies.[89] Four distinct image volumetric zones were defined: (1) internal hypodensity within the zone of contrast enhancement; (2) the region of contrast enhancement; (3) a zone of hypodensity peripheral to the contrast enhancement on CT scan; and (4) a volume defined by T_2

prolongation on MRI scans which extended beyond the CT-defined volume. The contrast-enhancing region corresponded to tumour tissue, whereas the surrounding hypodensity represented parenchyma infiltrated by isolated tumour cells, tumour tissue in low-grade gliomas, or oedema without tumour. Isolated tumour cells within the brain parenchyma may be found at the periphery of the T_2 abnormalitiy on MRI scans.[89]

From the clinical standpoint there is no definite convincing evidence for the superiority of whole-brain irradiation over "generous volume" irradiation. Many reports failed to demonstrate an advantage of whole-brain irradiation over more limited fields. Sheline used limited fields and reported a median survival of 10 months for patients with glioblastoma multiforme,[90] a survival time comparable to that obtained in the BTSG and RTOG–ECOG studies in which whole-brain irradiation was used. Others have found that treating less than the total intracranial contents does not compromise results.[68, 91, 93, 94] Urtasun et al., using CT scanning for treatment planning, found no extension of tumour beyond the volume of irradiation in the 30 per cent of patients who had an autopsy.[95] In a recent Brain Tumour Cooperative Group protocol (8001) a portion of the patients received 60.2 Gy to the whole brain with concomitant chemotherapy while others received 43 Gy to the whole brain with an additional 17.2 Gy boost to the tumour-bearing volume. There was no difference in survival between the two treatment options.[79] These results, however, are of questionable significance since 43 Gy is probably insufficient to treat even microscopic glioblastoma multiforme effectively. Whole-brain irradiation is no longer being employed for malignant gliomas in most cooperative group studies.

At UCSF, our approach has been to treat malignant gliomas with large margins for uncertainty of distance of tumour infiltration beyond that identified by available diagnostic techniques. At present we utilized a margin of at least 3 cm beyond the enhancing volume on CT scans and 1 cm beyond the T_2-weighted MRI, whichever volume is larger. Supporting this approach, in addition to the above, is a recent review of multiplictiy and recurrence sites in 1047 patients (409 with glioblastoma multiforme and 638 with anaplastic gliomas) treated at UCSF from 1976 to 1985. Only 1.1 per cent of patients presented with multiple lesions. Following treatment, 4.4 per cent of patients with glioblastoma multiforme and 8.6 per cent with anaplastic gliomas developed a second lesion. More than 90 per cent of patients who had failed therapy died of recurrence at the site of the original tumour.[96]

As discussed above, patients surviving for extended periods following high-dose radiation therapy to the brain may develop a syndrome of progressive dementia, ventricular enlargement and pathological changes suggesting radiation damage.[75] Limiting the irradiated volume is important if, without missing tumour that might be controlled if irradiated, it permits avoidance of injury to tissues that would cause significant morbidity, loss of function or death. At least until we are better able to control tumour at the primary site and patterns of failure in such patients can be assessed, there seems little reason to treat the whole brain with the attendant morbidity thereof.

Selection of the proper dose for malignant gliomas has also been a subject of controversy. The question of optimal dose has been addressed in controlled clinical studies by the BTSG and by the RTOG–ECOG. In these trials the individual daily dose was 1.80–2.0 Gy which was given five days per week to total doses ranging from 45 to 70 Gy. Walker et al. analysed the data from 621 patients treated in three successive BTSG studies. The patients were divided into three groups with median doses of 50, 55, and 60 Gy. Patients in the three dose groups were comparable with respect to population characteristics including sex, age, percentage of patients with glioblastoma multiforme, interval from first symptom of treatment, initial performance status, and percentage of patients receiving chemotherapy. There was a stepwise prolongation in survival with dose; the median survival for 50 Gy was 28 weeks, compared with 36 weeks for 55 Gy and 42 weeks for 60 Gy. The median life span for patients receiving 60 Gy was 1.3 times longer than those receiving 50 Gy ($p = 0.004$). Since 90 per cent of the patients in the BTSG study had glioblastoma multiforme, this dose–response relationship applies to glioblastoma multiforme but not necessarily to other malignant gliomas. As detailed earlier in this review, the RTOG–ECOG prospectively compared 60 Gy whole irradiation to a 60 Gy whole-brain plus a boost of 10 Gy to the tumour volume. Survival for the 70 Gy regimen was not significantly better than for the lower dose.[80]

In a limited non-randomized trial Salazar *et al.* used radiation doses to limited boost fields as high as 80 Gy following 50–60 Gy to the whole brain.[5, 98] For patients with grade IV astrocytomas, there was a progressive increase in median survival associated with an increase in median dose from 52 to 60 to 75 Gy. The median survival for the three dose groups was 30, 42, and 56 weeks, respectively. The difference in survival between 52 Gy and 75 Gy was statistically significant. For grade III astrocytomas, there was also a statistically significant increase in median survival when the dose was increased from 52 to 58 to 74.5 Gy. However, there was no improvement in overall survival or local tumour control in the higher dose groups.[98] Because the total number of patients in the study was very small, the radiation doses were increased chronologically, distribution of patients by histology changed over time, and there was no consideration of the distribution of prognostic factors among the various dose groups, this study is of little value. Furthermore, it should not be inferred that large volumes of normal brain can be treated to doses of 70 to 80 Gy without incurring a substantial risk of injury. Salazar *et al.* observed a steady decline in performance status accompanied by general debilitation in patients who received the higher-dose radiation therapy. Furthermore, in their autopsy material, they found peritumoural radionecrosis in the region of the high-dose boost therapy.[98]

Based on the BTSG and RTOG–ECOG trials, the optimum dose for glioblastoma multiforme appears to be about 60 Gy when the radiation is given with daily single fractions of 1.8–2.0 Gy, five times per week. Presumably, the optimum dose for anaplastic astrocytomas is similar, but this is yet unproven. These data, tempered by concern for the adverse effects of irradiation, have led us to limit the total dose to 60 Gy for either anaplastic astrocytoma or glioblastoma multiforme when the radiation is conventionally fractionated.

New directions

Several new approaches have been or are being examined in an attempt to improve the efficacy of radiation therapy for malignant gliomas. These include the use of radiation sensitizers, heavy particle radiotherapy, unconventional radiation fractionation schemes, and interstitial brachytherapy. The use of interstitial brachytherapy is currently undergoing extensive study at the UCSF and the findings to date are reviewed below. Hyperthermia in conjunction with radiotherapy is also being investigated but these results are too preliminary for consideration at present.

Hypoxic, but viable, cells may be found in regions of coagulation necrosis present in glioblastoma multiforme. Hypoxia protects cells from irradiation. Hypoxic cells are up to three times more resistant to irradiation by low LET radiations (e.g. X-rays) than well-oxygenated cells, and hence require much larger photon doses to produce the same degree of cell kill that is achieved in oxygenated cells. In an effort to overcome the effects of hypoxia, hyperbaric oxygen during irradiation,[99] hypoxic cell radiation sensitizers,[100] and high linear energy transfer (LET) radiations*[101] have been employed. To date, none of these approaches has resulted in an improvement in survival rates over those produced by conventional radiotherapy. Except for the Vienna Study Group trial[102] in which the observed improvement in median survival with misonidozole may be due to an unequal distribution of prognostic variables between treatment groups, clinical trials testing the hypoxic cell radiation sensitizing drug misonidazole have failed to show a benefit.[78, 95, 103, 104]

Neutron irradiation using doses presumably biologically equivalent to conventional photon radiotherapy gave survival rates similar to those for X-rays.[105-108] The neutron irradiation increased the local tumour control rate; however, many patients died of radiation-induced brain injury and survival rates were not improved. Autopsy findings in the neutron-treated patients revealed a high rate of local tumour control but also an unexpectedly high rate of diffuse degenerative changes in the white matter, probably due to underestimation of the relative biological effectiveness (RBE) of neutrons.[108-110] Similarly preliminary trials with heavy-ion radiotherapy have proved ineffective.

Halogenated pyrimidines are radiosensitizers that appear to act independently of the oxygen effect. When incorporated into DNA in place of thymidine before irradiation, they increase the radiation effect two- to three-fold. A differential effect between tumour and normal cells might be expected when the tumour cells undergo division more rapidly then the slowly dividing endothelial and stromal cells and the non-dividing normal glial cells.[111] The intravenous infusion before irradiation of halogenated pyrimidines, including 5-bromo-2-deoxyuridine (BUdR) and 5-iodo-2-deoxyuridine (IUdR), are under investigation in phase I–II studies.[112-114]

The radiation tolerance of normal glial and vascular tissues determines to a large extent the amount of radiation that can be delivered to a brain tumour. Compared with neoplastic glioma cells, these tissues exhibit a low or zero rate of cell division. The neoplastic glioma cells going through proliferation are more likely than normal cells to be exposed to radiation during the most radiosensitive phase of the cell cycle. The likelihood of exposure during such sensitive parts of the proliferation cycle is increased by delivering a greater number of fractions of radiation. It also is thought that with an increased number of (smaller) fractions, the less proliferative normal glial cells will have a greater capacity for repair of sublethal radiation injury than will glioma tissue; this assumes that the latter undergo proliferation at a more rapid rate. Furthermore, since the oxygen effect decreases with decreasing dose per fraction, increasing the number of fractions should yield a relatively greater effect on (radio-resistent) hypoxic tumour cells than on well-oxygenated normal cells. For these various reasons increasing the number of fractions, i.e. hyperfractionation, might be

*Hypoxia does not protect against high LET radiations.

expected to increase the difference between the survival of normal and tumour cells exposed to a given total radiation dose.[111]

The reported results for clinical trials employing hyperfractionated irradiation in patients with malignant gliomas have been variable.[111] Payne et al.,[93] Shin et al.,[115] and the BTSG[78] failed to find a significant improvement in the overall median survival; however, in each of these studies the total doses were relatively low. Others, however, have demonstrated a significant increase in both time to tumour progression and overall survival for patients treated with hyperfractionated radiation. Douglas and Worth treated 30 patients with astrocytoma grade III, astrocytoma grade IV, or glioblastoma multiforme with three 1 Gy fractions per day.[116] Survival with the hyperfractionated radiotherapy was significantly longer than that for conventionally treated historical controls. However, the small number of patients, use of historical control groups and failure to control prognostic variables make this trial difficult to interpret. Fulton et al. suggested that hyperfractionation plus acceleration (reduction of overall treatment time) may improve survival.[117] A regimen of 89 Gy three times per day (with or without misonidozole) to a total of 61.4 Gy (over 4.5 weeks) was compared with a course of 1.93 Gy once per day to a total of 58 Gy (over 6 weeks). The median survival for conventional fractionation was 29 weeks vs. 45 and 50 weeks for the two treatment options using multiple daily fractionation; the difference was significant ($p = 0.002$). Even though the survival time for patients receiving conventional fractionation was unusually low, this is the most convincing study of the value of hyperfractionation. The RTOG has designed its current studies to test the concept of hyperfractionation using 1.2 Gy twice per day, to total doses escalating upward until normal tissue tolerance has been reached; therefore, these studies should be able to assess clinically the possible advantages of hyperfractionation.[111] Wara and his colleagues have administered doses of 72 Gy at 1 Gy twice per day to patients with brain stem gliomas.[118] There have been no cases of radiation induced injury in 53 patients, but only two cases had an autopsy. A total dose of 78 Gy is currently being employed.

Interstitial brachytherapy has been employed at UCSF since 1980 for the treatment of recurrent, and, more recently, previously untreated malignant gliomas. The rationale is largely based on the observation that malignant gliomas recur locally rather than distantly and, therefore, should benefit from more intensive local therapy that avoids significant exposure of adjacent normal structures.[119] Also, compared with external beam radiotherapy the dose rates are relatively low, and hence, the theoretical advantages of hyperfractionation might be expected to extend to brachytherapy. Several radioactive isotopes have been employed for brain tumour brachytherapy. However, in recent years iodine-125 (^{125}I) and iridium-192 (^{192}Ir) have been used most frequently. We generally employ radioactive sources afterloaded into removable catheters inserted into the tumour. Such interstitial implantation is done using a CT-directed stereotaxic technique. CT stereotaxy allows detailed treatment planning and superior implant accuracy. Computer programs that yield implant coordinates for optimum isodose coverage are available for stereotaxic treatment planning.[119]

An analysis of the initial 41 patients with recurrent malignant gliomas treated by interstitial brachytherapy with doses of 80–120 Gy at UCSF revealed partial or complete responses of five to 53 months duration in 21 patients. Response was determined by either a reduction in tumour size on CT scan or clinical improvement with stable or decreasing dose of corticosteriods. Analysis of the response data showed that because of inability to differentiate tumour regrowth from focal radiation necrosis either clinically or by CT scan, the usual criteria for the evaluation of patients undergoing therapy cannot be used to evaluate the effects of high-dose re-irradiation brachytherapy. Response or failure to respond was not a reliable predictor of survival. Patients who showed clinical or CT evidence of progression or failure to respond, as judged by traditional criteria, often had focal necrosis and, after its removal, did well in terms of survival.[120] As of March 1986, 77 patients with recurrent malignant brain tumours had undergone interstitial implantation at UCSF with high activity (usually $\geq$ 40 mCi)[125] I sources. At the time of analysis 45 per cent of patients with anaplastic astrocytoma (AA) were alive (median follow-up 13 months) and 34 per cent of patients with glioblastoma multiforme (GBM) were alive (median follow-up 9 months). The two-year survival after retreatment for patients with recurrent AA was 49 per cent compared with 26 per cent for patients with GBM. Thirty-five per cent of the patients underwent post-implantation craniotomy. The time to reoperation ranged from nine to 80 weeks with a median of 34 weeks. The histopathological findings at reoperation were not predictive of outcome. Those patients undergoing reoperation however, had a significant improvement of survival compared with those patients not undergoing reoperation. Several patients who had necrosis but no histological evidence of active tumour have had survivals ranging up to more than six years after treatment for recurrent glioblastoma multiforme.[121]

Encouraged by the results in patients with recurrent malignant gliomas, a phase II study integrating interstitial implantation into the primary management of patients with malignant gliomas has been initiated.[121] Treatment consists of partial brain external-beam irradiation to a dose of 60 Gy in six to seven weeks combined with hydroxyurea (300 mg/m^2 q6h every other day) followed by an interstitial implant delivering an additional dose of 50 to 60 Gy to a volume 0.5 cm beyond the enhancing lesion on CT. Radiation therapy is followed by a one-year course of chemotherapy consisting of CCNU (110 mg/m^2, day 1), procarbazine (16 mg/m^2, days 8–21), and vincristine (1.4 mg/m^2, days 8–29). As of Januray 1987, 49 patients had been entered into this study. Although it is too early for more than a preliminary evaluation, at present the median survival for patients with anaplastic astrocytoma is 35 months and for glioblastoma multiforme 22 months. When compared with historical controls matched by age, performance status, and histology, patients with glioblastoma multiforme appear to have almost a doubling of median survival (13 *vs.* 22 months) but there is little improvement evident for patient with anaplastic astrocytomas.[122]

Summary

The available data on the use of radiation therapy for the low-grade astrocytoma suggest that postoperative radiation therapy favorably influences the outcome of patients harboring these neoplasms. Until recently there has been a total lack of randomized prospective trials evaluating the efficacy of radiation therapy for these tumours. Randomized studies which address many of the important issues in the treatment of low-grade astrocytomas have begun both in Europe and the United States. These studies examine the timing of radiation therapy (immediate *vs.*

delayed) radiation dose, the use of chemotherapy, and the quality of life using different treatment schemes. Retrospective studies, however, show that with current treatment regimens these "low-grade" astrocytomas, although slowly progressive, are highly lethal and that more effective treatment strategies will be needed, if survival is to be improved.

Randomized studies have demonstrated that, as measured by median and two- or three-year survival, postoperative conventional radiation therapy influences the outcome of patients with malignant gliomas favourably. In selected patients the addition of chemotherapy results in a prolongation of survival by increasing the number of long-term survivors. Additional randomized studies exploring optimally hyperfractionated (optimum fractionation, total dose and overall time) irradiation and interstitial irradiation are needed as well as continued exploration of new agents which selectively sensitize malignant gliomas to radiation therapy. Additionally, a better understanding of the mechanism of radiation injury could lead to the development of new radioprotective agents which would allow the delivery of more effective radiotherapy without the associated risk of prohibitive normal tissue injury.

Acknowledgements

This work was supported by PHS RTOG Grant #CA-21439 awarded by National Cancer Institute, DHHS.

The authors gratefully acknowledge Ms Margaret Britton for her excellent secretarial assistance.

References

1. Kramer S. The hazards of therapeutic irradiation of the central nervous system. *Clinical Neurosurgery*. 1968; **15**, 301-18.
2. Sheline GE, Wara WM, Smith V. Therapeutic irradiation and brain injury. *International Journal of Radiation Oncology, Biology, Physics*. 1980; **6**, 1215-28.
3. Leibel SA, Sheline GE. Tolerance of the central and peripheral nervous system to therapeutic irradiation. In: Lett JT, Altman KI, eds. *Advances in Radiation Biology*. New York: Academic Press, Inc., 1987: 257-88.
4. Deck MDF. Imaging techniques in the diagnosis of radiation damage to the nervous system. In: Gilbert HA, Kagan RA, eds. *Radiation Damage to the Nervous System. A Delayed Therapeutic Hazard*. New York: Raven Press, 1980: 107-27.
5. Salazar OM, Rubin P, McDonald JV, Feldstein ML. High dose radiation therapy in the treatment of glioblastoma multiforme: a preliminary report. *International Journal of Radiation Oncology, Biology, Physics*. 1976; **1**, 717-27.
6. Leibel SA, Sheline GE. Radiation therapy for neoplasms of the brain. *Journal of Neurosurgery*. 1987; **66**, 1-22.
7. Hindo WA, DeTrana FA III, Lee MS, Hendrickson FR. Large dose increment irradiation in the treatment of cerebral metastases. *Cancer*. 1970; **26**, 138-41.
8. Young DF, Posner JB, Chu F, Nesce L. Rapid-course radiation therapy of cerebral metastases: Results and complications. *Cancer*. 1974; **34**, 1069-76.
9. Hoffman WF, Levin VA, Wilson CB. Evaluation of malignant glioma patients during the post-irradiation period. *Journal of Neurosurgery*. 1979; **50**, 624-28.
10. Edwards MS, Wilson CB. Treatment of radiation necrosis. In: Gilbert HA,

Kagan AR, eds. *Radiation Damage to the Nervous System. A Delayed Therapeutic Hazard*. New York: Raven Press, 1980: 129-43.
11. Groothuis DR, Vick NA. Radionecrosis of the central nervous system: The perspective of the clinical neurologist and neuropathologist. In: Gilbert HA, Kagan AR, eds. *Radiation Damage to the Nervous System. A Delayed Therapeutic Hazard*. New York: Raven Press, 1980: 93-106.
12. Boldrey E, Sheline GE. Delayed transitory clinical manifestations after radiation treatment of intracranial tumours. *Acta Radiolociga (Therapy, Biology, Physics)*. 1966; **5**, 5-10.
13. Brant-Zawadzki MB, Anderson M, DeArmond SJ, Conley FK, Jahnke RW. Radiation-induced large intracranial vessel occlusive vasculopathy. *American Journal of Roentgenology*. 1980; **134**, 51-5.
14. Marus G, Levin CV, Rutherford SG. Malignant glioma following radiotherapy for unrelated primary tumours. *Cancer*. 1986; **58**, 886-94.
15. Fike JR, Sheline GE, Cann CE, David RL. Radiation necrosis. *Progress in Experimental Tumour Research*. 1984; **28**, 136-51.
16. Martins AN, Johnston IS, Henry JM, Stoffel TJ, DiChiro. Delayed radiation necrosis of the brain. *Journal of Neurosurgery*. 1977; **47**, 336-45.
17. Yoshii Y, Phillips TL. Late vascular effect of whole brain X-irradiation in the mouse. *Acta Neurochirugica*. 1982; **64**, 87-102.
18. Manz HJ, Woolley PV, Ornitz RD. Delayed radiation necrosis of brainstem related to fast neutron beam irradiation. *Cancer*. 1979; **44**, 473-79.
19. Ang KK, Van der Kogel AJ, van der Shueren E. Lack of evidence for increased tolerance of rat spinal cord with decreasing fractions doses below 2 Gy. *International Journal of Radiation Oncology, Biology, Physics*. 1985; **11**, 105-10.
20. Marks JE, Baylan RJ, Prassad SC, Blank WF. Cerebral radionecrosis: Incidence and risk in relation to disease, time, fractionation, and volume. *International Journal of Radiation Oncology, Biology, Physics*. 1981; **7**, 243-52.
21. Kornblith PL, Walker MD, Cassady JR. Neoplasms of the central nervous system. In: Devita VT Jr, Hellman S, Rosenberg, eds. *Principles and Practice of Oncology*. Philadelphia: Lippincott, 1982: 1181-1253.
22. Aristizabal SA, Boone ML, Laguna J. Endocrine factors influencing radiation injury of central nervous tissue. *International Journal of Radiation, Oncology, Biology, Physics*. 1979; **5**, 349-53.
23. Bloom JB, Kramer S. In: Black PMcL, Zervas NT, Ridgway EC, Martin JB, eds. *Secretory Tumours of the Pituitary Gland*. New York: Raven Press, 1984; 179-90.
24. Smith BM, McGinnis W, Cook J, Latourette H. Central nervous system changes complicating the use of radiotherapy for the treatment of a nasopharyngeal neoplasm in a diabetic patient. *Cancer*. 1979; **43**, 2239-42.
25. Cumberlin RL, Luk KH, Wara WM, Sheline GE, Wilson CB. Medullblastoma. Treatment results and effect on normal tissues. *Cancer*. 1979; **43**, 1014-20.
26. Bleyer WA. Neurologic sequelae of methotrexate and ionizing irradiaton: A new classification. *Cancer Treatment Reports*. 1981; **65**, (suppl.), 89-98.
27. Pratt RA, DeChiro G, Weed JC. Cerebral necrosis following irradiation and chemotherapy for metastatic choriocarcinoma. *Surgical Neurology*. 1977; **7**, 117-120.
28. Burger PC, Mahale MS Jr, Dudka L, Vogel FS: The morphologic effects of radiation administration therapeutically for intracranial gliomas. A post mortem study of 25 cases. *Cancer*. 1979; **44**, 1256-72.
29. Foo SH, Hiesiger E, Wise A, Ransohoff J, George A, Lin J, Newall, J. Quality of long term survival of treated patients with malignant glioma. *Proceedings of ASCO*, 1986; **5**, 136.
30. Mikhael MA. In: Gilbert HA, Kagan AR, eds. *Radiation Damage to the Nervous System*. New York: Raven Press, 1980; 59-91.

31. Davis PC, Hoffman JC, Pearl GS, Braun IF. CT evaluation of effects of cranial radiation therapy in children. *American Journal of Roentgenology*. 1986; **147**, 587–92.
32. Curnes JT, Laster DW, Ball MR, Moody DM, Witcofski RL. MRI of radiation injury to the brain. *American Journal of Roentgenology*. 1986; **147**, 119–24.
33. Curran WJ, Hecht-Levitt C, Nelson DF, Schut L, Zimmerman RA. Evaluation of MRI findings of radiation effects following cranial irradiation (meeting abstract). *American Journal of Clinical Oncology*. 1986; **9**, 101.
34. Packer RJ, Zimmerman RA, Bilaniuk LT. Magnetic resonance imaging in the evaluation of treatment related central nervous system damage. *Cancer*, 1986; **58**, 635–40.
35. Patronas NJ, DiChiro G, Brooks, RA, DeLaPaz RL, Kornblith PL, Smith BH, Rizzoli HV, Kessler RM, Manning RG, Channing M, Wolf AP, O'Connor C. [^{18}F] fluorodeoxyglucose and position emission tomography in the evaluation of radionecrosis of the brain. *Radiology*. 1982; **144**, 885–89.
36. Fike JR, Cann CE. Contrast medium accumulation and washout in canine brain tumours and irradiated normal brain: A CT study of kinetics. *Radiology*. 1984; **151**, 115–20.
37. Eiser C. Intellectual abilities among survivors of childhood leukaemia as a function of CNS irradiation. *Archieves of Diseases of the Child*. 1978; **53**, 391–95.
38. Kun LE, Mulhern RK, Crisco J. Quality of life in children treated for brain tumours. *Journal of Neurosurgery*. 1983; **58**, 1–6.
39. Danoff BF, Cowch S, Marquette C, Mulgrew L, Kramer S. Assessment of the long-term effects of primary radiation therapy for brain tumours in children. *Cancer*. 1982; **49**, 1580–86.
40. Hirsch JF, Renier D, Czernichow P, Benvenist L, Pierre-Kahn A. Medulloblastoma in childhood survival and functional results. *Acta Neurochirugica*. 1979; **48**, 1–15.
41. Esseltine DW, Tarshish E, Schulpen AE, Chevalier L, Whitehead VM. Cognitive function in long survivors of childhood acute lymphoblastic leukemia. *Proceedings of ASCO*. 1983; **2**, 74.
42. Meadows AT, Gordon J, Massari DJ, Littman P, Fergusson J, Moss K. Declines in IQ scores and cognitive dysfunctions in children with acute lymphocytic leukaemia treated with cranial irradiation. *Lancet*. 1981; **2**, 1015–1018.
43. Moss HA, Nannis ED, Poplack DG. The effects of prophylactic treatment of the central nervous system on the intellectual functioning of children with acute lymphocytic leukemia. *American Journal of Medicine*. 1981; **71**, 47–52.
44. Duffner PK, Cohen ME, Thomas P. Late effects of treatment on the intelligence of children with posterior fossa tumours. *Cancer*. 1983; **51**, 233–37.
45. Hochberg FH, Slotnick B. Neuropsychologic impairment in astrocytomas survivors. *Neurology*. 1980; **30**, 172–77.
46. Spunberg JJ, Chang GH, Goldman M, Auricchio E, Bell JJ. Quality of long-term survival following irradiation for intracranial tumours in children under the age of two. *International Journal of Radiation Oncology, Biology, Physics*. 1981; **7**, 727–36.
47. Tamaroff M, Salwen R, Miller DR, Murphy ML, Nir Y. Comparison of past therapy neuropsychologic performance in irradiation and nonirradiated children with acute lymphoblastic leukemia. *Proceedings of ASCO*. 1985; **4**, 165.
48. Ellison N, Bernath A, Kane R, Porter P. Disturbing problems of success: Clinical status of long-term survivors of small cell lung cancer (SCLC). *Proceedings of ASCO*. 1982; **1**, 149.
49. Licciardello J, Bromer R, Karp D, Hoffer S, Paquette D, Hong W. Delayed neurotoxicity (DN) after prophylactic cranial irradiation (PCXRT) or mediastinal irradiation with chemotherapy for patients with small cell lung cancer morbidity in long-term survivors of small cell carcinoma of lung. *Proceedings of ASCO*. 1983; **2**, 189.

50. Volk SA, Mansour RP, Gandara DR, Redmond J. Morbidity in long-term survivors of small cell carcinoma of the lung. *Proceedings of ASCO.* 1983; **2**, 185.
51. Maire J PH, Coudin B, Guerin J, Caudry M. Neuropsychologic impairment in adults with brain tumours. *American Journal of Clinical Oncology.* 1987; **10**(2), 156-62.
52. Bailey P, Cushing H. *A Classification of the Tumours of the Gliomas Group in a Histogenic Basis with a Correlated Study of Prognosis.* Philadelphia: JB Lippincott, 1926.
53. Rubinstein LJ. Tumours of the central nervous system. *Atlas of Tumour Pathology,* Series 2. Washington: DC Armed Forces Institute of Pathology, 1972; 7-17.
54. Russell DS, Rubenstein LJ. *Pathology of Tumours of the Nervous System.* Baltimore: Williams and Wilkins, 1977; 152-72, 226-44.
55. Burger PC, Vogel FS. *Surgical Pathology of the Nervous System and its Coverings.* New York: John Wiley and Sons, 1976; 191-222.
56. Kernohan JW, Mabon RF, Suien HJ, Adsun AW. A simplified classification of the gliomas. *Proceedings of Meetings of the Mayo Clinic.* 1949; **24**, 71-5.
57. Kernohan JW, Sayre GP. Tumours of the central nervous system. *Atlas of Tumour Pathology,* Section 10 Fascicle 35. Washington DC: Armed Forces Institute of Pathology, 1952.
58. Nelson JS, Schoenfeld D, Tsukada Y, Fulling K, Lamarche J, Peress N. Necrosis as a prognostic criterion in malignant supratentorial, astrocytic gliomas. *Cancer.* 1983; **52**, 550-54.
59. Svien HS, Mabon RF, Kernohan JW, Adson AW. Astrocytomas. *Proceedings of the Staff Meetings of the Mayo Clinic.* 1949; **24**, 54-64.
60. Laws ER, Taylor WF, Clifton MB, Okazaki H. Neurosurgical management of low-grade astrocytoma of the cerebral hemispheres. *Journal of Neurosurgery.* 1984; **61**, 665-73.
61. Fazekas JT. Treatment of grades I and II brain astrocytomas. The role of radiotherapy. *International Journal of Radiation Oncology, Biology, Physics.* 1977; **2**, 661-66.
62. Chang CH, Horton J, Schoenfeld D, Salazer O, Perez-Tamayo, Kramer S, Weinstein A, Nelson JS, Tsukada Y. Comparison of postoperative radiotherapy and combined postoperative radiotherapy and chemotherapy in the multidisciplinary management of malignant gliomas. *Cancer.* 1983; **52**, 997-1007.
63. Sheline, GE. The importance of distinguishing tumour grade in malignant gliomas: Treatment and prognosis. *International Journal of Radiation Oncology, Biology, Physics.* 1976; **1**, 781-86.
64. Lui HC, Davis RL, Vestnys P, Resser KJ, Levin VA. Correlation of survival and diagnosis in supratentorial malignant gliomas. *Journal of Neuro-oncology.* 1984; **2**, 268.
65. Sheline GE. The role of radiation therapy in the treatment of low-grade gliomas. *Clinical Neurosurgery.* 1986; **33**, 563-74.
66. Leibel SA, Sheline GE, Wara WM, Boldrey EB, Nielsen SL. The role of radiation therapy in the treatment of astrocytomas. *Cancer.* 1975; **36**, 1551-57.
67. Marsa GW, Goffinet DR, Rubinstein LJ, Bagshaw MA. Megavoltage irradiation in the treatment of gliomas of the brain and spinal cord, *Cancer.* 1975; **36**, 1781-89.
68. Scanlon PW, Taylor WF. Radiotherapy of intracranial astrocytomas: Analysis of 417 cases treated from 1960 through 1969. *Neurosurgery.* 1979; **5**, 301-8.
69. Dewit L, Van Der Schueren E, Ang KK, Van Den Bergh R, Dom R, Brucher JM. Low grade astrocytomas in children treated by surgery and radiation therapy. *Acta Radiologica.* 1984; **23**, 1-8.
70. Piepmeier JM. Observations on the current treatment of low-grade astrocytic tumours of the cerebral hemispheres. *Journal of Neurosurgery.* 1987; **67**, 177-81.
71. Bloom HJG. Intracranial tumours: Response and resistance to therapeutic endeavors, 1970-1980. *International Journal of Radiation Oncology, Biology, Physics.* 1982; **8**, 1083-113.

72. Wallner KE, Gonzales MF, Sheline GE, Wara WM, Edwards MSB. Treatment results of juvenile pilocytic astrocytoma. *Journal of Neurosurgery*, in press.
73. Walker MD, Alexander E, Hunt WE, MacCarty CS, Mahaley MS, Mealey J, Norrell HA, Owens G, Ransohoff J, Wilson CB, Gehan EA, Strike TA. Evaluation of BCNU and/or radiotherapy in the treatment of anaplastic gliomas. *Journal of Neurosurgery*. 1978; **49**, 333–43.
74. Kristiansen K, Hagen S, Kollevold T, Torvik A, Holme I, Nesbakken R, Hatlevoll R, Lindgren M, Brun A, Lindgren S, Notter G, Andersen AP, Elgen K. Combined modality therapy of operated astrocytomas grade III and IV. Confirmation of the value of postoperative irradiation and lack of potentiation of bleomycin on survival time: A prospective multicenter trial of the Scandinavian glioblastoma study group. *Cancer*. 1981; **47**, 649–52.
75. Shapiro WR. Therapy of adult malignant brain tumour: What have the clinical trials taught us? *Seminars in Oncology*. 1986; **13**, 38–45.
76. Walker MD, Green SB, Byar DP, Alexander E, Batzdorf U, Brooks, WH, Hunt WE, MacCarty CS, Mahaley MS, Mealey J, Owens G, Ransohoff J, Robertson JT, Shapiro WR, Smith KR, Wilson CB, Strike TA. Randomized comparisons of radiotherapy and nitrosoureas for the treatment of malignant glioma after surgery. *New England Journal of Medicine*. 1980; **303**, 1323–29.
77. Green SB, Byar DP, Walker MD, Pistenmaa DA, Alexander E, Batzdorf U, Brooks WH, Hunt WE, Mealey J, Odom GL, Paoletti P, Ransohoff J, Robertson JT, Selker RG, Shapiro WR, Smith KR, Wilson CB, Strike TA. Comparisons of carmustine, procarbazine, and high-dose methylprednisolone as additions to surgery and radiotherapy for the treatment of malignant glioma. *Cancer Treatment Reports*. 1983; **67**, 121–32.
78. Green SB, Byar DP, Strike TA, Alexander E, Brooks WH, Burger PC, Hunt WE, Mealey J, Odom GL, Paoletti P, Pistenmaa DA, Ransohoff J, Robertson JT, Selker RG, Shapiro WR, Smith KR. Randomized comparisons of BCNU, streptozotocin, radiosensitizer, and fractionation of radiotherapy in the post-operative treatment of malignant glioma. *Proceedings of ASCO*. 1984; **3**, 260.
79. Green SB, Byar DB, Strike TA, Burger PC, Mahaley MS, Mealey J, Pistenma DA, Ransohoff J, Robertson JT, Selker RG, Shapiro WR, VanGilder JD. Randomized comparisons of single or multiple drug chemotherapy combined with either whole brain or whole brain plus coned-down boost radiotherapy for the post-operative treatment of maglignant gliomas. *Proceedings of ASCO*. 1986; **5**, 135.
80. Nelson DF, Diener-West M, Horton J, Chang CH, Shoenfeld D, Nelson JS. Combined modality approach to treatment of malignant gliomas. Reevaluation of RTOG 7401/ECOG 1374 with long-term follow-up. *NCI Monograph*, in press.
81. Levin VA, Wilson CB, Davis R, Wara WM, Pischer TL, Irwin L. A phase III comparison of BCNU, hydroxyurea, and radiation therapy to BCNU and radiation therapy for treatment of primary malignant gliomas. *Journal of Neurosurgery*. 1979; **51**, 526–32.
82. Byar DP, Green SB, Strike TA. Prognostic factors for malignant glioma. In: Walker MD, ed. *Oncology of the Nervous System*. Boston: Martinus Nijhoff Publishers, 1983: 379–95.
83. Nelson DF, Nelson JS, Davis DR, Chang CH, Griffin TW, Pajak TF. Survival and prognosis with atypical or anaplastic features. *Journal of Neuro-oncology*. 1985; **99**, 99–103.
84. Concannan JP, Kramer S, Berry R. The extent of intracranial gliomas at autopsy and its relationship to techniques used in radiation therapy of brain tumours. *American Journal of Roentgenology*. 1960; **99**, 99–107.
85. Kramer S. Tumour extent as a determining factor in radiotherapy of glioblastomas. *Acta Radiologica* (Therapy Physics Biology). 1969; **8**, 111–7.

86. Salazar OM, Rubin P. The spread of glioblastoma multiforme as a determining factor in the radiation treated volume. *International Journal of Radiation Oncology, Biology, Physics.* 1976; **1**, 627-37.
87. Salazar OM, Rubin P, McDonald JV, Feldstein ML. Patterns of failure in intracranial astrocytomas after irradiation: Analysis of dose and field factors. *Amercian Journal of Roentgenology.* 1976; **126**, 279-92.
88. Hochberg FH, Pruitt A. Assumptions in the radiotherapy of glioblastomas. *Neurology.* 1980; **30**, 907-11.
89. Kelly PJ, Daumas-Duport C, Kispert DB, Kall BA, Scheithauer BW, Illig JJ. Imaging-based stereotaxic serial biopsies in untreated intracranial glial neoplasms. *Journal of Neurosurgery.* 1987; **66**; 865-74.
90. Sheline GE. Radiation therapy of primary tumours. *Seminars in Oncology.* 1975; **2**, 29-42.
91. Fossati F, Jucker C, Tosi G. Effect of field size and unconventional dose fractionation in the radiotherapy of malignant cerebral gliomas. In: Paoletti P, Walker MD, Butti G, et al., eds. *Multidisciplinary Aspects of Brain Tumour Therapy.* Amsterdam: North-Holland, 1979: 106-15.
92. Onoyama Y, Abe M, Yabumoto E, Sakamoto T, Nishidai T, Suyama S. Radiation therapy in the treatment of glioblastoma. *American Journal of Roentgenology.* 1967; **126**, 481-92.
93. Payne D, Simpson WJ, Keen C. Platts M. Malignant astrocytoma: Hyperfractionated and standard radiotherapy with chemotherapy in a randomized prospective clinical trial. *Cancer.* 1982; **50**, 2301-6.
94. Ramsey RG, Brand WN. Radiotherapy of glioblastoma multiforme. *Journal of Neurosurgery.* 1973; **39**, 197-202.
95. Urtasun R, Feldstein ML, Patington J, Tanasichuk H, Miller JDR, Russell DB, Agboola O, Mielke B. Radiation and nitromidazoles in supratentorial high grade gliomas: A second clinical trial. *British Journal of Cancer.* 1982; **46**, 101-7.
96. Choucair AK, Levin VA, Gutin PH, Davis RL, Silver P, Edwards MSB, Wilson CB. Development of multiple lesions during radiation therapy and chemotherapy in patients with gliomas. *Journal of Neurosurgery.* 1986; **65**, 654-58.
97. Walker MD, Strike TA, Sheline GE. An analysis of dose-effect relationship in the radiotherapy of malignant gliomas. *International Journal of Radiation Oncology, Biology, Physics.* 1979; **5**, 1725-31.
98. Salazar OM, Rubin P Feldstein ML, Pizzutiello R. High dose radiation therapy in the treatment of malignant gliomas: Final report. *International Journal of Radiation Onology, Biology, Physics.* 1979; **5**, 1733-40.
99. Chang CH. Hyperbaric oxygen and radiation therapy in the management of glioblastoma. *National Cancer Institute Monographs.* 1977; **46**, 163-9.
100. Gutin PH, Wara WM, Phillips TL, Wilson CB. Hypoxic cell radiosensitizers in the treatment of malignant brain tumours. *Neurosurgery.* 1980; **6**, 567-76.
101. Castro JR, Saunders WM, Tobias CA, Chen GTY, Curtis S, Lyman JT, Collier JM, Pitluck S, Woodruff KA, Blakely EA, Tenforde T, Char D, Phillips TL, Alpen EL. Treatment of cancer with heavy charged particles. *International Journal of Radiation Oncology, Biology.* 1982; **8**, 2191-98.
102. Stadler B, Karcher KH, Kogelnik HD, *et al.* Misonidazole and irradiation in the treatment of glioblastoma multiforme: Preliminary report of the Vienna study group. *International Journal of Radiation Oncology, Biology, Physics.* 1984; **10**, 1713-17.
103. Bleehen NM, Wiltshire CR, Plowman PN, Watson JV, Gleave JRW, Holmes AE, Lewin WS, Treip CS, Hawkins TD. A randomized study of misonidazole and radiotherapy for grade 3 and 4 cerebral astrocytoma. *British Journal of Cancer.* 1981; **43**, 436-42.
104. Nelson DF, Diener-West M, Weinstein AS, Schenfeld D, Nelson JS, Sause WT,

Chang CH, Goodman R, Carabell S. A randomized comparison of misonidazole sensitized radiotherapy plus BCNU for treatment of malignant glioma after surgery: Final report of RTOG study. *International Journal of Radiation Oncology, Biology, Physics.* 1986; **12**, 1793-800.
105. Catterall M, Bloom HJ, Ash DV, Walsh L, Richardson A, Uttley D, Gowing NFC, Lewis P, Chaucer B. Fast neutrons compared with megavoltage X-rays in the treatment of patients with supratentorial glioblastoma: A controlled protocol study. *International Journal of Radiation Oncology, Biology, Physics.* 1980; **6**, 261-66.
106. Duncan W, McLelland J, Jack JL, Arnott SJ, Gordon A, Kerr GR, Williams JR. Report of a randomized pilot study of the treatment of patients with supratentorial gliomas using neutron irradiation. *British Journal of Radiology.* 1986; **59**, 373-7.
107. Duncan W, McLelland J, Jack JL, Arnott SJ, Davey P, Gordon A, Kerr GR, Williams JR. The results of a randomised trial of mixed-schedule (neutron/photon) irradiation in the treatment of supratentorial grade III and grade IV astrocytoma. *British Journal of Radiology.* 1986; **59**, 379-83.
108. Griffin TW, Davis R, Laramore G, Hendrickson F, Rodrigues-Antunez A, Hussey D, Nelson J. Fast neutron radiation therapy for glioblastoma multiforme. *American Journal of Clinical Oncology.* 1983; **6**, 661-7.
109. Hornsey S, Morris CC, Meyers R, White A. Radiation biologic effectiveness for damage to the central nervous system by neutrons. *International Journal of Radiation Oncology, Biology, Physics.* 1980; **7**, 185-9.
110. Parker RG, Berry HC, Gerdes AJ, Soronen MD, Shaw CM. Fast neutron beam radiotherapy of glioblastoma multiforme. *American Journal of Roentgenology.* 1976; **127**, 331-5.
111. Nelson DF, Urtasun RC, Saunders WM, Gutin PH, Sheline GE. Recent and current investigations of radiation therapy of malignant gliomas. *Seminars in Oncology.* 1986; **13**, 46-55.
112. Phuphanich S, Levin E, Levin V. Phase I study of intravenous bromodeoxyuridine used concomitantly with radiation therapy in patients with primary malignant brain tumours. *International Journal of Radiation Oncology, Biology, Physics.* 1984; **10**, 1769-72.
113. Kinsella TJ, Russo, A Mitchell JB, Rowland J, Jenkins J, Schwade J, Myers CE, Collins JM, Speyer J, Kornblith P, Smith B, Kufta C, Glatstein E. A phase I study of intermittent intravenous bromodeoxyuridine (BUdR) with conventional fractionated irradiation. *International Journal of Radiation Oncology, Biology, Physics.* 1984; **10**, 69-76.
114. Kinsella TJ, Russo A, Mitchell JB, Russo A, Aiken M, Mortyn G, Hsu SM, Rowlands J, Glatstein E, Miller PJ, Moody J, Tanasichuk H, Mielke B, Johnson E, Curry B. The use of prolonged constant intravenous infusions of bromodeoxyuridine (BUdR) as a radiosensitizer. *Journal of Clinical Oncology.* 1984; **2**, 1144-50.
115. Shin KH, Muller PJ, Geggie PHS. Suprafractionation radiation therapy in the treatment of malignant astrocytoma. *Cancer.* 1983; **52**, 2040-3.
116. Douglas BG, Worth AJ. Suprafractionation in glioblastoma multiforme – results of a phase II study. *International Journal of Radiation Oncology, Biology, Physics.* 1982; **8**, 1782-94.
117. Fulton DS, Urtasun RC, Shin KH, Geggie PHS, Thomas H. Misonidazole combined with hyperfractionation in the management of malignant gliomas. *International Journal of Radiation Oncology, Biology, Physics.* 1984; **10**, 1709-12.
118. Wara, WM. Personal communication, 1987.
119. Leibel SA, Gutin PH. Stereotaxic interstitial implantation for the treatment of malignant brain tumours. In: Phillips TL, Wara WM, eds. *Radiation Oncology.* Vol. 2. New York: Raven Press, 1987: 73-90.
120. Gutin PH, Leibel SA, Wara WM, Chouchair A, Levin VA, Phillips TL,

Silver P, Da Silva V, Edwards M, Davis RL, Weaver KA, Lamb S. Recurrent malignant gliomas improved survival following interstitial brachytherapy with high activity iodine-125 sources. *Journal of Neurosurgery* 1987; **67**, 864–873.

121. Leibel SA, Gutin PH, Phillips TL, Wara WM, Levin V, Hannigan J, Silver P, Weaver K. The integration of interstitial implantation into the primary management of patients with malignant gliomas: Results of a phase II Northern California oncology group trial. *American Journal of Clinical Oncology*. 1987; **10**, 106.
122. Leibel SA, Gutin PH. Unpublished data, 1987.

13 Chemotherapy for malignant gliomas in adults

Edward J Dropcho and M Stephen Mahaley

Introduction

The poor prognosis of patients with glioblastoma multiforme and other malignant gliomas following surgery and radiation therapy has motivated the search for effective chemotherapy. This chapter is not meant to provide an exhaustive list of all chemotherapy trials for malignant gliomas, but rather to summarize the agents currently available and to outline regimens and methods of drug delivery which may provide future hope for patients.

Even a casual review of published chemotherapy trials for malignant gliomas reveals a large number of regimens and a rather broad range of reported efficacy. The number and diversity of trials attest to the absence of a chemotherapy regimen with dramatic effectiveness and acceptable toxicity[1,2]. The great majority of studies have been Phase I or II trials and have therefore involved relatively small numbers of patients. Unfortunately, many studies have not stratified or analyzed patients for several recently recognized prognostic variables. Extensive studies by the Brain Tumor Cooperative Group (BTCG)[3,4] and Radiation Therapy Oncology Group (RTOG)[5] have identified age, tumour histology, and performance status as patient factors which consistently have significant, independent impact on outcome. Patients with glioblastoma multiforme (GBM), as defined by the presence of gross or microcopic tumour necrosis, have median survival and two-year survival less than half that of patients with anaplastic astrocytomas (AA) or other malignant gliomas[4,6]. Survival is inversely correlated with age for adults with malignant gliomas, regardless of other factors. Unfortunately, most of these tumours occur in a "poor prognosis" age group, and GBM is at least five times more common than AA or other malignant gliomas. At the present time, age and tumour histology probably have more impact on patient outcome than any currently available chemotherapy regimen and must be taken into account when designing or interpreting trials.

Another source of difficulty in designing and interpreting chemotherapy trials for malignant gliomas is the assessment of response to treatment. Improvement in the clinical status of the patient is obviously the goal of any therapy, but neurological sign and symptoms are very difficult to quantify and are subject to bias on the part of patient and physician. The clinical status is also affected by a number of factors unrelated to the patient's tumour burden, such as cerebral oedema, corticosteroid treatment, seizures, and side effects of surgery and radiation therapy. The area of contrast enhancement in serial CT scans provides an objective measure of response but reflects only the portion of the tumour in which the blood-brain barrier is disrupted. In addition, the CT appearance is affected by corticosteroids[7] and can show misleading changes following radiation[8, 9] and surgery[10] unrelated to the tumour burden. Most recent studies have used a combination of the CT scan, neurological examination and performance status to define treatment response or failure, with the realization that the correlation between these criteria is good but not perfect[11, 12].

Duration of survival is the least subjective endpoint for treatment response and is the statistic most frequently reported in Phase III studies of newly diagnosed patients. The proportion of "long-term" (18- or 24-month) survivors is also a valuable statistic. As noted above, survival times are profoundly affected by patients' age, histology and pretreatment performance status. The amount of residual tumour following surgery[6, 13] and the dose of radiation[14] each also significantly affect survival. Survival is a less useful response endpoint in studies of patients with recurrent tumours, since patients have usually had a diversity of prior treatments and have already survived different periods following the initial diagnosis. Most studies of recurrent tumours report the percentage of responders as defined by clinical and radiological criteria, and/or the time to tumour progression or treatment failure. Unfortunately, there are no universally accepted, precise guidelines for defining "response" and "treatment failure," making comparisons between studies from different institutions somewhat tenuous[15, 16]. Most studies also include "disease stabilization" as a favorable response, although the biological significance of this state is unclear. Finally, patients who fail chemotherapy very early in the course of treatment are often considered "not evaluable" and excluded from statistical consideration, a practice which clearly biases the overall analysis.

When considering criteria for treatment response it is important to recall that preserving the quality of patients' survival is at least as important as prolonging of survival. The value of a treatment programme which modestly prolongs survival is debatable if it also produces toxicity which seriously disrupts the patients' personal interactions and function in society. These considerations are virtually impossible to quantify but should be kept in mind when assessing the "efficacy" of treatment.

Single-agent therapy

Nitrosoureas have been the most widely used chemotherapeutic agents for malignant gliomas. The usefulness of nitrosoureas for brain tumours is supported in theory by their low molecular weight and high degree of lipid solubility. Nitrosoureas have also been shown *in vitro* to be radiosensitizers[17]. The most extensive prospective studies of single-agent nitrosourea therapy have been carried out by the BTCG. In a randomized study of more than 500 newly diagnosed patients, the addition of intravenous BCNU (80 mg/m^2 for 3 days every 8 weeks) to surgery and radiation therapy significantly increased median survival from 40 weeks to 50 weeks.[3] In addition, BCNU significantly increased the percent of patients (up to 24 per cent) who survived 18 months or more after surgery. Procarbazine was shown to be as effective as BCNU. There was no evidence for chemotherapeutic activity of high-dose corticosteroids. Most recent regimens employing BCNU use 200 mg/m² as a single dose, as this is easier for patients and is more effective than a split dose *in vitro*[18]. Studies of nitrosoureas or procarbazine as single-agent therapy for patients with recurrent tumours have yielded objective response rates of up to 40 to 50 percent, with a median duration of response of approximately six months[19].

A relative advantage of nitrosourea therapy at the conventional dose of 200 mg/m² is the low incidence of serious toxicity. Acute side-effects are generally limited to nausea and vomiting. The most frequent dose-limiting side effect is myelosuppression which is delayed and cumulative, necessitating dose intervals of eight weeks and dose reductions in some successive courses. The most serious toxicity is a progressive, often fatal, fibrosing alveolitis[20]. The incidence of symptomatic pulmonary fibrosis in glioma patients receiving BCNU or other nitrosoureas varies from 4 to 30 per cent in different series[21, 22, 23]; risk is mainly related to cumulative dose of nitrosourea (up to 50 per cent after 1500 mg/m²)[21] and to the presence of preexisting lung disease. As a result, it is generally recommended that:

1) patients with significant pulmonary problems not receive nitrosoureas;
2) pulmonary function tests (especially diffusion capacity) should be performed periodically to detect presymptomatic toxicity;
3) nitrosoureas should be discontinued when the cumulative dose exceeds 1500 mg/m².

Several other nitrosoureas such as methyl-CCNU[24], ACNU[25], CCNU[19, 26, 27] and PCNU have been given to patients with newly diagnosed or recurrent tumours. PCNU has received particular attention because it was initially predicted to be superior to other nitrosoureas based on its lipophilicity, low molecular weight, and activity in preclinical studies[28]. Two studies of PCNU in patients with recurrent tumours have shown response rates of 21 per cent[28] and 38 per cent[29]; better responses were seen in patients who had not received prior chemotherapy. At this time there is no definite evidence that PCNU or any other nitrosourea is more effective than BCNU[1, 30]. All available nitrosoureas produce cumulative myelosuppression and carry the potential for serious pulmonary damage. The incidence of pulmonary fibrosis may be higher with BCNU than with other nitrosoureas[20]. PCNU is especially likely to produce cumulative thrombocytopenia[29], while nephrotoxicity has been associated with methyl-CCNU[31], and sudden bilateral visual loss has been reported in two patients receiving several courses of CCNU following radiation therapy[32].

Very high doses of intravenous (i.v.) BCNU have been combined with autologous bone marrow transplantation as a way of circumventing the dose-limiting myelotoxicity of conventionally administered nitrosoureas. Several small, nonrandomized studies have reported objective response rates of 30 to 80 per cent following 600 to 2850 mg/m² BCNU in "evaluable" malignant glioma patients, with the duration of response exceeding four years in occasional patients[33, 34, 35, 36, 37, 38]. Unfortunately, these high doses still produce significant myelosupression and have also caused life-threatening pulmonary fibrosis in up to 33 per cent of patients and hepatic necrosis in 10 to 20 per cent[33, 34, 37, 39]. In addition, several pathologically proven cases of fatal encephalomyelopathy have been reported in patients receiving as little as

1050 mg/m² BCNU, including patients who received no prior cranial RT[39, 40]. It is doubtful that the potential benefit of "megadose" i.v. BCNU will exceed its ability to cause severe toxicity.

Cisplatin is active against a number of solid tumours and has radiosensitizing activity[41]. The drug has very limited penetration across the intact blood-brain barrier (BBB) when given i.v. but has been shown to enter experimental and human brain tumours readily and also the oedematous brain around tumours[42, 43]. A pilot study of i.v. cisplatin (40 mg/m²/day for 3 days every 3 weeks) given during and after cranial RT to patients with newly diagnosed tumours showed a median survival of 53 weeks[44]. Response rates in patients with recurrent tumours who received monthly 60–100 mg/m² cisplatin have varied from 13 to 20 per cent[45, 46].

The systemic toxicity of cisplatin in brain tumour patients is generally similar to that observed in treatment of extraneural tumours and includes moderate to severe nausea and vomiting, nephrotoxicity, hypomagnesemia and occasional myelosupression[44]. The occurence of significant irreversible hearing loss in as many as 45 per cent of tumour patients suggests a possible potentiating effect of cranial RT on cisplatin ototoxicity[44]. Carboplatin (CBDCA) is less toxic to the ear and kidney than cisplatin but more myelosuppressive; its efficacy for recurrent tumours does not differ greatly from cisplatin[47]. Acute CNS toxicity of cisplatin has occurred in 16 to 25 per cent of patients and generally manifests as seizures and/or a transient worsening of preexisting neurological signs and symptoms[44, 46]. Fatal cerebral herniation has occurred within several hours of i.v. cisplatin infusion, possibly related to the high volumes of i.v. fluid administered concomitantly, to hyponatremia, or to direct neurotoxic effects of cisplatin[46, 48, 49].

Diaziquone (AZQ) is an alkylating agent which cross-links DNA strands and resembles the nitrosoureas in its low molecular weight, high lipid solubility and ability to readily cross the blood-brain and blood-tumour barriers[50, 51]. Intravenous AZQ has been extensively studied in nonrandomized phase II trials for patients with recurrent malignant gliomas (Table 13.1), with an average response rate of about 25 per cent. There is a trend toward poorer responses in patients who received and failed prior chemotherapy, but there does not seem to be a striking cross-resistance between AZQ and nitrosoureas. AZQ causes less acute nausea and vomiting than BCNU and has no appreciable pulmonary toxicity, but cumulative and occasionally profound myelosuppression often becomes dose-limiting. To date there are no published studies of AZQ in patients with newly diagnosed tumours.

The hexitol derivative dibromodulcitol (DBD) and its metabolite dianhydrogalactitol (DAG) cross the BBB and are active against several extraneural malignancies. The median survival time and time to progression for newly diagnosed patients given DBD were similar to that produced by i.v. BCNU in a Phase III randomized study[61]. The hexitols have been disappointing in single-agent studies of patients with recurrent tumours[62] but have been used as part of several combination regimens (see below).

Single-agent studies of the semisynthetic epipodophyllotoxins VM-26 (teniposide) and VP-16 (etoposide) have reported responses in 13 to 20 per cent of patients with recurrent tumours[63, 64, 65]. The use of high-dose i.v. VP-16 with autologous bone marrow transplantation has not significantly improved these results[66, 67, 68]. One study of high-dose VP-16 reported acute but transient neurological deterioration in 75 per cent of patients treated for recurrent tumours[68].

Table 13.1 Intravenous Diaziquone (AZQ) for recurrent tumors

Reference	Regimen	Number evaluable patients	Percent responders	Percent stable	Median time to progression (weeks)	Median survival (weeks)
52	17.5 mg/m^2/d × 2d q 4 wks	20	5	25	—	—
50	20 mg/m^2/d × 2d q 4 wks	28	21	36	33[1]	—
53	8 mg/m^2/d × 5d q 4 wks	20	25	30	54[1]	—
54	15 mg/m^2/d × 3d q 4 wks	12	42	—	—	—
55	30 mg/m^2 q 3 wks	27	14	25	—	46[1]
56	15–20 mg/m^2/wk × 4 wks	17	24	—	—	—
57	30–45 mg/m^2 q 3 wks	48	9	14	—	—
58	5.5 mg/m^2/d × 5d q 4 wks	23	35	—	—	—
59	25–30 mg/m^2 q 4 wks	93	26	—	—	—
60	25–45 mg/m^2 in 24-hr infusion q 3–4 wks	34	3	48	18	—

[1]reported for responders only

Combination therapy

The rationale behind combination chemotherapy for malignant gliomas includes:
1) the lack of dramatically effective single-agent therapy;
2) the growing evidence for tumour cell heterogeneity in malignant gliomas[69, 70], including *in vitro* chemosensitivity[71, 72]; and
3) the theoretical advantage of combining cell cycle nonspecific and cycle-specific agents. A cycle nonspecific drug (e.g. nitrosoureas, procarbazine, cisplatin) is initially given to reduce the total tumour cell population and to "recruit" remaining tumour cells into active division. This is followed by a drug specifically active on dividing cells (e.g., hydroxyurea, vincristine, 5-fluorouracil, epipodophyllotoxins). The cycle-specific drug hydroxyurea has received particular attention because of its radiosensitizing properties[73]. The pyrimidine analogue 5-fluorouracil (5-FU) readily crosses the BBB and has been shown to increase the cytotoxicity of BCNU in the rat 9L gliosarcoma model[74].

Representative Phase II and III studies of combination chemotherapy for newly diagnosed malignant gliomas are summarized in Table 13.2 and 13.3. None of the randomized studies has shown statistically significant increases in median survival over that obtained with single-agent nitrosoureas, and the Phase II studies have not offered clear advantages over the BTCG studies of BCNU alone[3, 24]. When the data from the Northern California Oncology Group study were analyzed according to the known prognostic variables for malignant gliomas, the addition of hydroxyurea to BCNU appeared to increase the median time to progression (MTP) for the "GBM" subgroup from 31 to 42 weeks[73]. The combination of procarbazine, CCNU and vincristine (PCV) may be superior to BCNU (as evaluated by MTP) for newly diagnosed patients with anaplastic gliomas other then "GBM"[78]. Unfortunately, the definition of glioblastoma multiforme in the latter two studies differs from that used by the BTCG and RTOG, making these data somewhat difficult to interpret.

Recent Phase II studies of combination chemotherapy for recurrent malignant gliomas are outlined in Table 13.4. The per cent of objective responses (not including "stable disease") for the larger studies is generally 20 to 40 percent, with MTP in responders of approximately six to seven months. Not surprisingly, patients with GBM appear less likely to respond than patients with AA or other malignant gliomas[85, 90, 91, 92]. There is also a trend toward fewer responses in patients who failed previous chemotherapy than in patients with tumour progression but no prior chemotherapy, but this has not been seen in all studies.

Intra-arterial therapy

The theoretical advantage of intra-arterial (i.a.) administration of cytotoxic drugs is the achievement of locally high concentrations in the tumour for a given amount of systemic exposure. Mathematical modelling has predicted up to a five-fold increase in the concentration-time integral for a given dose of drug administered intra-arterially versus intravenously. In addition, intra-arterial infusion has been predicted to produce as much as a ten-fold increase in peak drug concentration in brain[93, 94].

Favorable drug characteristics for intra-arterial use include:

Table 13.2 Combination chemotherapy for newly diagnosed patients: randomized studies

Reference	Regimen	Number evaluable patients	Percent responders	Percent stable	Median time to progression (weeks)	Median survival (weeks)	Notes
73	BCNU+HU vs BCNU	53 46	21 13	60 74	42[1] 50[2] 31[1] 73[2]	— —	[1]"glioblastoma" [2]other malignant glioma [3]chemotherapy given at recurrence
75	CCNU+VM-26 vs no chemotherapy[3]	61 55	— —	— —	39 —	58 55	
26	CCNU+PCB vs CCNu	58 56	28 41	— —	31 —	50 55	
76	CCNU+DBD vs CCNU	28 26	— —	— —	— —	60 57	increased myelo-suppression with CCNU+DBD
77	Methyl-CCNU+DTIC vs BCNU	136 165	— —	— —	— —	42 43	
78	CCNU+VCR+PCB+HU vs BCNU+HU	72 76	33 32	64 65	— —	— 68	
79	BCNU vs BCNU+PCB	25 26	— —	— —	42 26	65 65	
	vs BCNU+HU+PCB+VM-26	28	—	—	48	73	

Abbreviations: BCNU Carmustine, HU hydroxyurea, CCNU lomustine, PCB procarbazine, DBD dibormodulcitol, DTIC dacarbazine, VCR vincristine, VM-26 teniposide
Note: Chemotherapy was administered following surgery and in conjuction with radiation therapy.

Table 13.3 Combination chemotherapy for newly diagnosed patients: nonrandomized studies

Reference	Regimen	Number evaluable patients	Percent responders	Percent stable	Median time to progression (weeks)	Median survival (weeks)
80	BCNU+PCB+VCR	36	—	—	—	45
81	BCNU+CDDP	30	—	—	30	54
82	CCNU+DBD+PCB	38	—	—	—	55
83	5–FU+CCNU+HU+PCB+VCR+BCNU+misonidazole	64	23	73	41	—

Abbreviations: CDDP cisplatin, 5–FU 5–fluorouracil
Note: Chemotherapy was administered following surgery and in conjunction with radiation therapy

Table 13.4 Combination chemotherapy for recurrent tumours

Reference	Regimen	Number evaluable patients	Percent responders	Percent (weeks)	Median time to progression (weeks)	Median survival Notes
84	BCNU+5–Fu	29	31	52	27	—
85	CCNU+PCB+VCR	46	26	35	26[1]	—
86	DAG+VP-16	15	40	—	31	—
87	BCNU+triazinate	16	44	—	—	35
88	CDDP+AraC	13	23	38	—	11[1]
89	CCNU+VCR+PCB+HU+CDDP+DTIC+AraC	9	92	—	—	— 8 drugs in 1 day
90	BCNU+5–FU+HU+6–MP	29 GBM 45 non-GBM	17 31	38 40	23[1] 46[1]	— greater response in AA vs GBM
91	6–MP	20	15	35	26	84
92	BCNU+AZQ	42	24	17	48[1]GBM 68[1]AA	—
	PCB+AZQ	61	23	15	28[1]GBM 75[1]AA	—

Abbreviations: GBM glioblastoma multiforme, AA anaplastic astrocytoma, DAG dianhydrogalactitol, VP-16 etoposide, AraC cytarabine, 6-MP 6-mercaptopurine
[1] reported for responding or stable patients only

1) high capillary permeability (which for brain tumours means lipid solubility);
2) high extraction fraction (first-pass effect) in the target organ; and
3) rapid metabolism and/or excretion, resulting in less systemic toxicity per a given dose[94, 95, 96]. According to these criteria, nitrosoureas would appear to be nearly ideal agents for intra-arterial therapy of brain tumours. Increased delivery of BCNU after i.a. infusion has been confirmed in animal tumour models[97]. The increase in peak drug concentration provided by i.a. infusion may be especially important for nitrosoureas in light of their steep dose-response curves in experimental systems[18, 98].

Nonrandomized studies of single-agent i.a. therapy for new and recurrent malignant gliomas are summarized in Table 13.5 and 13.6. Trials of i.a. BCNU therapy for newly diagnosed patients have demonstrated median survival times which compare quite favorably with the 50 weeks generally reported for "conventional" i.v. BCNU. At least half of these patients have responded to i.a. BCNU alone, before receiving any RT. The number of patients is small compared to studies of i.v. BCNU and does not allow for analysis according to prognostic variables. Patients with recurrent tumours have shown a response rate to i.a. BCNU or PCNU of 22 to 47 per cent, with median prolongation of survival as long as 50 weeks in responders. Again, these data are derived entirely from small, nonrandomized trials.

Preliminary results from a randomized Phase III comparison of i.v. BCNU and i.a. BCNU conducted by the BTCG have been published[110]. After the accrual and randomization of nearly 300 newly diagnosed patients, no apparent survival advantage was observed for patients receiving i.a. vs. i.v. BCNU (with or without the addition of i.v. 5-FU).

Intra-arterial BCNU is associated with a slight risk of catheter-related thromboembolic complications[102], as well as with significant toxicity to the eye and brain. Nearly all patients have ipsilateral periorbital erythralgia during the drug infusion. Unilateral retinal vasculopathy characterized by haemorrhages and nerve fibre layer infarcts occurs in 25 per cent of patients receiving intracarotid BCNU; the incidence of total irreversible blindness may be as high as 18 per cent[100, 102, 111]. Ocular toxicity of i.a. BCNU may be potentiated by the ethanol diluent[100]. Selective infusion of BCNU into the internal carotid artery above the origin of the ophthalmic artery greatly reduces the incidence of retinal toxicity, although supraophthalmic BCNU infusion has been reported to cause optic tract damage[112] and subclinical changes in visual evoked potentials[113].

Neurotoxicity associated with i.a. BCNU or PCNU is characterized by a spectrum of changes ranging from asymptomatic findings on imaging studies to fatal brain necrosis. As many as 20 per cent of patients develop hypodensity of the ipsilateral hemispheric white matter within several days to weeks of infusion; this has occurred after as little as 415 mg/m^2 BCNU in two infusions[100, 101]. This apparent leucoencephalopathy remains subclinical in the majority of patients[100]. Transient symptoms such as focal seizures, confusion, and a worsening of focal deficits have occurred within 24 hours of intracarotid BCNU in 15 to 38 per cent of patients[99, 101, 114, 115, 116]. The incidence of transient neurological deterioration is even higher after i.a. PCNU[104]. Severe neurotoxicity is characterized by progressive lethargy and focal neurological deficits generally beginning within two to three months of an i.a. infusion and frequently resulting in shortened survival[116, 117, 118].

Table 13.5 Intra-arterial BCNU for newly diagnosed patients

Reference	Regimen	Number evaluable patients	Percent responders	Percent stable	Median time to progression (weeks)	Median survival (weeks)	Notes
99	BCNU 100 mg/m^2 × 4	15	75	—	—	67	pre-RT
100	BCNU 200–300 mg/m^2 q 6–8 wks	12	75	8	25	54	RT after progression; 42% 18-mo survivors
101	BCNU 240 mg/m^2 q 4–6 wks	49	—	—	—	57	18 supra-ophthalmic infusions
102	BCNU 400 mg q 4 wks × 4	28	44	—	—	37	pre-RT

Note: All patients received surgery and radiation therapy (RT)

Several autopsy reports of patients with severe BCNU neurotoxicity have featured confluent areas of coagulative necrosis of the white matter within the infused hemisphere, with foci of petechial hemorrhages, axonal swellings, and/or calcification. Fibrinoid necrosis of small vessels, fibrin thrombi, and telangiectasias are often prominent[116, 117, 118]. The overlying gray matter is relatively preserved. These changes closely resemble the pathology of "radiation necrosis"[119] and of fatal neurotoxicity of "megadose" i.v. BCNU[40]. The bulk of the neuropathologic evidence in humans and in animal models[120] implicates injury to small blood vessels as the primary pathogenetic event, although there may also be direct damage to myelinated fibres.

The incidence and severity of neurotoxicity following i.a. BCNU appear to be related to the cumulative dose of drug and to a possible synergistic interaction with concurrent cranial radiation. Most cases of permanent symptomatic leucoencephalopathy have occurred after cumulative i.v. doses of 300–600 mg/m^2 BCNU[110, 116]. Supraophthalmic BCNU infusion probably carries an increased risk of neurotoxicity relative to infusions below the ophthalmic artery, presumably due to increased drug delivery to the brain[101]. Hyperlucency of the ipsilateral hemispheric white matter on CT scans has been reported after a single supraophthalmic infusion of 200 mg/m^2 [121]. One factor which probably contributes to the neurotoxicity of i.a. BCNU and to the imperfect correlation between drug dose and toxicity is drug steaming. Striking non-uniformity of BCNU delivery following intracarotid infusion has been reported in rhesus monkeys[122], particularly at relatively slow rates of infusion. This effect may lead to lower than expected drug concentrations in some tumour areas, and simultaneous toxic concentrations of drug in normal brain. Unfortunately, high infusion rates are often limited by ocular and cephalic pain[99, 110].

The incidence of serious neurotoxicity is probably higher in newly diagnosed patients receiving i.a. BCNU in conjunction with RT than in patients treated at time of tumour recurrence, suggesting a synergistic effect between RT and the focally high brain concentrations of BCNU achieved by i.a. infusion[101, 116]. The reported incidence of severe neurotoxicity in "new" patients ranges from 10 per cent to 33 per cent after a cumulative i.a. BCNU dose of 400 mg/m^2 [102, 110, 116]. Severe neurotoxicity has been observed even when several cycles of i.a. BCNU are given prior to any radiation therapy[102]. It is becoming clear that toxicity to the brain itself, and not systemic toxicity, is the dose-limiting factor for intra-arterial BCNU therapy. The crucial question, as yet unanswered, is whether the neurotoxicity of this therapy is outweighed by improved length and quality of survival.

Cisplatin is theoretically not as ideally suited for intra-arterial therapy as are nitrosoureas, but studies in dogs[123] and humans[124, 125] have demonstrated increased delivery of i.a. cisplatin compared with i.v. infusion. This may be at least partially explained by the ability of i.a. cisplatin to open the BBB[126]. Two published studies of intracarotid cisplatin for recurrent malignant gliomas have reported a 30–35 per cent response rate, with stabilization of disease in another 25–35 per cent of patients[105, 107]. The toxicity of i.a. cisplatin varies widely in different studies. The reported incidence of visual loss varies from 3 per cent[107] to 75 per cent (3 of 4 patients)[113]; several patients developed bilateral visual loss following unilateral carotid infusion[105]. The reasons for the marked differences in incidence are not clear but may in part be related to the dose of cisplatin[105]. Acute bilateral deafness has occurred following intravertebral cisplatin, while 15–20 per cent of patients have mild to moderate bilateral hearing loss after intracarotid infusion[105, 107]. The most serious toxicity of i.a.

cisplatin has been acute neurological deterioration, manifesting as seizures and/or worsening of pre-existing focal deficits occurring within 48 hours after 5–33 per cent of infusions[105, 106, 111, 127]. Several of these patients received cisplatin in addition to other i.a. agents (see below), making it difficult to assign the toxicity to a single drug. There is a suggestion, however, that the incidence of transient neurotoxicity is related to the dose of cisplatin. As with i.v. cisplatin, fatal cerebral oedema and herniation has occurred within 24 hours after i.a. infusion[105, 107]. Despite this potential for severe acute toxicity, i.a. cisplatin to this date has not been shown to cause chronic brain injury or delayed leucoencephalopathy as seen with i.a. BCNU.

A study of i.a. AZQ in patients with recurrent tumours has reported a response rate of 10 per cent[108], with visual loss occuring in another 10 per cent. The intracarotid administration of VP-16 has not produced any improvement over the published results for the drug given intravenously[109].

Combination therapy consisting of two supraophthalmic infusions of BCNU and cisplatin followed by oral CCNU "maintenance" has been administered to patients with recurrent tumours[127, 128]. Several patients underwent surgical modification of the cerebral vasculature to result in the perfusion of the tumour by a single internal carotid artery. Objective responses occurred in 83 per cent of patients, although 16 per cent of patients developed acute, permanent post-treatment hemiplegia with extensive hypodensity of the hemispheric white matter ipsilateral to the infused artery.

A study of intra-arterial BCNU, cisplatin and VM-26 reported a response rate of 63 per cent for patients with recurrent tumours[111]. Complications included severe ocular toxicity (19 per cent) and permanent neurological deterioration (11 per cent); bilateral ototoxicity and transient respiratory depression were associated with vetebral artery infusions. This three-drug i.a. regimen has also been combined with i.v. vincristine, bleomycin, VM-26, MTX, and PCB to produce a response rate of 71 per cent in "fully evaluable" patients with recurrent tumours, but a disappointing MTP of 19 weeks[129].

Blood-brain barrier disruption

The major determinant of delivery of small, lipid-soluble drugs such as the nitrosoureas is local blood flow to the tumour, while the entry of larger, water-soluble molecules into brain (and brain tumours) depends mainly on the degree of breakdown of the blood-brain barrier (BBB). The importance of the BBB as a cause of restricted drug entry and consequent chemotherapeutic failure in malignant gliomas (and other brain tumours) has been a matter of considerable controversy. At the risk of oversimplifying a large body of literature, it can be said that the BBB is at least partially opened in malignant gliomas. Recent studies of experimental brain tumours have shown, however, that the integrity of the BBB varies significantly between different tumour models and between different regions of a given tumour[130]. This variability is often especially prominent in the periphery of a tumour and the oedematous brain adjacent to the tumour (BAT). The BAT frequently contains tumour cells which are actively proliferating and infiltrating into normal brain[131, 132] but may be protected from chemotherapeutic agents by an intact BBB.

These observations have led to efforts at increasing the delivery of water-soluble drugs by transient disruption of the BBB with intra-arterial hyperosmolar agents immediately prior to i.a. drug infusion. Quantitative autoradiography studies in animals have verified the ability of i.a. mannitol or arabinose to increase the permeability of normal brain capillaries. The ability of hyperosmolar BBB disruption to increase the capillary permeability of animal tumour models, however, varies greatly between different models and different regions of a given tumour[133, 134, 135]. BBB disruption will not increase drug delivery to tumour regions where the BBB is already broken down. Animal studies suggest that the relative advantage of BBB disruption would vary with the individual patient's tumour and be very difficult to predict in advance.

Another serious limitation to i.a. chemotherapy with BBB modification is the theoretical potential for serious neurotoxicity. Several potentially active agents (including 5-fluorouracil and cisplatin) have produced necrosis and haemorrhagic infarction in dogs when administered after osmotic BBB disruption[126]. This clearly limits the number of agents which could be administered in this fashion. In addition, quantitative autoradiographic studies of the entry of radiolabelled methotrexate (MTX) or aminoisobutyric acid into animal tumours have shown a much greater proportional increase in "drug" entry into the normal brain surrounding a tumour than into the tumour itself following BBB opening with hyperosmolar mannitol[134, 136]. As with i.a. therapy in general, the key question concerning BBB modification appears to be whether any increase in tumour cell kill will outweigh the toxic effects of high concentrations of drug in normal brain.

Pilot studies of BBB modification and i.a. MTX have included several patients with recurrent GBM[137, 138]. There have been no comparison studies to evaluate the added benefit of BBB modification over "conventional" i.a. chemotherapy. In a single nonrandomized Phase II study, GBM patients who received high-dose i.a. MTX after BBB disruption had a longer survival than historical controls given "conventional" therapy[139]. All patients were also given cyclophosphamide and procarbazine; the study did not address the question of whether BBB disruption actually added to the effectiveness of this combination regimen. Delayed leucoencephalopathy was not observed, but acute neurotoxicity included seizures (56 per cent of patients), transient focal deficits (58 per cent), and permanent motor deficits (8 per cent).

References

1. Kornblith PL, Walker MD: Chemotherapy for malignant gliomas. *Journal of Neurosurgery.* **68**, 1988; 1-17.
2. Schold SC, Shapiro WR, Vick NA, Walker MD: Chemotherapy for malignant gliomas? *Annals of Neurology.* 1989; **25**, 88-9.
3. Green SB, Byar DP, Walker MD, *et al.* Comparisons of carmustine, procarbazine, and high-dose methylprednisolone as additions to surgery and radiotherapy for the treatment of malignant glioma. *Cancer treatment Reports.* 1983; **67**, 121-32.
4. Burger PC, Vogel FS, Green SB, Strike TA: Glioblastoma multiforme and anaplastic astrocytoma: pathologic criteria and prognostic implications. *Cancer.* 1985; **56**, 1106-11.

5. Nelson JS, Tsukada Y, Schoenfeld D, et al. Necrosis as a prognostic criterion in malignant supratentorial, astrocytic gliomas. Cancer. 1983; **52**, 550–4.
6. Nelson DF, Nelson JS, Davis DR, et al. Survival and prognosis of patients with astrocytoma with atypical or anaplastic features. Journal of Neurological-oncology. 1985; **3**, 99–103.
7. Macdonald DR, Cairncross JG, Pexman JH, et al. Steroid-induced CT changes in patients with recurrent malignant gliomas (abstract). Neurology. 1987; 37 (Suppl 1)., 300–1.
8. Hoffman WF, Levin VA, Wilson CB: Evaluation of malignant glioma patients during the postirradiation period. Journal of Neurosurgery. 1979; **50**, 624–8.
9. Graeb DA, Steinbok P, Robertson WD. Transient early computed tomographic changes mimicking tumour progression after brain tumour irradiation. Radiology. 1982; **144**, 813–7.
10. Cairncross JG, Pexman JH, Rathbone MP, DelMaestro RF. Postoperative contrast enhancement in patients with brain tumour. Annals of Neurology. 1985; **17**, 570–2.
11. Salcman M, Levine H, Rao K: Value of sequential computed tomography in the multimodality treatment of glioblastoma multiforme. Neurosurgery. 1981; **8**, 15–19.
12. Mahaley MS, Mitchell WG, Whaley R, et al. The relative roles of neurological examination, functional abilities, and computed tomography in the definition of treatment failure in patients with anaplastic gliomas. Surgical Neurology 1983; **20**, 297–300.
13. Wood JR, Green SB, Shapiro WR. The prognostic importance of tumour size in malignant gliomas: a computed tomographic scan study by the Brain Tumour Cooperative Group. Journal of Clinical Oncology. 1988; **6**, 338–43.
14. Walker MD, Strike TA, Sheline GE. An analysis of dose-effect relationship in the radiotherapy of malignant gliomas. International Journal of Radiation, Oncology, Biology and Physics. 1979; **5**, 1725–31.
15. Wilson CB, Crafts D, Levin VA. Brain tumours: criteria of response and definition of recurrence. National Cancer Institute Monograph. 1977; **46**, 197–203.
16. Hildebrand J: Current status of chemotherapy of brain tumours. Progress in Experimental Tumour Research. 1985; **29**, 152–66.
17. Leenhouts HP, Chadwick KH, Deen DF. An analysis of the interaction between two nitrosourea compounds and X-radiation in rat brain tumour cells. International Journal of Radiation, Oncology, Biology and Physics. 1980; **7**, 169–81.
18. Rosenblum ML, Gerosa MA, Dougherty DV, Wilson CB. Improved treatment of a brain tumour model: advantages of single-over multiple-dose BCNU schedules. Journal of Neurosurgery, 1983; **58**, 117–382.
19. Wilson CB, Gutin P, Boldrey EB, et al. Single-agent chemotherapy of brain tumours. Archives in Neurology. 1976; **33**, 739–44.
20. Weiss RB, Poster DS, Penta JS: The nitrosoureas and pulmonary toxicity. Cancer Treatment Review. 1981; **8**, 111–25.
21. Aronin PA, Mahaley MS, Rudnick SA, et al. Prediction of BCNU pulmonary toxicity in patients with malignant gliomas: an assessment of risk factors. New England Journal of Medicine. 1989; **303**, 183–8.
22. Selker RG, Jacobs SA, Moore PB, et al. BCNU-induced pulmonary fibrosis. Neurosurgery, 1980; **7**, 560–5.
23. Weinstein AS, Diener-West M, Nelson DF, Pakuris E: Pulmonary toxicity of carmustine in patients treated for malignant glioma. Cancer Treatment Review. 1986; **70**, 943–6.
24. Walker MD, Green SB, Byar DP, et al. Randomized comparisons of radiotherapy and nitrosoureas for the treatment of malignant glioma after surgery. New England Journal of Medicine. 1980; **303**, 1323–29.

25. Takakura K, Abe H, Tanaka R, *et al.* Effects of ACNU and radiotherapy on malignant glioma. *Journal of Neurosurgery.* 1986; **64**, 53–7.
26. Eyre HJ, Quagliana JM, Eltringham JR, Frank J: Randomized comparisons of radiotherapy and CCNU versus radiotherapy, CCNU plus procarbazine for the treatment of malignant gliomas following surgery. *Journal of Neuro-oncology.* 1983; **1**, 171–7.
27. Trojanowski T, Peszynski J, Turowski K, *et al.* Postoperative radiotherapy and radiotherapy combined with CCNU chemotherapy for treatment of brain gliomas. *Journal of Neuro-oncology.* 1988; **6**, 285–91.
28. Levin VA, Resser KJ, *et al.* PCNU treatment for recurrent malignant gliomas. *Cancer Treatment Reports.* 1984; **68**, 969–72.
29. Feun LG, Stewart DJ, Leavens ME, *et al.* A phase II trial of PCNU (NSC 95466) in recurrent malignant brain tumours. *Journal of Neuro-oncology.* 1983; **1**, 45–8.
30. Edwards MS, Levin VA, Wilson CB. Brain tumour chemotherapy: an evaluation of agents in current use for phase II and III trials. *Cancer Treatment Reports* 1980; **64**, 1179–1205.
31. Schacht RG, Feiner HD, Gallo GR, *et al.* Nephrotoxicity of nitrosoureas. *Cancer.* 1981; **48**, 1328–34.
32. Wilson WB, Perez GM, Kleinschmidt-Demasters BK. Sudden onset of blindness in patients treated with oral CCNU and low-dose cranial irradiation. *Cancer.* 1987; **59**, 901–7.
33. Hochberg FH, Parker LM, Takvorian T, *et al.* High-dose BCNU with autologous bone marrow rescue for recurrent glioblastoma multiforme. *Neurosurgery.* 1981; **54**, 455–60.
34. Phillips GL, Fay JW, Herzig GP, *et al.* Intensive BCNU and cryopreserved autologous marrow transplantation for refractory cancer: a phase I-II study. *Cancer.* 1983; **52**, 1792–1802.
35. Mortimer JE, Hewlett JS, Bay J, Livingston RB. High dose BCNU with autologous bone marrow rescue in the treatment of recurrent malignant gliomas. *Journal of Neuro-oncology.* 1983; **1**, 269–73.
36. Fingert HJ, Hochberg FH. Megadose chemotherapy with bone marrow rescue. *Progress in Experimental Tumour Research.* 1984; **28**, 67–78.
37. Phillips GL, Wolff SN, Fay JW, *et al.* Intensive BCNU monochemotherapy and autologous marrow transplantation for malignant glioma *Journal of Clinical oncology.* 1986; **4**, 639–45.
38. Johnson DB, Thompson JN, Corwin JA, *et al.* Prolongation of survival for high-grade malignant gliomas with adjuvant high-dose BCNU and autologous bone marrow transplantation. *Journal of Clinical Oncology.* 1987; **5**, 783–89.
39. Wolff SN, Phillips GL, Herzig GP. High-dose carmustine with autologous bone marrow transplantation for the adjuvant treatment of high-grade gliomas of the central nervous system. *Cancer Treatment Reports.* 1987; **71**, 183–5.
40. Burger PC, Kamenar E, Schold SC, *et al.* Encephalomyelopathy following high-dose BCNU therapy. *Cancer.* 1981; **48**, 1318–21.
41. Murthy AK, Rossof AH, Anderson KM. Cytotoxicity and influence on radiation dose response curve of cis-diaminedichloroplatinum. *International Journal of Radiation, Oncology, Biology and Physics.* 1979; **5**, 1411–15.
42. Stewart DJ, Leavens M, *et al.* Human central nervous system distribution of cisdiamminedichloroplatinum and use as a radiosensitizer in malignant brain tumours. *Cancer Research.* 1982; **42**, 2474–79.
43. Stillman M, Lipschutz L, Sher P, *et al.* Pharmacokinetics of intravenous ^{195}Pt-cisplatin (CDDP) in experimental rat brain tumours as measured by quantitative autoradiography (QAR) (abstract). *Neurology.* 1986; **36** (Suppl 1), 292.
44. Feun LG, Stewart DJ, Maor M, *et al.* A pilot study of cis-diamminedichloroplatinum and radiation therapy in patients with high grade astrocytomas. *Journal of Neuro-oncology.* 1983; **1**, 109–13.

45. Stewart DJ, O'Bryan RM, AL-Sarraf M, *et al.* Phase II study of cisplatin in recurrent astrocytomas in adults: a Southwest Oncology Group study. *Journal of Neuro-oncology.* 1983; **1**, 145-7.
46. Macdonald DR, Cairncross JG, Rathbone MP: Cisplatin chemotherapy for recurrent brain tumours (abstract). *Journal of Neuro-oncology.* 1984; **2**, 287.
47. Walker RW. Carboplatin (CBDCA) in the treatment of recurrent gliomas (abstract). *Neurology.* 1988; **38** (Suppl 1), 390.
48. Cairncross JG, Walker RW, Posner JB. Cerebral herniation complicating cisplatin chemotherapy (abstract). *Neurology.* 1986; **36** (Suppl 1), 329.
49. Ritch PS. Cis-diamminedichloroplatinum-induced syndrome of inappropriate secretion of antidiuretic hormone. *Cancer.* 1988; **61** 488-50.
50. Curt GA, Kelley JA, Kufta CV, Smith BH: Phase II and pharmacokinetic study of diaziquone (NSC 182986) in high-grade gliomas. *Cancer Research.* 1983; **43**, 6102-5.
51. Savaraj N, Lu K, Fuen LG, *et al.* Intracerebral penetration and tissue distribution of AZQ (NSC 182986). *Journal of Neuro-oncology.* 1983; **1**, 15-19.
52. Aroney RS, Kaplan RS, Salcman M, *et al.* A phase II trial of AZQ in patients with recurrent primary or metastatic brain tumours (abstract). *Proceedings of American Society of Clinical Oncology.* 1982; **1**, 24.
53. Feun LG, Yung WK, Leavens ME, *et al.* A phase II trial of AZQ in recurrent primary brain tumours. *Journal of Neuro-oncology.* 1984; **2**, 13-17.
54. Schold SC, Friedman HS, Bjornsson TD, Faletta JM. Treatment of patients with recurrent primary brain tumours with AZQ. *Neurology.* 1984; **34**, 615-19.
55. Haid M, Khandekar JD, Christ M, *et al.* Aziridinylbenzoquinone in recurrent, progressive glioma of the central nervous system: a phase II study by the Illinois Cancer Council. *Cancer.* 1985; **56**, 1311-15.
56. Decker DA, Sarraf MA, Kresge C, *et al.* Phase II study of AZQ in the treatment of malignant gliomas recurrent after radiation. *Journal of Neuro-oncology.* 1985; **3**, 19-21.
57. Taylor SA, McCracken JD, Eyre HJ, *et al.* Phase II study of aziridinylbenzoquinone (AZQ) in patients with central nervous system malignancies: a Southwest Oncology Group study. *Journal of Neuro-oncology.* 1985; **3**, 131-4.
58. Maral J, Poisson M, Pertuiset BF, *et al.* Phase II evaluation of diaziquone (AZQ) in the treatment of human malignant glioma. *Journal of Neuro-oncology.* 1985; **3** , 245.
59. Eagan RT, Dinapoli RP, Cascino TL, *et al.* Comprehensive phase II evaluation of aziridinylbenzoquinone (AZQ, diaziquone) in recurrent human primary brain tumours. *Journal of Neuro-oncology.* 1987; **5**, 309-14.
60. Chaimberlain MC, Prados MD, Silver P, Levin VA. A phase I/II study of 24-hour intravenous AZQ in recurrent primary brain tumours. *Journal of Neuro-oncology.* 1988; **6**, 319-23.
61. Dinapoli RP, Cascino TL, Krook JE, *et al.* Randomized trial of radiation therapy (RT) plus BCNU versus RT plus dibromodulcitol (DBD) in high-grade astrocytoma: a collaborative trial of North Central Cancer Treatment Group and Mayo Clinic (abstract). *Neurology.* 1986; **36** (Suppl 1), 335.
62. Levin VA, Edwards MS, Gutin PH, *et al.* Phase II evaluation of dibromodulcitol in the treatment of recurrent medulloblastoma, ependymoma, and malignant astrocytoma. J *Neurosurgery.* 1984; **61**, 1063-68.
63. Spremulli E, Schulz JJ, Speckhart VJ, Wampler GL. Phase II study of VM-26 in adult malignancies. *Cancer Treatment Reports* 1980; 64, 147-9.
64. Tirelli U, D'Incalci M, Canetta R, *et al.* Etoposide (VP-16-213) in malignant brain tumours: a phase II study. *Journal of Clinical Oncology.* 1984; **2**, 432-7.
65. Cascino T, Dinapoli R, Krook J, *et al.* Phase II study of VM-26 and VP-16 in recurrent primary brain tumour: a collaborative trial of North Central Cancer Treatment Group and Mayo Clinic (abstract). *Neurology.* 1986; **36** (Suppl 1), 336.
66. Finn GP, Bozek T, Souhami RL, *et al.* High-dose etoposide in the treatment of relapsed primary brain tumours. *Cancer Treatment Reports.* 1985; **69**, 603-5.

67. Giannone L, Wolff SN. Phase II treatment of central nervous system gliomas with high-dose etoposide and autologous bone marrow transplantation. *Cancer Treatment Reports*. 1987; **71**, 759–61.
68. Leff RS, Thompson JM, Daly MB, *et al*. Acute neurologic dysfunction after high-dose etoposide therapy for malignant glioma. *Cancer*. 1988; **62**, 32–5.
69. Bigner DD. Biology of gliomas: potential clinical implications of glioma cellular heterogeneity. *Neurosurgery*. 1981; **9**; 320–6.
70. Shapiro JR, Shapiro WR: Clonal tumour cell heterogeneity. *Progress in Experimental Tumour Research*. 1984; **27**, 49–66.
71. Yung WK, Shapiro JR, Shapiro WR. Heterogeneous chemosensitivities of subpopulations of human glioma cells in culture. *Cancer Research*. 1982; **42**; 992–8.
72. Shapiro JR, Pu PY, Mohammed AN, *et al*. Regional heterogeneity in high grade human gliomas (abstract). *Proceedings of American Association for Cancer Research*. 1984; **25**, 375.
73. Levin VA, Wilson CB, Davis R, *et al*. A phase III comparison of BCNU, hydroxyurea, and radiation therapy to BCNU and radiation therapy for treatment of primary malignant gliomas. *Journal of Neurosurgery*. 1979; **51**, 526–32.
74. Gerosa MA, Dougherty DV, Wilson CB, Rosenblum ML: Improved treatment of a brain tumour model: sequential therapy with BCNU and 5-fluorouracil. *Journal of Neurosurgery*. 1983; **58**, 368–73.
75. EORTC Brain Tumour Group: Evaluation of CCNU, VM-26 plus CCNU, and procarbazine in supratentorial brain gliomas. *Journal of Neurosurgery*. 1981; **55**, 27–31.
76. Afra D, Kocsis B, Dobay J, Eckhardt S: Combined radiotherapy and chemotherapy with dibromodulcitol and CCNU in the postoperative treatment of malignant gliomas. *Journal of Neurosurgery*. 1983; **59**, 106–10.
77. Chang CH, Horton J, Shoenfeld D, *et al*. Comparison of postoperative radiotherapy and combined postoperative radiotherapy and chemotherapy in the multidisciplinary management of malignant gliomas. *Cancer*. 1983; **52**, 997–1007.
78. Levin VA, Wara WM, Davis RL, *et al*. Phase III comparison of BCNU and the combination of procarbazine, CCNU, and vincristine administered after radiotherapy with hydroxyurea for malignant gliomas. *Journal of Neurosurgery*. 1985; **63**, 218–23.
79. Mahaley MS, Whaley RA, Krigman MR, *et al*. Randomized Phase III trial of single versus multiple chemotherapeutic treatment following surgery and during radiotherapy for patients with anaplastic gliomas. *Surgical Neurology*. 1987; **27**, 430–2.
80. Comella G, Scoppa G, DeMarco M, *et al*. Radiotherapy and combination chemotherapy with carmustine, vincristine, and procarbazine (BVP) in primary brain tumours. *Journal of Neuro-oncology*. 1985; **3**, 13–17.
81. Yung WK, Martinez-Prieto JN, Castellanos AM, *et al*. Adjuvant chemotherapy with BCNU and CDDP for patients with malignant gliomas (abstract). *Neurology*. 1986; **36** (Suppl 1), 328.
82. Afra D, Kocsis B, Kerpel-Fronius S, Eckhardt S. Dibromodulcitol-based combined postoperative chemotherapy of malignant astrocytomas and glioblastomas. *Journal of Neuro-oncology*. 1986; **4**, 65–70.
83. Levin VA, Wara WM, Davis RL, *et al*. Northern California Oncology Group Protocol 6G91: response to treatment with radiation therapy and seven-drug chemotherapy in patients with glioblastoma multiforme. *Cancer Treatment Reports*. 1986; **70**, 739–43.
84. Levin VA, Hoffman WF, Pischer TL, *et al*. BCNU-5-fluorouracil combination therapy for recurrent malignant brain tumours. *Cancer Treatment Reports*. 1978; **62**, 2071–76.
85. Levin VA, Edwards MS, Wright DC, *et al*. Modified procarbazine, CCNU, and vincristine (PCV 3) combination chemotherapy in the treatment of malignant brain tumours. *Cancer Treatment Reports*. 1980; **64**, 237–41.
86. Eagan RT, Creagan ET, Bisel HF, *et al*. Phase II studies of dianhydrogalactitol-based combination chemotherapy for recurrent brain tumours. *Oncology*. 1981; **38**, 4–6.
87. Eagan RT, Dinapoli RP, Hermann RC, *et al*. Carmustine and Baker's antifol combina-

tion chemotherapy for primary brain tumours progressive after irradiation and chemotherapy. *Cancer Treatment Reports.* 1984; **68**, 431–34.
88. Stewart DJ, Richard MT, Benoit B, *et al.* Cisplatin plus cytosine arabinoside in adults with malignant gliomas. *Journal of Neuro-oncology.* 1984; **2**, 29–34.
89. Rozental J, Trump D, Finlay J, *et al.* Pilot study of eight-drugs-in-one-day chemotherapy for high-grade astrocytomas (abstract). *Journal of Neuro-oncology.* 1986; **4**, 115.
90. Levin VA, Phuphanich S, Liu HC, *et al.* Phase II study of combined carmustine, 5-fluorouracil, hydroxyurea and 6-mercaptopurine (BFHM) for the treatment of malignant gliomas. *Cancer Treatment Reports.* 1986; **70**, 1271–4.
91. Harris MI, Bruner JM, Feun LG, Yung WK: Phase II study of alternating BCNU and AZQ in recurrent malignant gliomas (abstract). *Neurology.* 1987; **37** (Suppl 1), 288.
92. Schold SC, Mahaley MS, Vick NA, *et al.* Phase II diaziquone-based chemotherapy trials in patients with anaplastic supratentorial astrocytic neoplasms. *Journal of Clinical Oncology.* 1987; **5**, 464–71.
93. Eckman WW, Patlak CS, Fenstermacher JD: A critical evaluation of the principles governing the advantages of intra-arterial infusions. *Journal of Pharmacokinetics and Biopharmacokinetics.* 1974; **2**, 257–85.
94. Fenstermacher JD, Cowles AL. Theoretic limitations of intracarotid infusions in brain tumour chemotherapy. *Cancer Treatment Reports.* 1977; **61**, 519–26.
95. Fenstermacher JD, Gazendam J. Intra-arterial infusions of drugs and hyperosmotic solutions as ways of enhancing CNS chemotherapy. *Cancer Treatment Reports.* 1981; **65** (Suppl 2), 27–37.
96. Collins JM: Pharmacologic rationale for regional drug delivery. *Journal of Clinical Oncology.* 1984; **2**, 498–504.
97. Levin VA, Kabra PM, Freeman-Dove MA: Pharmacokinetics of intracarotid artery ^{14}C-BCNU in the squirrel monkey. *Journal of Neurosurgery.* 1978; **48**, 587–93.
98. Rosenblum ML, Dougherty DA, Wilson CB: Rational planning of brain tumour therapy based on laboratory investigation: comparison of single and multiple-dose BCNU schedules. *British Journal of Cancer.* 1980; **41** (Suppl 4), 253–4.
99. West CR, Avellanosa AM, Barua NR, *et al.* Intraarterial BCNU and systemic chemotherapy for malignant gliomas: a follow-up study. *Neurosurgery.* 1983; **13**, 420–6.
100. Greenberg HS, Ensminger WD, Chandler WF, *et al.* Intra-arterial BCNU chemotherapy for treatment of malignant gliomas of the central nervous system. *Journal of Neurosurgery.* 1984; **61**, 423–9.
101. Hochberg FH, Pruitt AA, Beck DO, *et al.* The rationale and methodology for intra-arterial chemotherapy with BCNU as treatment for glioblastoma. *Journal of Neurosurgery.* 1985; **63**, 876–80.
102. Bashir R, Hochberg FH, Linggood RM, Hottleman K. Pre-irradiation internal carotid artery BCNU in treatment of glioblastoma multiforme. *Journal of Neurosurgery*, 1988; **68**, 917–19.
103. Johnson DW, Parkinson D, Wolpert SM, *et al.* Intracarotid chemotherapy with BCNU in 5 per cent dextrose in water in the treatment of malignant glioma. *Neurosurgery.* 1987; **20**, 577–83.
104. Stewart DJ, Grahovac Z, Russel NA, *et al.* Phase I study of intracarotid PCNU. *Journal of Neuro-oncology.* 1987; **5**, 245–50.
105. Feun LG, Wallace S, Stewart DJ, *et al.* Intracarotid infusion of cis-diamminedichloroplatinum in the treatment of recurrent malignant brain tumours. *Cancer.* 1984; **54**, 794–99.
106. Newton HB, Page MA, Junck L, Greenberg HS. Intra-arterial cisplatin for the treatment of malignant gliomas (abstract). *Neurology.* 1988; **38** (Suppl 1), 305.
107. Mahaley MS, Hipp SW, Dropcho EJ, *et al.* Intracarotid cisplatin chemotherapy for recurrent gliomas. *Journal of Neurosurgery.* 1989; **70**, 371–378.

108. Greenberg HS, Ensminger WD, Layton PB, et al. Phase I-II evaluation of intra-arterial diaziquone for recurrent malignant astrocytomas. *Cancer Treatment Reports.* 1986; **70**, 353-7.
109. Feun LG, Lee Y, Yung A, et al. Intracarotid VP-16 in malignant brain tumours. *Journal of Neuro-oncology.* 1987; **4**, 397-401.
110. Shapiro WR, Green SB. Reevaluating the efficacy of intra-arterial BCNU (letter). *Journal of Neurosurgery.* 1987; **66**, 313-15.
111. Stewart DJ, Grahovac Z, Benoit B, et al. Intracarotid chemotherapy with a combination of BCNU, Cisplatin, and VM-26 in the treatment of primary and metastatic brain tumours. *Neurosurgery.* 1984; **15**, 828-33.
112. Kapp JP, Parker JL, Tucker EM: Supraophthalmic carotid infusion for brain chemotherapy: experience with a single-lumen catheter and maneuverable tip. *Journal of Neurosurgery.* 1985; **62**, 823-5.
113. Kupersmith MJ, Frohman LP, Carr RE, et al. Visual dysfunction related to intra-arterial chemotherapy for gliomas (abstract). *Neurology.* 1985; **35** (Suppl 1), 114.
114. Madajewicz S, West CR, Park HC, et al. Phase II study of intra-arterial BCNU therapy for metastatic brain tumours. *Cancer.* 1981; **47**, 653-7.
115. Bremer AM, Kleriga E, Nguyen TQ, et al. Complications associated with intra-arterial BCNU administered in combination with vincristine and procarbazine for the treatment of malignant brain tumours. *Journal of Neuro-oncology.* 1984; **2**, 129-32.
116. Mahaley MS, Whaley RA, Blue M, Bertsch L. Central neorotoxicity following intra-carotid BCNU chemotherapy for malignant gliomas. *Journal of Neuro-oncology.* 1986; **3**, 297-314.
117. Kleinschmidt-DeMasters BK: Intracarotid BCNU leukoencephalopathy. *Cancer.* 1986; **57**, 1276-80.
118. Delattre JY, Rosenblum M, Shapiro WR. Fatal necrotizing encephalopathy complicating treatment of malignant gliomas with intraarterial BCNU and irradiation: a pathological study (abstract). *Annals of Neurology.* 1987; **22**, 162.
119. Sheline GE, Wara WM, Smith V. Therapeutic irradiation and brain injury. *International Journal of Radiation, Oncology, Biology and Physics.* 1980; **6**, 1215-28.
120. Omojola MF, Fox AJ, Auer RN, Vinuela FV. Hemorrhagic encephalitis produced by selective non-occlusive intracarotid BCNU injection in dogs. *Journal of Neurosurgery.* 1982; **57**, 791-6.
121. Foo SH, Choi IS, Berenstein A, et al. Supraophthalmic intracarotid infusion of BCNU for malignant glioma. *Neurology.* 1986; **36**, 1437-44.
122. Blaylock JB, Wright DC, Dedrick RL, et al. Drug streaming during intra-arterial chemotherapy. *Journal of Neurosurgery.* 1986; **64**, 284-91.
123. Madajewicz S, Kanter P, West C, et al. Plasma, spinal fluid, and organ distribution of cisplatinum following intravenous and intracarotid infusion (abstract). *Proceedings of the American Association of Cancer Research* 1981; **176**, 22.
124. Stewart DJ, Benjamin RS, Zimmerman S, et al. Clinical pharmacology of intraarterial cis-diamminedichloroplatinum (II). *Cancer Research.* 1983; **43**, 917-20.
125. Rottenberg DA, Dhawan V, Cooper AJ, et al. Assessment of the pharmacologic advantage of intra-arterial versus intravenous chemotherapy using ^{13}N-cisplatin and positron emission tomography (PET) (abstract). *Neurology.* 1987; **37** (Suppl 1), 335.
126. Neuwelt EA, Glasberg M, Frankel E, Barnett P: Neurotoxicity of chemotherapeutic agents after blood-brain barrier modification: neuropathological studies. *Annals of Neurology.* 1983; **14**, 316-24.
127. Kapp JP, Vance RB: Supraophthalmic carotid infusion of cisplatin and BCNU for malignant gliomas (abstract). *Journal of Neuro-oncology.* 1986; **4**, 110.
128. Kapp JP, Vance RB: Supraophthalmic carotid infusion for recurrent glioma: rationale, technique, and preliminary results for cisplatin and BCNU. *Journal of Neuro-oncology.* 1985; **3**, 5-11.

129. Stewart DJ, Grahovac Z, Hugenholtz H, *et al*. Combined intraarterial and systemic chemotherapy for intracerebral tumours. *Neurosurgery*. 1987; **21**, 207-14.
130. Groothuis DR, Molnar P, Blasberg RG: Regional blood flow and blood-to-tissue transport in five brain tumour models: implications for chemotherapy. *Progress in Experimental Tumour Research*. 1984; **27**, 132-53.
131. Burger PC, Dubois PJ, Schold SC, *et al*. Computerized tomographic and pathologic studies of the untreated, quiescent, and recurrent glioblastoma multiforme. *Journal of Neurosurgery*. 1983; **58**, 159-169.
132. Kelly PJ, Daumas-Duport C, Kispert BA, Kall BA. Imaging-based stereotaxic serial biopsies in untreated intracranial glial neoplasms. *Journal of Neurosurgery*. 1987; **66**, 865-74.
133. Nakagawa H, Groothuis D, Blasberg RG. The effect of graded hypertonic intracarotid infusions on drug delivery to experimental RG-2 gliomas. *Neurology*. 34: 1571-1581, 1984; **34**, 1571-81.
134. Hiesinger EM, Voorhies RM, Basler GA, *et al*. Opening the blood-brain and blood-tumour barriers in experimental rat brain tumours: the effect of intracarotid hyperosmolar mannitol on capillary permeability and blood flow. *Annals of Neurology*. 1986; **19**, 50-9.
135. Warnke P, Groothuis D, Nakagawa H, *et al*. Capillary permeability of experimental brain tumours after hyperosmotic blood-brain barrier disruption (abstract). *Journal of Neuro-oncology*. 1986; **4**, 105.
136. Warnke PC, Blasberg RG, Groothuis DR. The effect of hyperosmotic blood-brain barrier disruption on blood-to-tissue transport in ENU-induced gliomas. *Annals of Neurology*. 1987; **22**, 300-5.
137. Neuwelt EA. Therapeutic potential for blood-brain barrier modification in malignant brain tumour. *Progress in Experimental Tumour Research*. 1984; **28**, 51-60.
138. Neuwelt EA, Hill SA, Frenkel EP. Osmotic blood-brain barrier modification and combination chemotherapy: concurrent tumour regression in areas of barrier opening and progression in brain regions distant to barrier opening. *Neurosurgery*. 1984; **15**, 362-5.
139. Neuwelt EA, Howieson J, Frenkel EP, *et al*. Therapeutic efficacy of multiagent chemotherapy with drug delivery enhancement by blood-brain barrier modification. *Neurosurgery*. 1986; **19**, 573-82.

14 Biological response modifier therapies for patients with malignant gliomas

G Yancey Gillespie and M Stephen Mahaley

Introduction

In the last 10 years, new therapeutic approaches for a wide variety of diseases and disorders have evolved around the application of an expanding spectrum of agents collectively known as biological response modifiers. The term biological response modifier (BRM) has come to include an extremely heterogenous group of substances (and their application) each of which has been shown to evoke an immunological and/or a non-immunologic response on behalf of the host. In most instances, the type(s) of responses defined represent only a small portion of those that are actually evoked and these restricted definitions often mirror the expertise and interests of the investigator. Biological response modifiers are of increasing interest as the fourth modality of therapy for certain infectious diseases, immunological disorders, cancer and idiosyncratic diseases thought to have an immunological basis. The principal rationale for BRM therapy lies in the belief that a BRM derived from "natural sources" should provide precisely the type of measured, biological control to treat successfully a disease process and that these natural products, although in unnatural concentration, should be less harmful to patients than chemically synthesized chemotherapeutic agents. This concept, together with the advent of recombinant DNA technology, has fostered an expanding new industry seeking to provide heretofore unheard-of quantities of biologically active peptides and proteins that govern basic biological response mechanisms. Attempts have been made to classify biological response modifiers based on their nature or on the principal type of response observed. A general classification scheme that recognizes both immunological and non-immunological effects of BRMs or BRM therapies is presented in Table 14.1.

Classifications

Biological response modifier therapy represents a challenge to classification if one attempts to identify the relation, if any, of an agent and its application within the

Table 14.1 A classification of biological response modifiers

Immunological
Restorative/non-specific immunotherapy agents
Adoptive immunotherapy
Passive immunotherapy
Active immunotherapy
Non-immunological
Chemoprotective agents
Radioprotective agents
Chemopreventatives
Nutritional agents

context of classical immunotherapeutic approaches. This challenge exists due to the desire of many investigators to identify those mechanisms that underlie BRM therapy. Classification becomes somewhat easier to conceptualize if one presumes that the most striking effects of BRMs are due largely to stimulation/augmentation of the immune system. Broadly, various therapies employing BRM agents can be considered to be a form of immunotherapy; however, not all BRM agents have effects consistent with positive or negative modulation of the immune system (Table 14.1). Furthermore, it must be borne in mind that BRM agents may have multiple effects, only some of which result in immune response modulation. In keeping with the focus of immunological modulation as a major effect of BRM therapy, non-immunological BRM effects or therapies (i.e., chemo- or radioprotective agents, chemopreventatives or nutritional agents) will not be reviewed here.

Accepting this restriction, it is possible to classify various immune modulatory BRM approaches within four generally accepted modalities: (1) restorative or non-specific immunotherapy; (2) adoptive immunotherapy; (3) passive immunotherapy; and (4) active immunotherapy (Table 14.2). Restorative (non-specific) immunotherapy encompasses the largest number of approaches involving BRM agents. Each of these represents an attempt to stimulate or boost in a non-specific way the deficient immune capabilities of cancer patients with one or more agents. Grouped here also are attempts to remove suppressive substances or inappropriate circulating antibodies by extracorporeal depletive techniques. The latter method will not be discussed here.

Adoptive immunotherapy is defined as the administration of sensitized immune cells, either autologous or allogeneic, in an attempt to transfer specific immunity to a patient with absent or weak immunological reactivity. Prior to the ready availability of recombinant lymphocyte growth factors, principally Il-2, this was technically impractical. In theory one would have to rely chiefly on mitogens (e.g., phytohaemagglutinin or concanavalin A) to stimulate lymphocytes *in vitro* in the absence or presence of antigen prior to transfusing these activated lymphocytes back into the patient. The possibility of strong host *vs.* graft or graft *vs.* host reactions would prevent the use of allogeneic lymphocytes in adoptive therapy, further limiting the source of effector cells. However, now that T-cell growth factor (Il-2) has been cloned and is available as an investigational agent from at least three major biotechnology firms, various approaches of adoptive immunotherapy are being seriously evaluated in a large number of clinical settings, the most obvious example

Table 14.2 Examples of immunological biological response modifiers

Type	Effect(s)	Examples
Restorative		
Augmenting agents	Non-specific stimulation of immune defence functions	Microbial agents or fractions, synthetic activators or inducers
Lymphokines and cytokines	Immunomodulation, direct or indirect antitumour actions	Interferons, interleukins, thymosins, lymphotoxins, tumour necrosis factor, transfer factors
Depletive therapy	Removal or absorption of suppressive factors	Immunoabsorption, plasmapheresis
Adoptive immunotherapy		
Autochthonous or allogeneic leucocytes	Systemic or intralesional infusion of immune-related effector cells	Mitogen- or lymphokine-activated killer cells
Passive immunotherapy		
Specific antitumour antibody therapy	Direct tumour cell killing by immunological means or by drug/radioisotope localization	Heterologous serum or monoclonal anti-bodies, human monoclonal antibodies
Active immunotherapy		
Allogeneic or autochthonous tumour cells	Invoke immune responses against patient's tumour *in situ*	Cultured or fresh glioma cell preparations with or without adjuvants

of which is lymphokine-activated killer (LAK) cell therapy.

Passive immunotherapy, the humoral immune response equivalent of adoptive immunotherapy, is based on administration of serum or specific antitumour antibodies rather than cellular immune components. Early attempts with polyclonal antisera revealed specific tumour localization but these encouraging studies were frustrating and disappointing due to the lack of sufficient quantities of absorbed antibodies for therapeutic evaluation. Monoclonal antibody technology which can provide unlimited quantities of highly specific antibodies has fostered a renewed interest in this potentially important immunotherapy arena.

Active immunotherapy requires active immunization with tumour-related antigens in an effort to increase the patient's ability to generate an antitumour response (cellular and/or humoral immune reactivity) specific for the patient's autochthonous neoplasm. This may involve autochthonous or allogeneic tumour-associated or tumour-specific antigens and quite frequently requires microbiological BRMs incorporated as strong adjuvants in order to elicit immunological responsiveness.

Restorative immunotherapeutic approaches

This type of therapy quite frequently employs microbiological organisms or their active components in an attempt to arouse or heighten activity of immune-related cells non-specifically. The rationale lies in the belief that non-specific systemic immunological activation will result in immune recognition of tumour antigens as foreign with subsequent focused antitumour responses. This non-specific arousal is presumed to facilitate escape of immune-related cells from whatever suppressive control or insufficient stimulation has prevented an appropriate antitumour response. With regard to the possibility that there is a lack of appropriate, strong or continuous stimulation, some investigators have shown that the interaction of immune-related cells in patients with brain tumours may be weak due to an inability to secrete sufficient lymphokines (immune response soluble messengers). This deficit is further compounded by the observation that mitogenic activation of peripheral blood T lymphocytes is dramatically impaired and appears to be principally due to a functional deficiency of the helper T lymphocyte subset[41]. This deficiency appears to be attributable to a paucity of high-affinity cell surface receptors for interleukin-2[134]. There appear to be relatively normal numbers of low affinity receptor molecules, but these alone are not sufficient for normal mitogenic responsiveness of T lymphocytes. In view of this, natural biological agents such as various cytokines (interferons, interleukins, thymosins) have also been used in a broad attempt to startle immune-related cells into action or to supplement low or absent levels of these essential immune soluble messengers.

Mircrobial/synthetic agents

Restorative immunotherapy with microbial/synthetic agents alone in patients with malignant brain tumours has been uniformly disappointing from the standpoint of efficacy (Table 14.3). In general, however, these agents have been relatively safe and well tolerated which suggests that there could be some benefit gained with little risk by combining restorative immunotherapy with other immunotherapeutic modalities. Among microbial agents used for restorative immunotherapy in patients with malignant brain tumours are: BCG (*bacille Calmette-Geurin*), BCG-cell walls (BCG-CW), *Corynebacterium parvum*, OK-432 and mumps virus. In a series of 13 patients, DeCarvalho et al.[31] were not able to ascribe any efficacy from giving 0.5 ml of BCG organisms intradermally per week for three to four treatments together with other therapy. Berquist et al.[8] reported treatment of one patient with recurrent glioma with BCG-CW with no indication of efficacy. Selker et al.[41] treated six patients with anaplastic gliomas with *C. parvum* (5 mg/m^2) given intravenously one to two times/month. There were no neurological improvements, no increases in delayed hypersensitivity responses (DHR) to *C. parvum* and no increases in PHA responsiveness. OK-432, also known as Picibanil, is an inactivated (heat and penicillin-treated), lyophilized preparation of the low-virulence strain (Su) of *Streptococcus pyogenes* (group A) originally developed by Okamoto et al.[119]. It has been studied extensively in Japan as a non-specific immunostimulator for patients with cancer. Ishizawa (56) treated 13 patients with gliomas (five with glioblastoma multiforme) but no efficacy data were reported. Likewise, Shibata et al.[142] reported a randomized controlled trial of 24 patients with gliomas who were treated with Picibinal in addition to radiation therapy and ACNU chemotherapy. Efficacy of this adjuvant immunotherapy was not observed. Mumps virus vaccination has been tried in six patients with lower grade gliomas and three patients showed some form of clinical improvement[192].

Levamisole, a synthetic antihelminthic, has been studied in two groups of

Table 14.3 Restorative immunotherapy attempts in patients with malignant glioma

Agent	Administration specifics	Number of patients	Efficacy	Reference
Bacterial				
bacille Calmette-Guerin BCG organisms (10^9/me)	0.5 ml intradermally/week × 3-4 weeks plus other therapies	13	None	31
BCG-cell wall	5 mg intralesional	1	None	8
C. parvum	5 mg/m^2, intravenous × 1-2/month	6	None (no immune profile changes)	141
OK-432	—	13	None	56
OK-432	0.5 KE × 3d, 1 KE × 3d, 2 KE daily, intradermal	24	None	142
Viral				
Mumps virus vaccine	—	6	Three patients showed response	192
Synthetic				
Levamisole	—		No improvement in T-cell function	22
Levamisole	2.5 mg/kg orally/day × 3, twice/month	100	None	82
Levamisole	(Same regimen)	6	None	47
Cytokine				
Thymosin α-1	300-900 μg/m^2, subcutaneous 2×/week × 4 weeks	14	No changes in total lymphocytes or T-cells	7

KE = unit of OK-432 activity.

patients. Mahaley et al.[82] reported the largest series of 100 patients in a prospective study in which patients who had surgical resection of a significant portion of their tumours were randomized to receive levamisole or not at the beginning of a standard adjunctive course of whole brain radiotherapy and BCNU chemotherapy. In a serial examination of immune profiles, there was no improvement in T-cell function and no efficacy as determined by overall survival times. A similar protocol of therapy, evaluated concurrently in the avian sarcoma virus (ASV)-induced glioma model in F344 rats, also failed to show any significant prolongation in expected survival[82]. In a later study, Fischer et al.[47] confirmed Mahaley's observation of a lack of efficacy of levamisole therapy in six patients with glioblastoma multiforme. Despite the lack of efficacy when used alone, levamisole stimulation was included as part of Phase I[83] and Phase III (Mahaley et al., unpublished data) trials of active immunotherapy of malignant brain tumours in 20 and 152 patients, respectively, with no evidence of serious systemic toxicity. Against the background of other biological stimulation in these last two trials, it would be extremely difficult to attribute any efficacy to this form of immunostimulation.

Interferons

Interferon was a term applied originally to a protein that induces protection in eukaryotic cells against viral infection. Interferons constitute at least three separate families of closely related glycoproteins with antiviral, immunoregulatory and antiproliferative properties. It is these last two properties that underlie the current interest in interferons as antineoplastic agents. Multiple species of human interferons have been shown to differ in molecular weight, antigenic composition and other properties. A revised nomenclature based on antigenic relation has designated the three major families or classes as: alpha- (IFNα), beta- (IFNβ) or gamma- (IFNγ) interferons. These three major clases of human interferons also correspond to those defined by an operational classification based on the cell of origin and the inciting stimulus that generates IFN production (Table 14.4). Alpha-interferons are a complex group of which there are at least 23 allelic loci of which 14 code for functional proteins comprised of 165 or 166 amino acids each. Genes coding for these various forms are localized to linkage group IX. These IFNαs are charac-

Table 14.4 Classification of interferons

Type	Inducing agents	Physicochemical characteristics	Cell sources
IFN-alpha (IFNα)	Viruses, dsRNAs, microbial agents, organic polymers, foreign cells	19–24 000 dalton protein, acid-stable, 14 different subtypes, weak species-specificity	B and null lymphocytes, macrophages
IFN-beta (IFNβ)	Viruses, dsRNAs microbial agents, organic polymers, foreign cells	19–24 000 dalton glycoprotein, acid-stable, 1 major type, moderate species-specificity	Fibroblasts, epithelial cells
IFN-gamma (IFNγ)	Specific antigens, T lymphocyte mitogens, activated T lymphocytes, calcium ionophores, phorbol esters	17–25 000 dalton monomer glycoprotein, functional unit is tetramer, acid-labile, strong species specificity	T lymphocytes

teristically produced as a result of viral insult; examples of the cell types responding include null lymphocytes, B lymphocytes and macrophages. For seveal years since the discovery of IFNβs, it was believed that there were just two major allelic forms of IFNβ, with the β-1 form comprising 90–95 per cent of the IFNβ produced by mesenchymal (fibroblasts) and epithelial cells in response to viral infection. IFNβ, also encoded on linkage group IX, is a 166 amino acid protein with about 30 per cent homology to some of the IFNαs. T lymphocytes are principally responsible for production of "immune" (IFNγ) interferon as a result of stimulation with antigens or mitogens. There appears to be only one major alleleic form of IFNγ, encoding a protein of 146 amino acids[125].

Until the recent advances in recombinant DNA technology, IFN for clinical evaluation was usually produced by, and purified from, peripheral blood leucocytes, cultured fibroblasts or lymphoblastoid cell lines stimulated with virus. Interferon produced by cells in response to virus or other stimuli commonly contains more than one type and is identified by the predominant component.

Alpha interferon Human IFNα has been shown to affect the growth of human glioma cells *in vitro*[18, 111] and in nude mice[17] variably (Table 14.5). Fidler *et al.*[46] have shown that hybrid molecules made from two different allelic forms (B and D) have direct antiproliferative effects on a variety of cell lines including those derived from glioblastomas. Of interest was the observation that the antitumour activity of these interferons was not enhanced by addition of mononuclear phagocytes to the cultures. A number of different groups[12, 52, 53, 86, 104–106, 118, 137] have evaluated the clinical applica-

Table 14.5 Preclinical studies of interferons in malignant glioma models

Model system	Application specifics	Effects	Reference
IFNα			
In vitro assays	100 U/ml HuIFNα(Leu)	Growth delay of U-251 Mg cell line up to 3 weeks	111
	100 U/ml + 300 rad	Additive growth delay	
In vitro assays	1000 U/ml HuIFNα(Leu)	No growth inhibition of 5 glioma cells in monolayers or spheroids	18
Gliomas implanted in nude mice	2 × 10⁴ U/day HuIFNα(Leu) × 23 days	Growth retardation in only 1 of 5 glioma	18
IFNβ			
In vitro assays	10–1000 U/ml	Block of glioma cells in S phase (dose-dependent)	76

Table 14.5 Cont'd

Model system	Application specifics	Effects	Reference
In vitro assays	3×10^6 U/day	Growth inhibition. Increased cytotoxicity of patients' PBL 7 days after beginning therapy	177
In vitro assays	5×10^2 to 5×10^4 U/ml	Dose-dependent growth inhibition; induction of glial maturation	66
In vitro assays	3–3000 U/ml	Dramatic morphological change; growth inhibition, diploid cells 100-fold less sensitive	26
In vitro assays	100–1000 U/ml	Growth inhibition	187
In vitro assays	1000 U/ml	Growth inhibition	189
In vitro assays	IFNβ encapsulated in liposomes	Growth inhibition of glioma cell lines with liposome-IFNβ > free IFNβ	62
In vitro assays		Growth inhibition of glioma cell lines	98
Two human glioma cell lines implanted in nude mice	6×10^5 U/day $\times$ 29 days	Regression of tumour growth	167
IFNβ			
Nude mice implanted with glioma tissue		Retardation of tumour growth	107, 108
Glioblastoma multiforme implanted in nude mouse	5×10^6 U/kg/day $\times$ 21 days	Growth inhibition	109
Nude mice implanted with glioma tissue	1000 U	Growth inhibition	189
Intrathecal injection in nude mice		Growth inhibition of glioma cell lines in CSF of mice	98

Table 14.5 Cont'd

Model system	Application specifics	Effects	Reference
IFNβ versus IFNα			
In vitro assays on glioma biopsy tissue	4–1000 U IFNα/ml or 4–1000 U IFNβ/ml	RNA and protein synthesis inhibited by HuIFNβ > HuIFNα Ly, low doses of HuIFNβ increased proliferation	13
In vitro assays	50 U rIFNα/ml vs. 50 U rIFNβ/ml	No inhibition Growth inhibition, cell line differences	193
IFNα versus IFNγ			
Immunofluorescence	rIFNγ	HLA-DR increase no antigen change	127
	rIFNα		
In vitro assays	rIFNγ	Growth inhibition no inhibition	
	rIFNα		
IFNγ			
In vitro assays with human glioma cell lines	rHuIFNγ 10–500 U/ml (dose-related)	Increase in HLA-DR antigen and mRNA transcripts glioma-mediated MLR augmented	166
In vitro assays with human glioma cell lines	HuIFNγ	Specific cytotoxicity of lymphocytes activated by IFNγ and Il-2	14, 15
Interferon and chemotherapy			
Glioblastoma multiforme implanted in nude mice	HuIFNγ + adriamycin or HuIFNγ + ACNU	Either combination gave inhibition of tumour growth	109
Interferon and radiation			
Glioblastoma multiforme implanted in nude mice	HuIFNβ plus 390–650 rad	Inhibition of tumour growth	109

tion and efficacy of human IFNα alone and with other therapies (Table 14.6). Salford et al.[137] first reported the use of IFN in two brain tumour patients in which daily administration of low doses (4×10^6 U) for prolonged periods (up to three months) by both intracranial and intramuscular routes simultaneously was without toxicity. In the largest clinical series, Mahaley et al.[86] reported CT scan evidence of response in seven of 17 patients with recurrent gliomas who received 900×10^6 U/m² of

Table 14.6 Reported trials of interferon therapy for malignant glioma

Type of interferon	Administration specifics		Route	Number of patients	Efficacy (responses)	Reference
	Dose					
Alpha Interferons						
Leucocyte	4 MU/day/route × 2–3 months		IT and IM	2	NR	137
Leucocyte	0.05–3 MU/day		IM	8	2	53
Leucocyte	1–6 MU/day; 12–25 MU total		IT	6	2	106
Leucocyte	3–9 MU/day; 2190 MU over 30+ months		IM	12	1	12
Leucocyte	9 MU × 3/week; 160 MU/3–11 weeks		IT	3	1	118
Lymphoblastoid	3–6 MU/day		IM	3	1	105
Lymphoblastoid	10–30 MU/m^2/day; 900 MU/8 weeks		IV or IM	17	7	86
Recombinant (Leu)	1–50 MU/day		IM	5	NR	121
Recombinant A	3–50 MU/day		IM	9	2	105
Recombinant	59–107 MU for 52–94 days		IT	4	NR	52
Beta Interferons						
Hu-IFNβ	1–6 MU/day; 240–360 MU/8 weeks		IV	54	12	138
Hu-IFNβ	1–6 MU/day; 336 MU/8 weeks		IV or IT	24	11	102, 103
Hu-IFNβ	0.3–3 MU/day; 10.5–171 MU/2–15 months		IV and IT	7	5	102, 103
			IT only	14	8	103
Hu-IFNβ	3–9 MU/day; 1638 MU/24 weeks		IV	3	0	107
			IT	4	1	
Hu-IFNβ	3 MU/day; 10.5–192 MU/2 months		IV & IT	5	0	122
Hu-IFNβ	0.3–6 MU/day		IT	20	8	105
Hu-IFNβ	2–69 MU/week × 4; 2–276 MU/4 weeks		IV	3	NR	15

Table 14.6 Cont'd

Type of interferon	Administration specifics		Route	Number of patients	Efficacy (responses)	Reference
	Dose					
Hu-IFNβ	10 MU/day × 10 and 1 MU every other day; 300 MU IV and 15 MU IT		IV ITu	12	0	38
Hu-IFNβ$_{ser}$	90 MU/week × 3 for 0.2–5 months		IV	10	2	193, 194
Hu-IFNβ$_{ser}$	90–540 MU 3 times/week 0.2–5 months		IV	18	6	195
Gamma Interferons						
Recombinant	0.07–0.12 MU every 3 days × 8 months		IT	3	1	154
Recombinant	2 mg/m², twice/week for 8 week, repeat × 2		IV	15	1	88
Combination therapies						
Hu-IFNβ plus Hu-IFNα	0.3–6 MU/day 0.3–6 MU/day		IM or IV	20	9	104
Hu-IFNβ plus 60–70 Gy and 100–150 mg ACNU × 1	1–3 MU/day		IV or ITu	9	5	188, 189
Hu-IFNβ$_{ser}$ plus radiotherapy plus BCNU	45 MU		ITu	15	NR	45

MU = 1 × 10⁶ U. IV = intravenous, ITu = intratumoural, IT = intrathecal, IM = intramuscular, NR = not reported.

IFNα intravenously or intramuscularly over an eight-week treatment period. Otsuka et al.[123] was the only group to report high titre serum antibodies formed in one of five patients treated with very high doses (as much as 14×10^9 total units over 44 weeks) of recombinant human IFNα.

Beta interferon Beta interferon was the first of the interferons to be extensively studied clinically in patients with gliomas (Table 14.6). As seen in Table 13.5, IFNβ has been shown to inhibit replication of human glioma cells *in vitro*[62, 66, 76, 98, 175, 187, 189] and in nude mice[107, 109, 110, 167, 189]. In addition, exposure of human glioma cells *in vitro* to human IFNβ encapsulated in liposomes produced a greater cytotoxic effect then was seen with free IFNβ[62]. The first clinical trials with human IFNβ for recurrent gliomas were conducted in Japan (Table 14.6) using intravenous as well as intrathecal or intratumoural routes of administration. Responses were reported in 12 of 54 patients treated intravenously[138], in 11 of 24 patients receiving IFNβ intravenously or intrathecally[102, 103] and in eight of 20 treated intrathecally or intratumorally[105]. Earlier work[105] had suggested that a combined route of intravenous and intratumoural was more effective (five responses of seven patients) compared with intratumoural alone (eight of 14 responding). Smaller groups of patients have been treated subsequently by several investigators[15, 38, 45, 107, 193-195] with less impressive responses. Yoshida et al.[189] has reported treating nine cases of recently diagnosed brain tumours with radiotherapy, ACNU and IFNβ with four complete responses and one partial response. However, in this report, the criteria for response were not clearly defined. Yung et al.[193-195] also reported preliminary results of a clinical trial of a recombinant form of IFNβ which has been genetically modified to substitute a serine residue for a cysteine residue at position 17. This piece of genetic engineering was performed to make the molecule more stable; it appears to be an innocuous change in that the biological activities of the IFNβ$_{ser}$ do not seem to be altered from those of native IFNβ. At the time of the report 16 patients with recurrent anaplastic astrocytomas were accrued to a protocol that planned biweekly intravenous doses escalating from 90×10^6 IU to 540×10^6 IU. Doses of 360×10^6 IU had been achieved with moderate toxicities. Two patients showed evidence of tumour regression, with one patient in complete remission at 12 months. In a larger study with unmodified human IFNβ, Yoshida et al.[188, 189] compared responses in two groups treated postoperatively for malignant glioma. Thirty-three patients were treated with radiation and ACNU chemotherapy only, while 25 patients received IFNβ in addition. Objective tumour regression was reported in 35.7 per cent of patients in the first group compared with 57.1 per cent of patients in the latter group.

Gamma interferon Gamma interferon has been shown *in vitro* to increase the HLA-DR antigens on glioma cell surfaces[127, 166] and to activate lymphocytes to produce specific toxicity in the presence of Il-2[14]. Smith et al.[154] reported using intraventricular IFNγ beginning two months after postoperative radiotherapy in three patients with gliomas. One patient was observed to have a gradual reduction in tumour size over a nine-month period based on CT scan changes. Because of the proximity to radiotherapy, it is not clear that this one response was due to the IFNγ alone.

Because glioma patients appear to be severely immunosuppressed, it was hoped that IFNγ might be an affective therapeutic agent in that it has been shown to stimulate various components of the immune response. In addition, recombinant IFNγ has been shown to stimulate the production of human tumour necrosis factor by human peripheral blood monocytes *in vitro*[140], an effect not produced by IFNα stimulation. In a recently completed Phase I trial[88], 15 patients with recurrent gliomas smaller than 50 cm^3 by CT scan were treated for an eight- week period using a recombinant IFNγ (2 mg/m^2 twice weekly). The results of this study were disappointing, with only one patient (with an oligodendroglioma that was the smallest tumour treated) responding with a decrease in CT tumour volume of more than 25 per cent in the absence of an increase in steroids. Eleven patients showed evidence of tumour progression within the eight-week treatment period and the median survival for the group was 24 weeks. Toxicities observed were those anticipated. In one patient vascular hypotension was sufficiently severe to abandon further IFNγ therapy after three treatments. In view of the disappointing results of IFNγ as a single agent in this selected group of 15 patients, it is not obvious that further single agent trials with IFNγ are warranted. However, IFNγ may be more effective when administered with other cytokines or chemotherapeutic agents.

Combination interferon therapies In a comparison of the three types of interferon in nude mice bearing six different human gliomas as xenografts, IFNα and IFNβ appeared to have equally effective antitumour activities, whereas IFNγ was ineffective. None was as effective as ACNU or vincristine chemotherapy, however. In combination with ACNU chemotherapy and radiotherapy, the effectiveness of IFNβ was enhanced if it was given after radiation therapy[109]. Interestingly, mouse IFNγ was effective against mouse gliomas in C57BL mice, suggesting species differences that could incorrectly predict therapeutic effectiveness for this biological response modifier.

IFNγ is reported to enhance the antitumour cell effects of tumour necrosis factor in assays *in vitro*, presumably by incresing the numbers of cell surface receptors for tumour necrosis factor. The use of IFNγ in any therapy must also take into consideration its ability to enhance antigen expression on glioma cells (*supra vide*) and its capacity to enhance slightly glioma cell growth *in vitro* at low doses (Gillespie, *et al.*; unpublished observations). Piguet *et al.*[127] has reported some efficacy when IFNγ was used in combination with other interferons.

Interleukins

The term interleukin (Il) is relatively new and was chosen to represent those soluble immune messengers that specifically stimulate immune-related cells to amplify a specific immune response through proliferation and/or differentiation into immune effector cells. As individual interleukins have been identified through conventional biochemical/biophysical analyses or as the result of gene cloning technology, classification has resulted in an identifying numerical progression. There are now six universally accepted distinct "interleukins", Il-1 to Il-6, with many more candidates waiting for indisputable proof of individuality.

Il-1, also knows as endogenous pyrogen, exists in at least two allelic forms; Il-1β (the predominant form) and Il-1α, each coded by separate genes of seven exons each with both genes located in linkage group 2[37]. Il-1 is a true immunostimulant that can regulate functional responses of immune-related cells (T and B lymphocytes, macrophages) non-specifically. In addition, Il-1 has been shown to induce other lymphokines and cytokines and to potentiate their activities. Il-1 also has direct antiproliferative and cytotoxic effects on some, but not all tumour cells[43]. Profound immunomodulatory activity coupled with its antitumour cytotoxic activity would make Il-1 an excellent candidate as an anticancer BRM. However, Il-1 is perhaps the most potent of the interleukins with profound neurological, metabolic and endocrinological systemic toxicities. Its principal mode of action appears to be its capacity to induce synthesis of prostaglandins, especially PGE_2 which mediate a variety of important physiological changes. Of major concern is the severe hypotension and capillary leak syndrome that can result from elevated prostaglandins secretion produced as a result of *in vivo* administration of Il-1. Paradoxically, Guilian, *et al.*[51] have recently reported that amoeboid microglia of the CNS in rats produce an Il-1 activity. This is consistent with previous reports from this group and others that normal astrocytes respond to Il-1 by proliferation and that some malignant glial cell lines produce Il-1 constitutively in culture. However, because the potent BRM effects of Il-1 could yield life-threatening toxicities, it is unlikely that Il-1 will be used soon to treat patients *in vivo*. Il-1 has been shown in animal studies to augment an antitumour immune response by increasing the number of Il-2 inducible lymph node cells in sites draining tumours[91]. This suggests that the lymphokine potentiating effects of Il-1 may make it useful for *in vitro* modulation of various immune-related cell responses prior to auto-adoptive therapy.

Il-2 or T-cell growth factor has already become the most useful interleukin for BRM-related therapeutic endeavours. To date, the focus has been on evaluating the use of Il-2 *in vivo* alone and in combination with LAK cells generated *in vitro*[50]. Il-3 principally causes differentiation and proliferation of mast cells and may have only limited usefulness in glioma therapy. Il-4 was originally known as B-cell growth factor and may become an essential ingredient in the effort to stimulate specifically the B lymphocytes of brain tumour patients *in vitro* prior to their use in generating human–human hybridomas secreting cells. It has recently been shown to synergize with Il.2 in the induction human antiglioma monoclonal antibodies.

Interleukin-5 is also a B-cell growth/differentiation factor produced by T lymphocytes[64]. It was originally designated T-cell replacing factor (TRF) or B-cell growth factor-II (BCGF-II) due to its capacity to promote proliferation of resting normal B-cells with differentiation into immunoglobulin-secreting of cytotoxic T lymphocytes[165]. Despite their identification, the precise role of each of the interleukins (Il-1, Il-2, Il-4 and Il-5) involved in B-cell growth and differentiation is still uncertain. Interleukin-6 is perhaps the most intriguing of this group. It was originally designated $IFN\beta_2$ due to its weak antiviral activity but it developed a large number of descriptive names ($IFN\beta_2$, B-cell stimulating factor-2, inducible 26 kD protein or hepatocyte-stimulating factor) based on biological activities. Its gene was independently cloned in three laboratories and the sequences proved that the various biological activities were due to the same biochemical entity. Il-6 shares many immunoregulatory properties in common with Il-1, yet has its own unique activities.

Interleukin-2 as a single agent One of the major side-effects of Il-2 administration has been a "capillary leak" syndrome leading to anasarca and multiple organ system dysfunction, most notably interstitial pulmonary oedema[75, 132] together with decreased systemic vascular resistance. Since therapeutic efficacy predicted for Il-2 in animal models is proportionate to dose, this represents a serious limitation to Il-2 based therapy. Rosenstein et al.[133] explored Il-2 induced vascular leakage of proteinaceous fluids in mice and determined that immunosuppressive pretreatment (cyclophosphamide, corticosteroids or whole body irradiation) markedly reduced transudation in lungs, liver, spleen, lymph nodes and thymus. In contrast to normals, nude mice (immunologically compromised) did not experience vascular leak syndrome when treated with Il-2. Ellison et al.[42] demonstrated that Il-2 (10^5 U/kg) given intravenously to cats as a single bolus injection produced significant increases in blood–brain barrier permeability as indicated by endogenous IgG or exogenous horseradish peroxidase extravasated in brain parenchyma. Not all of these effects were due to Il-2 as some alterations were also seen with the vehicle solution alone. However, taken together, these data suggest that host lymphoid elements mediate this symptom directly or indirectly. The best candidate as the pharmacological mediator of this side-effect is Il-1, based on its role as a potent vasodilator and inducer of capillary leakage mentioned earlier. Rather than give Il-2 as a bolus dose, West et al.[179] have presented evidence from clinical trials in which 48 patients with advanced cancer were given lower doses of Il-2 by constant infusion. Using this technique they were able to avoid the severe fluid retention and cardiopulmonary mobidity while preserving an antitumour effect in 15 of the 40 patients who completed at least one cycle of therapy. Alternatively, Vetto et al.[175] have shown that intravenous dexamethasone (mg every six hours) ameliorated some of the toxic side-effects (dyspnoa, confusion, fever, raised serum creatinine and bilirubin levels) in patients receiving Il-2. The influence of corticosteroids on the efficacy of this thrrerapy has yet to be determined, a significant concern in patients for whom brain oedema is routinely controlled with corticosteroid therapy. Denicoff et al.[33] observed severe behavioural changes that required acute intervention in 15 of 44 cancer patients treated with Il-2 during LAK cell therapy. An additional 22 patients developed severe cognitive changes (disorientation, cognitive deterioration). These neuropsychiatric toxicities, also reported for other forms of BRM therapy (IFNα, IFNγ) were time and dose-related and eventually resolved with cessation of treatment.

As if the obvious life-threatening toxicities (fever, chills, tachycardia, hypotension, vomiting, diarrhoea, fluid retention) reported for patients receiving high-dose Il-2 and LAK cell therapy were not serious enough, there are other more insidious side-effects, such as severe hypovitaminosis C[90]. Ascorbic acid levels dropped by 80 per cent after five days of high dose (10^5 U/kg every eight hours) Il-2 intravenous therapy and remained severely depleted during subsequent infusions of LAK cells and Il-2. Plasma levels returned to normal one month after the end of therapy. It did not appear that the ascorbate was being excreted and serum pantothenate and vitamin E levels were not affected. Importantly, patients who responded to Il-2/LAK therapy had a much less severe chronic depletion of serum ascorbate. Ascorbic acid is felt to be important to cell-mediated immune function and becomes depleted during physiologially stressful events.

Il-2 has been reported as a single agent for malignant glioma therapy in one study[57-59] involving four of 10 patients. Dosages of 10^4 to 10^6 Il-2 units were administered intraoperatively by multiple intracerebral injections into the area surrounding the resected tumour cavity. No toxicities were noted and too few patients were studied to provide any indication of efficacy. Based on its principal biological action as a T-cell growth factor, Il-2 has been used primarily to produce (non-specifically) activated killer lymphocytes for "LAK cell" adoptive immunotherapy (*infra vide*). In most cases, Il-2 is given concomitantly with LAK cells and adjunctively thereafter to prolong or maintain LAK cell activity *in vivo*.

Thymosins

The thymosins represent a closely-related family of over 20 polypeptide hormones capable of inducing both maturation and/or differentiation of prothymocytes and stimulation of different T lymphocyte subsets with hepler, suppressor or cytotoxic capabilities. Two of these thymic hormone preparations, thymosin fraction 5 and thymosin alpha 1, have been most widely studied clinically in patients with advanced cancer of colon, breast, kidney and lung. Thymosin fraction 5 containing this diverse group of small polypeptides (2 000–15 000 daltons) was chromatographically prepared from thymic extracts. Several polypeptides have been isolated and sequenced and of these, thymosin alpha-1 (28 amino acids, 3100 daltons) has been synthesized and the gene cloned. It was the first of the purified polypeptides available for clinical evaluation. The documented immunosuppression of patients with malignant glioma has served as the impetus to evaluate this BRM as an immunorestorative agent. In 1981, Ommaya *et al.*[120] reported a Phase I trial of thymosin in patients with malignant glioma. Baskies and Chretien[7] treated 14 patients with recurrent gliomas with 300–900 µg/m^2 given twice a week for four weeks but observed no improvement in total lymphocyte or T lymphocyte levels. The failure to observe any sustained or evanescent immune enhancement is consistent with a larger body of data in patients with other types of advanced cancer[36]. In the absence of more convincing evidence of immunological augmentation, it is not obvious that further clinical trials with thymic hormones as single agents are warranted. However, the thymosins may have a role to play in combined chemotherapy–immunotherapy studies, provided that it is evaluated using a prospective, randomized trial design.

Other cytokines

Tumour necrosis factor-alpha and -beta represent two of the newer cytokines that have not yet been reported as being used in patients with brain tumours. Tumour necrosis factor-alpha (TNFα), also known as cachectin, is principally a product of activated macrophages and has strong cytocidal activities against a wide variety of human tumour cells. Likewise, tumour necrosis factor-beta (TNFβ) is a product of activated lymphocytes and has been known for some time as lymphotoxin. TNFα and TNFβ bind to the same cell surface receptor[1] and have indistinguishable biological activities. Both TNFs have been cloned and their genes are apparently located in tandem in association with the major histocompatibility gene complex in both mouse[112] and man[156]. Receptors for TNFα and TNFβ are regulated by γ-interferon and show a moderate degree of species specificity[155]. Rutka *et al.*[135] described pleomorphic effects of human recombinant TNFα on human normal and malignant glia and rat glioma cell lines in *in vitro* proliferation studies. Some gliomas were markedly inhibited, some were moderately inhibited and others were slightly inhibited. One of three normal glial cell lines actually showed increased proliferation. The numbers of receptors for TNF were highest on the cells most sensitive and lowest on those least affected. Mori et al.[100] reported that human recombinant TNFα was cytostatic for three of five glioma cell lines tested *in vitro* at 100 to 1 000 U/ml. Moreover, when TNFα was given daily for seven days at 10 000 U/0.05 ml to nude mice bearing human glioma xenografts, tumour size was observed to decrease with haemorrhage and necrosis present in most tumours two weeks after therapy. Given the ability of IFNγ to enhance TNF receptor expression, it might be possible to increase the sensivity of TNF resistant cells as well as gain a further therapeutic advantage by combined therapy with TNF and IFNγ[69, 176].

Passive serotherapy with antiglioma antibodies

Major hurdles to be overcome in passive antiglioma antibody therapy are those of producing "functionally- or operationally-specific" antibodies to glioma antigens and devising rational methods to deliver these antibodies within the tumour bed in diagnostically and/or therapeutically useful quantities. In theory, the most appropriate glioma antigens for targeting would be those expressed constitutively (or after biomodulation) on the surface of most, if not all, malignant cells, but absent from normal adult cells. While there have been no confirmed reports of a truly glioma-specific antigen, much progress has been made in defining, with both exhaustively

Table 14.7 Passive immunotherapy clinical trials in patients with brain tumours

Type of antibody therapy	Efficacy and localization results	Number of patients (gliomas)	Reference
Polyclonal			
Rabbit (intracarotid or intravenous)	No efficacy shown; Localization of ^{131}I-ab seen in all patients with mean 4.2 tumour: brain ratio	11 (11)	28–30, 78–81
Monoclonal			
Mouse UJ13A (intravenous)	Localization of ^{131}I-MoAb in all 8 patients; 3.1 to 12.8 tumour: brain ratios; no efficacy reported	8 (7)	129
Mouse 81C6 (intravenous or intracarotid)	Localization of ^{131}I-mab seen in all patients with mean 5.0 tumour: brain ratio	9	25
Mouse UJ13A Mouse UJ181.4 Mouse F8-11-13 Mouse Mel 14 (intrathecal or intraventricular)	Localization of ^{131}I-mab seen in 5 of 6 patients with leptomeningeal tumours of different types; efficacy noted in 4 of 5 patients given therapeutic doses	6	67, 68
Human LGL1-1D6 (intravenous)	Localization of ^{131}I-MoAb in 8 of 12 patients No indication as to efficacy	12 (12)	147, 148

adsorbed polyclonal antisera and carefully characterized monoclonal antibodies, a wide spectrum of glioma-associated antigens including those that are neuroectodermal tumour-associated, normal CNS-associated, extracellular matrix proteins and biochemically identified markers (reviewed in refs. 23, 47, 70, 90, 184). Complicating the search for suitable glioma "target" antigen(s) are the observations that there are complex and heterogenous patterns of cross-reactivities between CNS tumour cells and lymphoid cells (reviewed in refs. 47, 90, 184) The exquisite specificites of monoclonal antibodies may yet serve in the eventual identifications of the precise relations of these antigens. Nonetheless, there are "operationally or functionally specific" glioma-associated antigens (e.g., oncofetal markers, growth factor receptors) expressed by some glial tumours that might be targeted safely in adults. Specific antibodies have been used to vector a wide range of chemical and biological antitumour agents to malignant cell surfaces. Among these agents are radioisotopes[26, 63, 67, 68, 74], polyhedral boron for neutron-capture therapy[6], photo-reactive substances[95], bacterial or plant toxins[168, 195, 196] and interferons[3]. Perhaps the clearest example of the impact and potential of monoclonal antibodies for glioma therapy derives from comparisons with earlier clinical studies using polyclonal antiglioma antisera.

Polyclonal antisera

The first study of radiolabelled antibody localization in 11 patients with malignant gliomas was conducted by Day[28-30], Mahaley[78-81] and co-workers. In these studies individual rabbit antisera were prepared, purified and radiolabelled from tumour tissue removed at original surgery. Patients who were re-operated for progressive disease received radiolabelled antibodies three to seven days prior to surgery. Surgically removed recurrent tumour tissues were analysed by gamma scintillation counting and autoradiography to determine the extent of tumour localization by paired, radiolabelled antibodies from specifically immune or non-immune rabbits. Immunoscintigraphy was also conducted on several of these patients. These studies successfully demonstrated low but significant localization in each case, even in portions of the tumour distal to the internal carotid artery injection site. However, there appeared to be no advantage of intracarotid over intravenous administration, although binding to tumour parenchyma was slightly greater with intracarotid injection. The percentage of injected dose of specific antibodies that was seen to localize ranged from 0.00025-0.01035 per cent of injected dose/g of tumour with tumour tissue-blood ratios of 0.26 to 6.81. Autoradiographs clearly demonstrated specificlocalization in and around tumour cells. However, this was a limited trial for several practical reasons: (a) the great amount of effort put into preparing exhaustively adsorbed specific rabbit antisera to each patient's tumour; (b) the finite, very small amount of antibody that was obtained (less than 0.02 per cent of total rabbit immunoglobulin); (c) the relatively low levels of localization seen, and; (d) the unknown consequences of repeated treatments with heterologous antibody[79, 80]. Today, monoclonal antibody techniques have obviated many of the theoretical and practical technical difficulties that have made passive serotherapy heretofore impractical. The principal remaining questions are: (a) whether or not tumour-specific monoclonal antibodies (MoAbs) that are functionally specific for gliomas can be generated and (b) whether or not localization of these antibodies can be achieved in quantities sufficient for therapeutic use.

Murine monoclonal antibodies

The literature on mabs produced from spleens of mice and rats immunized against glioma antigens is rapidly expanding as evidenced in several excellent review articles[20, 24, 34, 48, 70, 92, 117, 182]. These provide in-depth descriptions of the specificities and cross-reactivities of these MoAbs, some of which are in preclinical and clinical trials for treatment of malignant glioma. A few of the more recent studies are mentioned below to give an overview of the theory, application and problems of MoAbs as antibrain tumour agents.

Specificities and cross-reactivities Stavrou et al.[159-161] have produced mouse mabs to rat MNU-induced glioma cells and have determined that one of these, 14AC1, was capable of inhibiting growth of rat glioma cells *in vitro* and drastically reduced the number of lung metastases of pretreated and intravenously injected glioma cells. This monoclonal has also been shown to suppress growth of rat gliomas in nude mice as indicated by the longer latency period and a smaller tumour size compared with controls. However, termination of monoclonal antibody treatment led to increased tumour growth. Using ^{131}I-labelled 14AC1 whole mab or F(ab')$_2$ fragments, they found that the F(ab')$_2$ fragments appeared superior to whole molecules for immunoscintigraphy in nude mice bearing rat glioma xenografts. F(ab')$_2$ fragments had a more rapid tumour permeation, a shorter blood clearance and a markedly reduced background.

Saya et al[139] have produced a syngeneic rat IgM MoAb (FR77) by immunizing Fischer 344 rats with syngeneic 9L/R$_3$ glioma cells. In addition to its strong binding to 9L/R$_3$ glioma cells, MoAb FR77 was reactive with 9L and 6C glioma cells, but not with rat fibroblasts. Using biotinylated FR77 on formalin-fixed tissue sections, they demonstrated binding to intracerebrally implanted 9L/R$_3$ glioma cells with no binding to normal adult rat brain parenchyma or to a panel of other normal rat tissues. The antigen, thought to be a neutral glycolipid, appears on some fetal rat brain cells and is located predominantly in glioma cell cytoplasm. ADCC studies demonstrated weak but definite killing, which suggests that a portion of the antigen is associated with the cell surface. Interestingly, the antibody also crosses species boundaries in that it binds selectively to some human malignant gliomas.

Lee et al.[71, 72] have characterized four syngeneic rat mabs raised to a cloned avian sarcoma virus-induced glioma cell line of F344 rat origin. The mabs appeared to recognize the same epitope (or spatially juxtaposed epitopes) on some, but not all, rat and mouse neurogenic tumous of viral or chemical carcinogen origin. The failure of the antibodies to identify the antigen on all clones of positive cell lines provides yet another example of the phenotypic heterogeneity among gliomas. The antigen was tentatively identified as a small (300-600 daltons molecular weight) peptide non-covalently associated with a (binding) polypeptide on the glioma cell surface.

de Vellis and co-workers[35, 124] have described production of mab 217c by immunizing mice with the C6 rat glioma cell line. This mab recognizes a single polypeptide with a molecular weight of 64 000[77] that is expressed on the surface of at least three rat glial tumour cell lines (C6, TOP-ET-1, BD-ST-1) but is not on normal rat tissues or cultured glial cells.

McKolanis et al.[93] have produced mouse mabs against the TE-671 medulloblastoma cell line that recognize two groups of cell types; neither group includes astrocytic tumours. One group includes Purkinje cells, neurons of cerebellar cortex internal granular layer, most medulloblastomas and some nueroblastomas or cell lines of neuroectodermal origin. The second group includes reactivity to some but not all medulloblastomas. These antibodies may be useful in helping to define better the primitive neuroectodermal tumours seen in children.

While most of these approaches try to take advantage of the "antigen-resolving" power of the hybridoma method, an alternative strategy for producing appropriate antiglioma monoclonals is to identify by standard biochemical means substances unique to human gliomas as starting immunogens[48]. Mansson et al. have identified novel glycolipids in a human glioma cell line xenograft[89] and a panel of monoclonals have been produced (Bigner, personal communication) which may eventually have both diagnostic and therapeutic applications.

Localization The second major consideration after defining MoAbs with appropriate specificities is the question of how localization at the tumour site is to be maximized. In contrast to low molecular weight chemotherapeutic agents in which localization appears to be dependent more on lipid solubility than size, it is the large size of MoAbs (150 000–1 000 000) that restricts entry into the tumour compartment from the blood stream. Compared with low molecular weight drugs, even the relatively smaller albumin (68 000 MW)[114] or horseradish peroxidase (44 000 MW) protein molecules are remarkably diminished in tumour permeation. Bullard et al.[19] have examined various routes of administration of mabs with or without disruption of the blood–brain barrier in normal rats. In comparing interhemispheric, interregional and brain–blood ratios, they could find no advantage of intracarotid over intravenous administration of MoAbs, regardless of whether the barrier was disrupted by prior intracarotid hyperosmolar perfusion. Disruption of the blood–brain barrier did produce significant elevation of MoAb localization in all regions of the brain, with a greater effect seen in the hemisphere ipsilateral to the intracarotid hyperosmolar perfusion. Neuwelt et al.[115] have reported three cases of melanoma metastatic to the CNS in which localization of Fab fragments of two different mouse MoAb was compared before and after osmotic modification of the blood–brain barrier. There was no significant localization of either tumour-specific or non-specific radiolabelled Fab fragments prior to disruption of the barrier. After osmotic disruption there was increased uptake in the tumour-bearing (disrupted) hemisphere; however, distinct, persistent localization in the tumour was not achieved since more than 90 per cent of the radiolabelled Fab fragments cleared the disrupted hemisphere within 72 hours.

These limited observations serve to emphasize the importance of carefully selecting a preclinical model when trying to develop useful strategies in improving localization. For example, Blasberg et al.[9] carefully quantified localization kinetics of radiolabelled mouse MoAb 81C6 in athymic mice bearing subcutaneous or intracerebral implants of the human glioma cell line, D54 Mg. In contrast to the difficulty in localizing MoAb reported by Neuwelt et al. (115; see above), the 81C6 mabs specifically accumulated in both tumour sites, due largely to a long plasma half-life of the mouse immunoglobulin (in mice) coupled with a lack of significant barrier restriction. Using immunosuppressed rats bearing intracranial xenografts of the D54 Mg human glioma cell line, Lee et al.[73] found a significant advantage of intracarotid over intravenous administration of MoAb 81C6 which was further increased for Fab and F(ab')$_2$ fragments. These animals also did not require disruption of the blood–brain barrier. Thus, in xenografts there appear to be insignificant differences in the blood vessel permeabilities of intracerebral and subcutaneous implantation sites. Even under these artifical circumstances, however, studies by Wikstrand et al.[185] using a panel of six MoAbs specifically reactive with the D54 Mg cell line emphasized that in vitro reactivity on a MoAb does not necessarily predict its in vivo localization potential. It would appear then that the real value of the glioma xenograft model is to serve as a predictor of failure to localize for candidate mabs prior to clinical applications. Further, the heterogeneity of MoAb localization even in this relatively permeable model supports the concept that panels of monoclonals will be needed for clinical diagnostic and therapeutic procedures.

Richardson et al.[129] have studied localization of ^{131}I-labelled MoAb UJ13A in eight patients initially diagnosed with malignant gliomas. Uptake was assessed by scintigraphic analysis and by gamma scintillation counting of tumour tissue resected between three and 16 days later. Tumour localization was evident by immunoscintigraphy and by tumour-to-normal brain ratios ranging from 3.1 to 12.8; however, the percentage of injected dose/g of tissue was low, ranging from 0.00036 to 0.0043 for tumour and from 0.000045 to 0.00035 for normal brain.

In summary, there is an increasing number of encouraging reports[15, 16, 22, 32, 126, 160, 183, 185] from in vivo localization studies of MoAbs in gliomas and that access of MoAbs to brain and tumour can be enhanced with blood–brain barrier disruption procedures. A major obstacle that remains to multiple therapeutic administrations of murine monoclonals is the avoidance or circumvention of the human antimouse antibody (HAMA) response in patients.

Human monoclonals

While it has now become relatively uncomplicated to produce mouse MoAbs to xenogeneic human tumour cell antigens, it has also become increasingly obvious that those with desirable antiglioma specificities are extraordinarily rare. It could be that tumour-specific antigens may be difficult for a xenogeneic system to recognize against a background of normal antigens. For this and other reasons, production of human mabs may provide the capability of recognizing relatively weak human tumour antigens. Human MoAbs would also obviate one of the major problems with multiple administration of mouse or rat MoAbs to patients; namely, the elicitation of a human antimurine antibody (HAMA) response. This HAMA response can develop after one injection of mouse mab and can effectively neutralize subsequent doses of mouse MoAb. Human MoAb should not elicit the same strong antiglobulin response, although an anti-idiotypic response may be eventually generated against the human mab. Sikora et al.[146, 147] have produced a panel of eight antiglioma human MoAbs in 23 fusion attempts using intratumoural lymphocytes. One of these antibodies has been used for specific localization studies in 12 patients with gliomas[148, 149]. Evidence of specific localization was obtained in eight patients 45 hours after administration of 1 mg of ^{131}I-labeled MoAb LGL1-1D6 antibody. Three patients have now been implanted subcutaneously with a special chamber that permits continuous release of human antiglioma MoAb while preventing egress and metastasis of the human hybridoma cells[149].

Adoptive immunotherapy

Adoptive immunotherapy can take two distinct routes with regard to the mechanisms used to sensitize the effector cells; namely, specific adoptive immunotherapy versus non-specific lymphokine-activated killer (LAK) cell production. Specific adoptive immunotherapy involves the administration of authochthonous lymphocytes that have been specifically stimulated *in vitro* with authochthonous tumour cells to generate an expanded population with a highly restricted cytotoxic activity. This is to be contrasted with LAK cell therapy which is non-specific in that no attempts are made to stimulate the effector cells with any specific (glioma) antigen. LAK cell activity is a composite effect of stimulating all mononuclear leucocytes non-specifically which is a technically simpler procedure that requires fewer days in culture to generate a non-specifically cytotoxic cell population. This may account for the rapid and broad clinical application of LAK cell therapy (reviewed ref. 50).

Specific adoptive immunotherapy

While specific adoptive immunotherapy in glioma patients has yet to be reported, its efficacy has been readily demonstrated in preclinical animal models. Yamasaki et al.[186] cloned a T lymphocyte cell line that was specifically cytotoxic toward the murine malignant glioma cell line 203-glioma. This cell line was maintained in culture by repeated restimulation with Il-2 and maintained its specific activity over an 18-month continuous culture period. Further, they demonstrated, using a Winn assay, that at a 10:1 ratio with 203-glioma cells, effective neutralization of tumour growth was achieved. In mice inoculated intracranially with 203-glioma cells, effective protection against lethal tumour growth could be achieved with intravenous administration of the cloned cytotoxic cells as late as seven days after tumour inoculation. In a preclinical study, Miyatake et al.[99] stimulated peripheral blood lymphocytes from a glioma patient and induced two human T lymphocyte cell lines that express glioma-specific cytotoxic activity. The PBL were co-cultured with the patient's own tumour cells and Il-2. Both autologous and allogeneic glioma cells were killed by these two cytotoxic T-cell lines with minimal reactivity towards non-glioma tumour cells and mitogen-activated autologous lymphoblasts. These studies provide evidence that it is possible to generate specific antiglioma cytotoxic T lymphocytes *in vitro* that could be expanded for antiglioma therapy. Despite its technical difficulties, specific adoptive immunotherapy may yet prove to be superior to LAK cell therapy because it generates a population of antigen-specific cytotoxic lymphocytes as well as memory T lymphocytes from which more effector cells can arise.

LAK cell therapy

Perhaps the most widely used application of adoptive immunotherapy today is that with LAK cells activated *in vitro* with Il-2. LAK cells are peripheral blood leucocytes that have been activated by *in vitro* culture with mitogens and/or Il-2 (reviewed in ref. 6650). These cells are non-specifically cytotoxic to tumour cells but with a broader range of specificity than the natural killer lymphocyte that occurs naturally in the peripheral blood. An increasing body of data attests to the fact that the nature of the LAK cell remains an enigma. It has been suggested that the LAK cell is not a specific cell type, but may represent a collection of stimulated peripheral blood leucocytes that manifests a polyspecific cytotoxic response to fresh tumour cells *in vitro*. For the time being, it may be more accurate to refer to this as LAK activity, rather than attempt to associate the cytotoxic activity with a specific cell type. In the hunt for the LAK cell many characteristics have been uncovered. LAK cells have been distinguished from NK cells on the basis of surface phenotype, target cell range, resistance to the lysosomotropic agent L-leucine-O-methyl ester and cell density. Ramsdell and Golub[128] have shown that $CD3^-$, Fcg receptor$^-$, low density LAK can be generated from human thymocytes, indicating that the precursor population may be of an immature nature. Tilden *et al.*[169] have identified two effector cell types generated from peripheral blood using FACS sorting to enrich for LAK precursors and effectors. Precursor cells and most of the effector activity were associated with a $CD5^-$, $CD16^+$ non-T lymphocyte population, with a small amount of activity present in $CD5^+$, Leu-7^+ T cells. Classically, LAK activity is tested against a battery of tumour cell lines, such as DAUDI cells, which are insensitive to NK killing to demonstrate which of the two activities the effector population possesses. LAK cytotoxic activity can be blocked by the monoclonal antibody to the LFA-1 antigen. Thus, it would appear that there are significant differences between NK lymphocytes and LAK cells.

There have been several reports of LAK cell therapy in patients with malignant gliomas (see Table 14.9). In most instances, the route of administration has been

Table 14.8 Preclinical studies of II-2/LAK cell therapy for brain tumours

Experimental system	Experimental details	Observations	Reference
In vitro studies			
Human	Autologous LAK cells	Killed glioma cells	57–59
	Autologous PBL plus rll-2	Killed both fresh and cell line gliomas	
Human	PBL plus IL-2	Killed human glioma cells	99
Human (5 glioma patients)	PBL (5×10^6) plus rll-2 (10 U/ml)	Less IFNγ production and less LAK cell killing against glioma cell lines than normal donor LAK	143, 144
Human (glioma patients)	Mitogen-activated PBL supernates	Suppression of DNA/RNA synthesis of glioma cells	94
Mouse	LAK	Killed mouse glioma cells; trypsin or chymotrypsin treatment of glioma cells reduced cytotoxicity	57, 60

intraoperative injection into the tumour cavity or tumour bed. This has been felt to be necessary to ensure adequate localization of the effector lymphocytes in proximity to the tumour cells. However, this route of adoptive immunotherapy administration has a significant history pre-dating the "LAK cell era". Intratumoural injection of large numbers of peripheral blood leucocytes in brain-tumour patients without serious toxicities was reported by Young et al.[191]. Of the 17 patients with glioblastoma who received 10^7 to 10^9 autologous fresh non-activated leucocytes, eight sustained clinical improvement and were alive 17 months following treatment. This same group now has extended their experience by treatment of over 30 patients with malignant gliomas using intracerebral LAK cell therapy intraoperatively with subsequent Il-2 given intravenously[93]. Jacobs et al.[57-59] reported results of preclinical research with the 9L glioma model in rats (Table 14.8) in conjunction with phase I clinical trials in 10 patients, four of whom received 10^4 to 10^6 units of Il-2 alone, five who received 5×10^7 to 10^{10} LAK cells alone and one who received 10^6 units of Il-2 and 3×10^9 LAK cells simultaneously (Table 14.9). All infusions in patients were given intraoperatively by multiple intracerebral injections into the area surrounding the resected tumour cavity without untoward toxicities. In separate in vitro functional assays of LAK cells from six of the treated patients and four who were not treated, LAK cells from eight of these patients were strongly cytotoxic towards autologous or allogeneic glioblastoma cells but did not kill autologous PBL or other normal cells. A similar pattern of tumour-associated cytotoxicity was demonstrated for rat LAK cells tested against 9L glioma cells. Modification of target cell surfaces by hydrolytic enzymes or chemical reduction revealed that proteolysis by trypsin or chymotrypsin had a major negative effect on tumour cell killing by LAK cells[60]. This would suggest that LAK cells may recognize a polypeptide epitope on tumour cells that is absent from normal cell surfaces. Ingram et al.[54, 55, 61] have reported preliminary data concerning a clinical Phase I trial in 39 brain-tumour patients (18 with glioblastoma multiforme) treated intracranially with LAK cells produced by a variation of the Rosenberg technique. Patients' peripheral blood lymphocytes were initially stimulate with PHA for 48 hours before adding Il-2 to maintain proliferation over a two-week culture interval. Escalating doses of these LAK cells (1.1×10^8 to 3.8×10^9) were given. Eight patients were treated more than once but none of the patients was given Il-2 in addition to the LAK cells or subsequently. With 30 of 39 patients still alive at the time of the report, they were able to document the minimal toxicity associated with this treatment modality. There was no report of in vitro studies to determine the cytotoxic activities of the LAK cells given.

The use of tumour infiltrating lymphocytes (TIL) for LAK cell generation in humans[170] has been suggested due to good results in animal model systems[131]. The rationale is that immune-related cells infiltrating the tumour bed are more likely to represent specifically activated effector cells than would peripheral blood leucocytes, the current favourite source of LAK cells. This concept finds support in old reports of perivascular infiltration seen in gliomas (reviewed in refs. 85, 87) as well as more recent attempts to identify the immune-related cells infiltrating gliomas. Saito et al.[136] examined glioma tissue from eight patients using avidin–biotin immunohistochemical staining of frozen sections with a panel of monoclonal antibodies. Stained cells were quantified microscopically which revealed a marked predominance of T over B lymphocytes with helper T (T_H)-cell to

Table 14.9 Reported trials of adoptive immunotherapy for malignant glioma

Source of leucocytes	Administration specifics	Number of patients	Efficacy (responses)	Reference
Non-LAK cell trials				
Autologous leucocytes	Intratumoural ($6-22 \times 10^6$)	3	NR	171-173
Autologous leucocytes	Intracavitary	10	NR	164
Autologous peripheral blood leucocytes	Intratumoural (10^7-10^9)	17	9 stable or with improvement at 17 months	191
Autologous peripheral blood lymphocytes	Intrathecal (10^6-10^9)	4	No efficacy	113
Autologous peripheral blood lymphocytes	Intratumoural	9	No efficacy proven	56
Autologous peripheral blood lymphocytes	Intratumoural (10^7-10^9)	4 recurrent	No efficacy	162
LAK cell trials				
Autologous LAK cells	Intratumoural 10^8-10^{10} or/and 10^4-10^6 U rIl-2	10	None proven	57-59
Autologous PBL	Intracisternal $1-2 \times 10^8$ 500 U Il-2r/ 100 ml + 500 U rIl-2 IV	1 (gliomatosis)	CSF cleared; improvement clinically	143, 144
Autologous leucocytes	Intrathecal $2.1-6.7 \times 10^9$	11	Median survival 28 weeks	174
Autologous ASL and LAK plus rIl-2	Plasma clot × 2 10^9 ASL + 10^7 LAK 2×10^6 U rIl-2 × 2	10	Median survival 13 weeks	27
Autologous ASL + Il-2	Plasma clot 10^9 ASL, 10^6 U Il-2	39	Median survival 26 weeks	54, 55
Autologous LAK plus rIl-2	Intratumoural $1-4 \times 10^2$ PBL + $2-4 \times 10^8$ rIl-2 2-3 times/ week, 2 months	14	Four responses by CT scan	190

Table 14.9 Cont'd

Source of leucocytes	Administration specifics	Number of patients	Efficacy (responses)	Reference
Autologous cytotoxic T lymphocytes	Intratumoural 5×10^7 CTL Twice/wk, 4–10 weeks	5	2 responses; median survival 18 weeks	65
Autologous LAK cells plus rIl-2	Intraparenchymal $1–15 \times 10^9$ plus 10^6 U rIl-2 Intracavitary rIl-2 $\times 3$ days, repeat @ 2 weeks	20	8 responders; mean time-to-failure 25 weeks	94
Autologous LAK cells plus Il-2	Intratumoural $2.7–20 \times 10^9$ plus $6.3–45 \times 10^4$ U/kg	7	No responses	5

cytotoxic/suppressor T ($T_{C/S}$) cell ratios ranging from 0.2 to 3.6. Peripheral blood levels and ratios of T lymphocytes were not determined. In a semiquantitative comparison of monoclonal antibody staining for T lymphocyte subsets in brain tissue from six glial and eight non-glial tumours, von Hanwehr et al.[176] reported a similar range of T_H : $T_{C/S}$ ratios with a perceived greater tendency for occurrence of the $T_{C/S}$ phenotype. Miescher et al.[96] have determined the phenotype, clonogenic potential and cytotoxic activities of TIL extracted from glioma tissue. TIL recovered by density gradient centrifugation of disaggregated glioma tissue were small, non-activated (HLA-DR-, IL-2r-) T (T11+) cells which had strikingly depressed proliferative responses to mitogenic lectins (PHA, con-A, TPA). By clonal dilution analysis, TIL were 10- to 50-fold less responsive than peripheral blood lymphocytes. TIL microcultures that did proliferate were either T_H (41 per cent) or $T_{C/S}$ (51 per cent) phenotype with only 7 per cent containing a mixture of T_H and $T_{C/S}$ cells. TIL microcultures from three patients were tested for cytotoxic activity against autologous and allogeneic tumour cells; most were cytolytic either in a natural killer-like fashion or in a glioma-associated fashion. The poor proliferative responsiveness of glioma-derived TIL does not bode well for those attempting to use these as a source of activated LAK cells for therapeutic purposes.

One of the major criticisms of LAK cell therapy has been that the blastic cells are not thought to home on to the tumour site, another reason for intratumoural injection of LAK cells. In an important report, Migliori et al.[97] have shown in a mouse model system that LAK cells can be made to home on to areas of normal tissue or to implanted tumours if the lymphocyte-recruiting factors Il-1, tumour necrosis factor or bacterial LPS were injected into those sites. Presumably these agents that attract tissue infiltration by normal immune-related inflammatory cells will also work for LAK cells. Sarcoma-bearing mice injected intralesionally with LPS prior to Il-2/LAK cell therapy survived longer than tumour-bearers injected intralesionally with saline.

Production of LAK cells is labour-intensive because of its requirement for large volume tissue culture and carries with it increased risk for the patient with regard to potential for microbial contamination of the cultured cells. Muul et al.[101] have described an automated closed system which was developed for production of human LAK that significantly reduces the contamination potential while providing essentially identical yields of LAK cell numbers and activity.

Active immunotherapy

Active immunotherapy can be generally defined as a method or methods that facilitate the ability of a patient's immune system to recognize, to interact with and attack his tumour cells in an antigen-specific fashion. In general application, extensive animal studies have shown that this can best be achieved through multiple injections of prepared autologous or homologous tumour cells or cross-reacting

Table 14.10 Reported trials of active immunotherapy for malignant glioma

Immunotherapy preparation	Number of patients	Efficacy	References
Live autologous glioma cells (injected subcutaneously)	5	None	11
Live autologous glioma cells (injected subcutaneously)	6	None; 2/6 developed DHR	49
Live autologous glioma cells (injected with extract plus Freund's adjuvant or BCG)	28	Survival improved; (?) 1 case of EAE	171–173
Live irradiated autologous glioma cells (injected subcutaneously)	62	None	10
Killed autologous glioma cells (10^6 neuroaminidase-treated cells injected intradermally with 10^7 BCG cells + 0.1 ml PPD)	5	None	2
Live irradiated homologous glioma cells (10^8 tissue culture cells injected subcutaneously + 500 μg BCG cell walls; levamisole given *per os*)	19	Prolonged survival of 9 patients	83, 84
Live homologous glioma cells (10^7 tissue culture cells injected subcutaneously + 500 μg BCG-CW)	3	Prolonged survival of 2 patients	20
Live autologous/homologous glioma cells (10^8 cells injected subcutaneously after treated with glycolipid + muramyl dipoptide adjuvant)	1	Not reported	39

antigenic material to "immunize" patients with neoplastic disease. This therapeutic approach has had perhaps the longest history of any BRM therapy for patients with gliomas (Table 13.10). Bloom et al.[11] conducted the first therapeutic attempt by subcutaneous implantation of autologous tumour cells in a patient with malignant astrocytoma. Serological assays did not indicate the complement-fixing antibodies were elicited nor was there any other evidence that an antitumour response was generated. To make matters worse, viable tumour cells grew at the implantation sites. Grace et al.[49] reported a year later a similar trial in six brain tumour patients, none of whom developed antiglioma antibodies. However, two patients did develop delayed hypersensitivity skin test responses to tumour extracts. In two other patients, unfortunately, viable tumour cells grew at the implant sites. Later, other investigators conducted a randomized prospective study in which 27 of 62 malignant glioma patients were treated with irradiated autologous tumour cells following cytoreductive surgery and postoperative irradiation[10]. Ten patients received more than one injection but none had more than three injections. Intradermal skin testing with autologous tumour extracts failed to elicit any responses from the immunized patients and there was no difference in survival between the immunized and non-immunized patient groups. Trouillas and Lapras[171] randomized 65 malignant glioma patients into four treatment groups: (a) 17 patients received no postoperative therapy; (b) 20 patients received postoperative irradiation; (c) 18 patients received postoperative irradiation and immunotherapy with autologous tumour cells emulsified in Freund's complete adjuvant; (d) 10 patients received postoperative immunotherapy alone. During the two-year course of this study, the 28 immunotherapy patients received between four and 10 serial immunizations with evidence of antitumour reactivity. Specifically, 25 of these patients developed cutaneous hypersensitivity responses to autologous tumour extracts with some sera samples showing cytotoxic antibodies against glioma cells in complement-dependent *in vitro* assays. In a later report of 20 patients immunized similarly, postimmunization sera from 14 patients showed diffuse immunoprecipitation reactions with extracts of autologous tumour and fetal brain, but not adult normal brain or meningioma extracts. Bullard et al.[19] reported a Phase I active immunotherapy trial with five patients conducted at the National Hospital for Nervous Diseases in London. Three of the five patients were given serial immunization with viable, HLA-mismatched glioma cell lines mixed with a BCG cell wall adjuvant in addition to standard chemotherapy of CCNU, vincristine and procarbazine. Two of the three serially immunized patients showed serological evidence of response to the immunizing cell line without developing untoward systemic reactions as noted clinically or at autopsy. At the sametime, Mahaley et al.[83] conducted a Phase I active immunotherapy trial in which the same glioma cell lines (D54 Mg and U251 Mg) were used to immunize serially 20 patients who were concomitantly treated with radiotherapy and BCNU chemotherapy postoperatively. The differences in this latter study were threefold: (1) the glioma cells were lethally irradiated (20 000 rads): (2) the patients also received levamisole orally as a further immunostimulant; and (3) patients were selected for this trial by meeting three criteria of immunocompetence, namely both blood lymphocyte and T lymphocyte levels to be at least 50 per cent of normal and cutaneous hypersensitivity response to at least one of four standard recall antigens. Serological analysis of serum samples collected monthly during immunization revealed striking responses by all patients to Class III antigens (e.g., fetal bovine serum antigens acquired passively through *in vitro* culture) and in most patients to Class II antigens (cross-reactive with other tumour types) in addition to HLA antigens expressed on the glioma cells[84]. In a few patients there was evidence after extensive absorption of low but significant antibody reactive against Class I tumour antigen(s) on the immunizing glioma cell line. As in the previous trial there was no indication of untoward systemic reactioon and, although the two groups were small, there was a suggestion of improved survival of patients receiving the U251 Mg cell line compared with that of the D54 Mg cell line group or 58 patients in a previous trial involving levamisole immunostimulation only in addition to an identical regimen of postoperative radiotherapy and BCNU chemotherapy[83]. Based on the findings from these two Phase I trials, Mahaley and co-workers initiated and are nearing completion of accrual of 100 patients to a collaborative randomized, prospective Phase III trial utilizing lethally irradiated U251 Mg glioma cells. In view of the fact that only one of 11 patients developed strong serological reactivity to Class I glioma cell antigens[84], the question arises as to whether or not it is important to use autologous cells for immunization. Eggers *et al.*[39] reported one case of autologous and homologous tumour-cell immunization of a patient with a diagnosis of glioblastoma multiforme in which the tumour cells were coupled to adjuvant compounds to make them more immunogenic. They used both muramyl dipeptide (the active granuloma-inciting agent of mycobacterium) and an analogue of cord factor, a glycolipid of mycobacterium that also induces granuloma formation. Although no serological data regarding the antigens that may have been recognized were reported, they did report that the cytotoxic activity of peripheral blood lymphocytes appeared to be T-cell-mediated. During the course of therapy, the patient's glioma cell line ceased growing *in vitro* and homologous glioma cells were used for immunization. Immunity, as measured by peripheral blood lymphocyte cytotoxicity assays, declined and this form of therapy was discontinued. Further studies will be warranted to determine the importance of autologous versus homologous tumour cells as well as the value of the adjuvants in improving the immunogenicity of injected glioma cells.

Other methods for improving the immunogenicity of tumour cells include modification of the cell membrane. Stavrou *et al.*[157, 158] chemically modified several different cell lines derived from rat MNU-induced gliomas with either trinitrobenzene sulphfonic acid (TNBS) or dimethyl sulphate (DMS). Multiple immunization of syngeneic rats with these "haptenized" glioma cells resulted in relatively specific cytotoxic antisera for unmodified glioma cells. This method was used to generate syngeneic rat MoAbs to these glioma cells[159]. It has not been tried clinically. Shinitzky and Skornick have published several papers[145, 150-153] describing modification of tumour cells by incorporation of cholesteryl hemisuccinate (CHS) into the cell membrane. This has been shown to increase membrane viscosity[145] and is thought to promote expression of (latent) tumour-associated antigens. Immunotherapeutic vaccination of naive mice with irradiated, CHS-treated tumour cells afforded protection to subsequent challenges with unmodified viable tumour cells. In clinical trials, most immunocompetent cancer patients expressed increased skin test reactivity to autologous, irradiated tumour cells which had been treated with CHS compared with tumour cells that had not been CHS-modified. Active immunotherapy of 21 patients with CHS-treated autologous tumous cells only led to seven responses and stable disease in nine[153]. This has not been attempted in patients with gliomas. In contrast to the observations of Shinitzky and

Skornick, Rong and Sindelar[130] determined that CHS-treated tumour cell vaccines were not effective in protecting against tumour challenges in five different syngeneic tumour models. Until human glioma-associated or glioma-specific antigens are identified, development and assessment of effective glioma vaccines will remain at a relative standstill.

Coda

In attempting to review as broad a topic as the history and future directions of biological response modifier therapy in patients with malignant gliomas, it quickly becomes obvious that the lists of agents and applications to elicit immunological responses are growing endlessly and faster than each agent can be adequately evaluated. We are seeking that "magic bullet" that will enable us to target glioma cells broadly and provide significantly improved therapeutic efficacy for this desperately devastating disease. Perhaps different combinations of treatment modalities that are being explored in non-gliogenous tumour systems may eventually find applicability in brain tumour therapy. Thermoimmunotherapy is but one example of a novel treatment modality that combines local hyperthermia (LH) with immunomodulation using *Propionibacterium granulosum* KP-45 in patients with advanced prostatic or breast cancer[163]. Thermoimmunotherapy has resulted in a increased number of responders compared with patients receiving LH alone. In preclinical trials in mice however, Baker *et al.*[4] found that the non-specific immune stimulant levamisole was antagonistic to the action of hyperthermia in controlling local tumour growth and extending animal survival. Despite these contradictions, which are inevitble between biological model systems and clinical reality, BRM therapies may yet prove to be the deciding factor as an adjunct to current modalities of surgery, radiotherapy and chemotherapy for malignant gliomas. The powerful methodological tools available today in the form of monoclonal antibody and recombinant DNA technologies significantly improve the possibility that successful efficacious antiglioma therapy will evolve quickly.

Acknowledgements

This work was supported in part by USPHS research awards CA29125 (GYG), CA30479 (GYG), NS 20023 (MSM) and CA 13148 (MSM).

References

1. Aggarwal BB, Eessalu TE, Hass PE. Characterization of receptors for human tumour necrosis factor and their regulation by γ-interferon. *Nature*. 1985; **318**, 665–7.
2. Albright L, Seab, JA, Ommaya AK. Intracerebral delayed hypersensitivity reactions in glioblastoma multiforme patients. *Cancer*. 1977; **39**, 1331–6.
3. Alkan SS, Miescher-Grander S, Braun DG, Hochkeppel HK. Antiviral and antiproliferative effects of interferons delivered via monoclonal antibodies. *Journal of Interferon Research*. 1984; **4**, 355–63.
4. Baker D, Sager H, Constable W. The influence of levamisole and hyperthermia on the incidence of metastases from an X-irradiated tumour. *Cancer Investigations*. 1986; **4**, 287–92.

5. Barba D, Oldfield EH, Saris SC, Rosenberg SA, Hamilton JM. Phase II immunotherapy of cystic primary brain tumours with Interleukin-2/LAK cells. *Proceedings of the American Society for Clinical Oncology.* 1988; **7**, 82.
6. Barth, RF, Johnson CW, Wei WZ, Carey WE, Soloway AH, McGuire J. Neutron capture using boronated monoclonal antibody directed against tumour-associated antigens. *Cancer Detection and Prevention.* 1982; **5**, 315-23.
7. Baskies AM, Chretien PB. Thymosin alpha-1 in malignant gliomas: Augmentation of immune reactivity in a phase I study. *Surgical Forum.* 1982; **33**, 522-34.
8. Berquist BJ, Mahaley MS Jr, Steinbok P, Dudka L. Treatment of a brain tumour with BCG cell wall preparation. *Surgical Neurology.* 1980; **13**, 197-201.
9. Blasberg RG, Nakagawa H, Bourdon MA, Groothuis DR, Patlak CS, Bigner DD. Regional localization of a glioma-associated antigen defined by monoclonal antibody 81C6 *in vivo*: Kinetics and implications for diagnosis and therapy. *Cancer Research.* 1987; **47**, 4432-43.
10. Bloom HJG, Peckham MJ, Richardson AE, Alexander PA, Payne PM. Glioblastoma multiforme: A controlled trial to assess the value of specific active immunotherapy in patients treated by radical surgery and radiotherapy. *British Journal of Cancer.* 1973; **27**, 253-67.
11. Bloom WH, Carstaris KC, Crompton MR, McKissock W. Autologous glioma transplantation. *Lancet.* 1960; **ii**, 77-8.
12. Boethius J, Blomgren H, Collins VP, Greitz T, Strander H. The effect of systemic human interferon-alpha administration to patients with glioblastoma multiforme. *Acta Neurochirugica.* 1983; **68**, 239-51.
13. Bogdahn U. Chemosensitivity of malignant brain tumours. *Journal of Neuro-oncology.* 1983; **1**, 149-66.
14. Bogdahn U, Fleischer B, Rupniak HTR, Epstein LB. Interferon in specific T-cell mediated cytotoxicity in human gliomas. *Antiviral Research, The Biology of the Interferon System.* Heidelberg, October 21-25. 1984; 84.
15. Bogdahn U, Fleischer B, Hilfenhaus J, Rothing HJ, Krauseneck P, Mertens HG, Przuntek H. Interferon-β in patients with low-grade astrocytomas. A Phase I study. *Journal of Neuro-oncology.* 1985; **3**, 125-30.
16. Bourdon MA, Wikstrand CJ, Furthmayr H, Matthews TJ, Bigner DD. Human glioma – mesenchymal extracellular matrix antigen defined by monoclonal antibody. *Cancer Research.* 1983; **43**, 2796-2805.
17. Bourdon MA, Coleman RE, Blasberg RG, Groothuis DR, Bigner DD. Monoclonal antibody localization in subcutaneous and intracranial human glioma xenografts: paired-label and imaging analysis. *Anticancer Research.* 1984; **4**, 133-40.
18. Bradley NJ, Darling JL, Oktar N, Bloom HJG, Thomas DGT, Davies AJS. The failure of human leukocyte interferon to influence the growth of human glioma cell populations: *in vitro* and *in vivo* studies. *British Journal of Cancer.* 1983; **48**, 819-25.
19. Bullard DE, Bourdon M, Bigner DD. Comparison of various methods for delivering radiolabeled monoclonal antibody to normal rat brain. *Journal of Neurosurgery.* 1984; **61**, 901-11.
20. Bullard DE, Thomas DGT, Darling JL, Wikstrand CJ, Diengdoh JV, Barnard RO, Bodmer JG, Bigner DD. A preliminary study utilizing viable HLA mismatched cultured glioma cells as adjuvant therapy for patients with malignant gliomas. *British Journal of Cancer.* 1985; **51**, 283-9.
21. Bullard DE, Bigner DD. Applications of monoclonal antibodies in the diagnosis and treatment of primary brain tumours. *Journal of Neurosurgery.* 1985; **63**, 2-16.
22. Caciagli P, Acerbi G, Ciccarelli R, D'Angelo C, Iovenitti P, Caciagli F. Surveys on the immune system in patients with glioblastoma. *Proceedings of the American Society for Clinical Oncology.* 1980; **1**, 44.
23. Cairncross JG, Mattis MJ, Beresford HR, Albino AP, Houghton AN, Lloyd KO,

Old, LJ. Surface antigens of human astrocytoma defined by monoclonal antibodies. Identification of astrocytoma subsets. *Proceedings of the National Academy of Sciences of the USA.* 1982; **79**, 5641–5.
24. Coakham HB, Garson JA, Brownell B, Kemshead JT. Diagnosis of cerebral neoplasms using monoclonal antibodies. *Progress in Experimental Tumour Research.* 1985; **29**, 57–77.
26. Cook AW, Carter WA, Nidzgordki F, Akhtar L. Human brain tumour-derived cell lines: growth rate reduced by human fibroblast interferon. *Science.* 1983; **219**, 881–3.
27. Cruse Carol, Lillehei Kevin. Personal communication, 1987.
28. Day ED, Lassiter S, Woodhall B, Mahaley JL, Mahaley MS Jr. The localization of radioantibodies in human brain tumours. I. Preliminary exploration. *Cancer Research.* 1965; **25**, 773–8.
29. Day ED, Lassiter S, Mahaley MS Jr. The localization of radioantibodies in human brain tumours. III. Radioiodination of pre-purified localizing antibody. *Journal of Nuclear Medicine.* 1965; **6**, 38–52.
30. Day ED, Rigsbee L, Wilkins R, Mahaley MS Jr. Localization of anti-brain radio-antibodies in rat brain. *Journal of Immunology.* 1967; **98**, 62–6.
31. DeCarvalho S, Kaufman A, Pineda A. Adjuvant chemo-immunotherapy in central nervous system tumours. In: Salmon SE, josen SE, eds. *Adjuvant Therapy of Cancer.* Amsterdam: Elsiever/North Holland, 1977; 495–502.
32. de Muralt B, de Tribolet N, Diserens AC, Carrel S, Mach JP. Reactivity of anti-glioma monoclonal antibodies for a large panel of cultured glioma and other neuroectoderm derived tumours. *Anticancer Research.* 1983; **3**, 1–6.
33. Denicoff KD, Rubinov DR, Papa MZ, Simpson C, Seipp CA, Lotze MT, Chang AE, Rosenstein D, Rosenberg SA. The neuropsychiatric effects of treatment with interleukin-2 and lymphokine-activated killer cells. *Annals of Internal Medicine.* 1987; **107**, 293–300.
34. de Tribolet N, de Muralt B, Buchetter F, Mach JP, Schreyer M, Carrel S. Monoclonal antibodies to glioma tumour antigens. In: Wright GL Jr, ed. *Monoclonal Antibodies and Cancer,* Immunology Series 23, New York: Marcel Dekker, 1984; 81–120.
35. de Vellis J, Peng WW, Pixley SKR, Tiffany-Castiglioni E. Oligodendroglial, astroglial and glial tumour-associated antigens defined by monoclonal antibodies. *Protides and Biological Fluids.* 1983; **30**, 99–102.
36. Dillman RO, Beauregard J, Royston I, Zavanelli MI. Phase II trial of thymosin fraction 5 and thymosin alpha 1. *Journal of Biological Response Modification.* 1987; **6**, 263–7.
37. Dinarello, CA. Biology of interleukin-1. *FASEB Journal.* 1988; **2**, 108–15.
38. Duff TA, Borden E, Bay J, Phepmeier J, Sielaff K. Phase III trial of interferon-β for treatment of recurrent glioblastoma multiforme. *Journal of Neurosurgery.* 1986; **64**, 408–13.
39. Eggers AE, Tarmin L, Gamboa ET. *In vivo* immunization against autologous glioblastoma-associated antigens. *Cancer Immunology and Immunotherapy.* 1985; **19**, 43–5.
40. Eisenthal A, Rosenberg SA. Cross linking of antiB16 melanoma monoclonal antibodies to LAK cells. *Proceedings of the American Association for Cancer Research.* 1986; **27**, 361.
41. Elliot LH, Brooks WH, Roszman TL. Activation of immunoregulatory lymphocytes obtained from patients with malignant gliomas. *Journal of Neurosurgery.* 1987; **67**, 231–6.
42. Ellison MD, Povlishock JT, Merchant RE. Blood–brain barrier dysfunction in cats following recombinant interleukin-2 infusion. *Cancer Research.* 1987; **47**, 5765–70.
43. Endo Y, Matsushima K, Oppenhein JJ. Mechanism of *in vitro* antitumour effects of Interleukin 1 (IL-1). *Immunobiology.* 1986; **172**, 316–22.
44. Epenetos AA, Courtnay-Luck N, Pickering D, Hooker G, Durbin H, Lavendar JP, McKenzie CG. Antibody guided irradiation of brain glioma by arterial infusion of

radioactive monoclonal antibody against epidermal growth factor receptor and blood group A antigen. *British Medical Journal.* 1985; **290**, 1463-6.
45. Fetell MR, Housepian EM, Oster MW, Fisher PB, Cote DN, Moser FG, Sisti MB. Intratumoral administration of β-interferon in glioblastoma: phase I study. *Neurology.* 1987; **37**, 334.
46. Fidler IJ, Heicappell R, Saiki I, Grutter MG, Horisberger AA, Neush J. Direct antiproliferative effects of recombinant human aplha B/D hybrids on human tumour cell lines. *Cancer Research.* 1987; **47**, 2020-7.
47. Fischer SP, Lindermuth J, Hash C, Shenkin HA. Levamisole in the treatment of glioblastoma multiforme. *Journal of Surgical Oncology.* 1985; **28**, 214-6.
48. Fischer DK, Chen TL, Narayan RK. Immunological and biochemical strategies for the identification of brain tumour-associated antigens. *Journal of Neurosurgery.* 1988, **68**, 165-80.
49. Grace JT Jr, Perese DM, Metzgar RS, Sasabe T, Holdridge B. Tumour autograft responses in patients with glioblastoma multiforme. *Journal of Neurosurgery.* 1961; **18**, 159-67.
50. Grimm EA. Human lymphokine-activated killer cells (LAK cells) as a potential immunotherapeutic modality. *Biochimica et Biophysica Acta.* 1986; **865**, 267-79.
51. Guilian D, Baker TJ, Shih LC, Lachman LB. Interleukin 1 of the central nervous system is produced by ameboid microglia. *Journal of Experimental Medicine.* 1986; **164**, 594-604.
52. Hamada H, Asakura T, Maeda Y, Yokoyama S, Niiro M. A study on the direct antitumoural effect of interferon-α on human glioma. *Japanese Journal of Cancer Chemotherapy.* 1986; **13**, 464-71.
53. Hirakawa K, Ueda S, Nakagawa Y, Suzuki K, Fukuma S, Kita M, Imanishi J, Kishida T. Effect of human leukocyte interferon on malignant brain tumours. *Cancer.* 1983; **51**, 1976-81.
54. Ingram M, Shelden SH, Jacques S, Skillen RG, Bradley WG, Techy GB, Freshwater DB, Abts RM, Rand RW. Preliminary clinical trial of immunotherapy for malignant glioma. *Journal of Biological Response Modification.* 1987; **6**, 489-98.
55. Ingram M, Jacques S, Freshwater DB, Techy GB, Shelden H, Helsper JT. Salvage immunotherapy of malignant glioma. *Archives of Surgery.* 1987; **122**, 1483-6.
56. Ishizawa A. Immunotherapy for malignant gliomas. *Neurologia Medico-Chirugica (Tokyo).* 1981; **21**, 179-91.
57. Jacobs SK, Wilson DJ, Melin G, Parham CW, Holcomb B, Kornblith PL, Grimm EA. Interleukin-2 and lymphokine activated killer (LAK) cells in the treatment of malignant glioma: clinical and experimental studies. *Neurological Research.* 1986; **8**, 81-7.
58. Jacobs SK, Wilson DJ, Kornblith PL, Grimm EA. Interleukin-2 and autologous lymphokine-activated killer cells in the treatment of malignant glioma. *Journal of Neurosurgery.* 1986; **64**, 743-9.
59. Jacobs SK, Wilson DJ, Kornblith PL, Grimm EA. Interleukin-2 or autologous lymphokine-activated killer cell treatment of malignant glioma: Phase I trial. *Cancer Research.* 1986; **46**, 2101-4.
60. Jacobs SK, Parham CW, Holcomb B, Ikejiri B, Kornblith PL, Grimm EA. Lymphokine activated killer (LAK) cell mediated killing of human glioma: Effect of pretreating glioma with various membrane modifying agents. *Journal of Neurooncology.* 1987; **5**, 5-10.
61. Jacques Deane, Ingram Marylou (Huntington, California). Personal communication, 1987.
62. Kato K, Yoshida J, Kageyama N, Kojima N, Yagi K. Liposome-entrapped human interferon-β, its pharmacokinetics and antitumour activity against malignant glioma. *Journal of Interferon Research.* 1986; **6** (suppl.), 131.
63. Kemshead JT, Goldman A, Jones D, Pritchard J, Malpas JS, Gordon I,

Malone JF, Hurley GD, Breatnach F. Therapeutic application of radiolabelled monoclonal antibody UJ13A in children with disseminated neuroblastoma–A phase I study. *Advances in Neuroblastoma Research,* New York: Alan R. Liss, Inc., 1985; 533–44.
64. Kinashi T, Harada N, Severinson E, Tanabe T, Sideras P, Konsisi M, Azuma A, Tominaga A, Bergstedt-Linqvist S, Takahashi M, Matsuda F, Yaoita Y, Takatsu K, Honjo T. cDNA for T cell-replacing factor and identity with B-cell growth factor II. *Nature.* 1986; **324**, 70–3.
65. Kitahara T, Watanabe O, Yamamura A, Makin H, Watanabe T, Suzuki G, Okumura K. Establishment of interleukin 2 dependent cytotoxic T lymphocyte cell line specific for autologous brain tumour and its intracranial administration for therapy of the tumour. *Journal of Neuro-oncology.* 1987; **4**, 329–36.
66. Korosue K, Takeshita I, Mannoji H, Fukui M. Interferon effects on multiplication, cytoplasmic protein and GFAP content, and morphology in human glioma cells. *Journal of Neuro-oncology.* 1983; **1**, 69–76.
67. Lashford LS, Mosely R, Davies AG, Richardson R, Kemshead JT, Coakham HB. A pilot study of ^{131}I monoclonal antibodies in the therapy of leptomeningeal tumours. *Proceedings of the American Society for Clinical Oncology.* 1987; **6**, 280.
68. Lashford LS, Mosely R, Davies AG, Richardson R, Kemshead JT, Coakham HB. The pharmacokinetics of intrathecally administered radiolabeled monoclonal antibodies in patients and animal models. *Proceedings of the American Association Cancer Research.* 1987; **28**, 387.
69. Lee SH, Aggarwal BB, Rinderknecht E, Assisi F, Chiu H. The synergistic antiproliferative effect of γ-interferon and human lymphotoxin. *Journal of Immunology.* 1984; **133**, 1083–6.
70. Lee Y, Bigner DD. Aspects of immunobiology and immunotherapy, and uses of monoclonal antibodies and biological response modifiers in human gliomas. In: Vick NA, Bigner DD, eds. *Neurooncology.* Neurological Clinics of North America, 1985; **3**; 901–17.
71. Lee Y, Wikstrand CJ, Bigner DD. Glioma-associated antigens defined by monoclonal antibodies against an avian sarcoma vires-induced rat astrocytoma. *Journal of Neuroimmunology.* 1986; **13**, 183–202.
72. Lee Y, Matthews TJ, Pizzo S, Abernethy JL, Bigner DD. Partial purification and characterization of a murine glioma-associated antigen defined by syngeneic rat monoclonal antibodies. *Journal of Neuroimmunology.* 1986; **13**, 203–16.
73. Lee Y, Bullard DE, Wikstrand CJ, Zalutsky MR, Muhlbaier LH, Bigner DD. Comparison of monoclonal antibody delivery to intracranial glioma xenografts by intravenous and intracarotid administration. *Cancer Research.* 1987; **47**, 1941–6.
74. Lee Y, Bullard DE, Zalutsky MR, Coleman RE, Wikstrand CJ, Friedman HS, Colapinto EV, Bigner DD. Therapeutic efficacy of antiglioma mesenchymal extracellular matrix ^{131}I-radiolabeled murine monoclonal antibody in a human glioma xenograft model. *Cancer Research.* 1988; **48**, 559–66.
75. Lotze MT, Matory YL, Rayner AA, Ettinghausen SE, Seipp CA, Rosenberg SA. Clinical effects and toxicity of interleukin 2 in patients with cancer. *Cancer.* 1986; **58**, 2764–72.
76. Lundblad D, Lundgren E. Block of a glioma cell line in S by interferon. *International Journal of Cancer.* 1981; **27**, 749–54.
77. Luner SJ, De Vellis J. Immunoprecipitation of a M_r 64 000 glial tumour-associated antigen by monoclonal antibody 217c. *Cancer Research.* 1986; **46**, 863–5.
78. Mahaley MS Jr, Day ED. Immunological studies of human gliomas. *Journal of Neurosurgery.* 1965, **23**, 363–70.
79. Mahaley MS Jr, Mahaley JL, Day ED. The localization of radioantibodies in human brain tumours. II. Radioautography. 1965; **25**, 779–93.
80. Mahaley MS Jr, Day ED, Bigner DD. Problems inherent to the *in vivo* localization

of anti-brain tumour antibodies. *Annals of the New York Academy of Science.* 1969; **159**, 451–60.
81. Mahaley MS Jr. Experiences with antibody production from human glioma tissue. *Progress in Experimental Tumour Research.* 1972; **17**, 31–9.
82. Mahaley MS Jr, Steinbok P, Aronin P, Dudka L, Zinn D. Immunobiology of primary intracranial tumours. V. Levamisole as an immune stimulant in patients and in the ASV glioma model. *Journal of Neurosurgery.* 1981; **54**, 220–7.
83. Mahaley MS Jr, Bigner DD, Dudka LF, Wilds PR, Williams DH, Bouldin TW, Whitaker JN, Bynum JM. Immunobiology of primary intracranial tumours. Part 7: Active immunization of patients with anaplastic glioma cells: a pilot study. *Journal of Neurosurgery.* 1983; **59**, 201–7.
84. Mahaley MS Jr, Gillespie GY, Gillespie RP, Watkins PJ, Bigner DD, Wikstrand CJ, MacQueen JM, Sanfilippo F. Immunobiology of primary intracranial tumours. Part 8: Serological responses to active immunization of patients with anaplastics gliomas. *Journal of Neurosurgery.* 1983; **59**, 208–16.
85. Mahaley MS Jr, Gillespie GY. Immunotherapy of patients with glioma: Fact, fancy and future. *Progress in Experimental Tumour Research.* 1984; **28**, 118–35.
86. Mahaley MS, Urso MB, Whaley RA, Williams TET, Guaspari A, Selker RG. Immunobiology of primary intracranial tumours: Part X. Therapeutic efficacy of interferon in the treatment of recurrent gliomas. *Journal of Neurosurgery.* 1985; **63**, 719–25.
87. Mahaley MS Jr, Gillespie GY. Immunologic considerations of patients with brain tumours. In: Walker MD, ed., *Oncology of the Nervous System.* Boston: Martinus Nijhoff Publishers, 1983; 151–65.
88. Mahaley MS Jr, Bertsch L, Cush S, Gillespie GY. Systemic gamma interferon therapy for recurrent gliomas. *Journal of Neurosurgery.* 1988; In press.
89. Mansson JE, Fredman P, Bigner DD, Molin K, Rosengren B, Friedman HS, Svennerholm L. Characterization of new gangliosides of the lactotetraose series in murine xenografts of a human glioma cell line. *FEBS Letters.* 1986; **201**, 109–13.
90. Marcus SL, Dutcher JP, Paietta E, Ciobanu N, Strauman J, Wierik PH, Hutner SH, Frank O, Baker H. Severe hypovitaminosis C occurring as the result of adoptive immunotherapy with high-dose interleukin 2 and lymphokine-activated killer cells. *Cancer Research.* 1987; **47**, 4208–412.
91. Mathews HL, Beno DW, Hornung RL. Augmentation of the tumour immune response with interleukin-1. *Federation Proceedings.* 1987; **46**, 1504.
92. McComb RD, Bigner DD. The biology of malignant gliomas – a comprehensive survey. *Clinical Neuropathology.* 1984; **3**, 93–106.
93. McKolanis JR, Nishio S, Takei Y, Ragab A. Monoclonal antibodies to a medulloblastoma cell line exhibit restricted reactivity to normal central nervous system tissue. *Federation Proceedings.* 1987; **46**, 1059.
94. Merchant RE, Merchant LH, Cook SHS, McVicar DW, Young HF. Intra-lesional infusion of lymphokine activated killer (LAK) cells and recombinant interleukin-2 (rIL-2) for the treatment of patients with malignant brain tumours. *Neurosurgery.* 1988; In press.
95. Mew D, Wat CK, Towers GHN, Levy JG. Photoimmunotherapy: Treatment of animal tumours with tumour-specific monoclonal antibody-hematoporphyrin conjugates. *Journal of Immunology.* 1983; **130**, 1473–7.
96. Miescher S, Whiteside TL, de Tribolet N, von Fliedner V. In situ characterization, clonogenic potential and antitumour cytolytic activity of T lymphocytes infiltrating human brain tumours. *Journal of Neurosurgery.* 1988; **68**, 438–48.
97. Migliori RJ, Gruber SA, Sawyer MD, Hoffman R, Ochoa A, Bach FH, Simmons RL. Lymphokine-activated killer (LAK) cells can be focused at sites of tumour growth by products of macrophage activation. *Surgery.* 1987; **102**, 155–62.

98. Miyao Y, Shimizu K, Okamoto Y, Matsui Y, Tsuda N, Yamada M, Tamura K, Mogami H. Antitumour efficacy of recombinant interferon-beta on human glioma. *Ganseki Tokyo Kagaku Ryoho.* 1987; **14**, 490-4.
99. Miyatake S, Handa H, Yamashita J, Yamasaki T, Ueda M, Namba Y, Hanaoka M. Induction of human glioma specific cytotoxic T-lymphocyte lines by autologous tumour stimulation and interleukin 2. *Journal of Neuro-oncology.* 1986; **4**, 55-64.
100. Mori T, Yoshida T, Sugiyama S, Hori S, Kuwano M. An experimental study on antitumour activity of recombinant human tumour necrotic factor (TNF) against malignant glioma cells. *Journal of Neuro-oncology* 1987; **5**, 177.
101. Muul LM, Nason-Burchenal K, Carter CS, Cullis H, Slavin D, Hyatt C, Director EP, Leitman SF, Klein HG, Rosenber SA. Development of an automated closed system for generation of human lymphokine-activated killer (LAK) cells for use in adoptive immunotherapy. *Journal of Immunological Methods.* 1987; **101**, 171-81.
102. Nagai M, Arai T. Interferon therapy for malignant brain tumours: Present and future. *No Shinkei Geka.* 1982; **10**, 463-76.
103. Nagai M, Arai T, Kohno S, Kohase M. Local application of interferon to malignant brain tumours. *Texas Reports on Biological Medicine.* 1982; **41**, 603-98.
104. Nagai M, Arai T, Kohno S, Iizuka E. Current status of interferon therapy on malignant brain tumour. *Gan No Rinsho.* 1983; **29**, 608-15.
105. Nagai M, Arai T. Clinical effect of interferon in malignant brain tumours. *Neurosurgical Reviews.* 1984; **7**, 55-64.
106. Nakagawa Y, Kirakawa K, Ueda S, Suzuki K, Fukuma S, Kishida T, Imanishi J, Amagai T. Local administration of interferon for malignant brain tumours. *Cancer Treatment Reports.* 1983: **67**, 833-5.
107. Nakamura O, Teramoto A, Yamamoto H, Ochiai C, Takakura K, Maruo K, Ueyamma Y, Shimamura K. Effect of human fibroblast interferon on malignant brain tumours. *No To Shinkei* 1983; **35**, 905-11.
108. Nakamura O. Antineoplastic effect of hu-IFN-beta. *Neurogical Surgery.* 1985; **13**, 503-8.
109. Nakamura O, Maruo K, Ueyama Y, Nomura K, Takakura K. Interactions of human fibroblast interferon with chemotherapeutic agents and radiation against human gliomas in nude mice. *Neurological Research.* 1986; **8**, 152-6.
110. Nakamura O, Matsutani M, Takakura K. Antineoplastic effect of interferons on malignant brain tumours in athymic nude mice. *Journal of Neuro-oncology.* 1987; **5**, 179.
111. Nederman T, Benediktsson G. Effects of interferon on growth rate and radiation sensitivity of cultured, human glioma cells. *Acta Radiologica Oncologica.* 1982; **21**, 231-34.
112. Nedosperov SA, Hirt B, Shakhov AN, Dobryin VN, Kawashima E, Accolla RS, Jongeneel CV. The genes for tumour necrosis factor (TNF-alpha) and lymphotoxin (TNF-beta) are tandemly arranged on chromosome 17 of the mouse. *Nucleic Acids Research.* 1986; **14**, 7713-25.
113. Neuwelt EA, Clark K, Kirkpatrick JB, Toben H. Clinical studies of intrathecal autologous lymphocyte infusions in patients with malignant gliomas: A toxicity study. *Annals of Neurology.* 1978; **4**, 307-12.
114. Neuwelt EA, Specht D, Hill SA. Permeability of human brain tumour to ^{99m}Tc-glucoheptonate and ^{99m}Tc-albumin. Implications for monoclonal antibody therapy. *Journal of Neurosurgery.* 1986; **65**, 194-8.
115. Neuwelt EA, Specht HD, Barnett PA, Dahlborg SA, Miley A, Larson SM, Brown P, Eckerman KF, Hellstrom KE, Hellstrom I. Increased delivery of tumour-specific monoclonal antibodies to brain after osmotic blood-brain barrier modification in patients with melanoma metastatic to the central nervous system. *Neurosurgery.* 1987; **20**, 885-95.

116. Nobuhara M, Kanamori T, Ashida Y, Horisawa Y, Harada Y, Asami T. Basic study of interferon-beta: Part IV. Antitumour effect on nude mouse-transplanted human tumours. *Gan To Kagaku Ryoho.* 1986; **13**, 2117–22.
117. Nowak TP: Monoclonal antibodies: Prospects for specific immunotherapy for gliomas. *American Journal of Clinical Oncology.* 1987; **10**, 278–80.
118. Obbens EAMT, Feun LG, Leavens ME, Savaraj N, Stewart DJ, Gutterman JU. Phase I clinical trial of intralesional or intraventricular leukocyte interferon for intracranial malignancies. *Journal of Neuro-oncology,* 1985; **3**, 61–7.
119. Okamoto H, Shoin S, Koshimura S, Shimizu R. Studies on the anticancer and streptolysin S-forming abilities of hemolytic streptococci. *Japanese Journal of Microbiology.* 1967; **11**, 323–36.
120. Ommaya AK, Reed J, Walters CL, Meeker WR, Weiss JF. Thymosin for brain tumour therapy. A phase I trial in patients with malignant gliomas. In: *Abstracts of the AANS meeting.* 1981, 90.
121. Otsuka S, Suda K, Yamashita J. Interferon therapy and natural killer activity in patients with brain tumours. *Gan To Kagaku Ryoho.* 1983; **10**, 46–52.
122. Otsuka S, Handa H, Yamashita J, Suda K, Takeuchi J. Single agent therapy of interferon for brain tumours: correlation between natural killer activity and clinical course. *Acta Neurochirugica.* 1984; **73**, 13–23.
123. Otsuka S, Handa H, Yamashita J. High titer of interferon (IFN)-neutralizing antibody in a patient with glioblastoma treated with IFNα. *Journal of Neurosurgery.* 1984; **61**, 591–3.
124. Peng WW, Bressler JP, Tiffany-Castiglioni E, de Vellis J. Development of a monoclonal antibody against a tumour-associated antigen. *Science.* 1982; **215**, 1102–4.
125. Pestka S, Langer JA, Zoon KC, Samuel CE. Interferons and their actions. *Annual Reviews of Biochemistry.* 1987; **56**, 727–77.
126. Phillips J, Alderson T, Sikora K, Watson J. Localization of malignant glioma by a radiolabelled human monoclonal antibody. *Journal of Neurology, Neurosurgery and Psychiatry.* 1983; **46**, 388–92.
127. Piguet V, Carrel S, de Tribolet N. Heterogeneity of the induction of HLA-DR expression by human immune interferon on glioma cell lines and their clones. *Journal of the National Cancer Institute.* 1986; **76**, 223–8.
128. Ramsdell FJ, Golub SH. Generation of lymphokine-activated killer cell activity from human thymocytes. *Journal of Immunology.* 1987; **139**, 1446–53.
129. Richardson RB, Davies AG, Bomne SP, Staddon GE, Jones DH, Kemshead JT, Coakham HB. Radioimmunolocalization of human brain tumours: biodistribution of radiolabelled monoclonal antibody UJ13A. *European Journal of Nuclear Medicine.* 1986; **12**, 313–20.
130. Rong GH, Sindelar WF. Experiments evaluating antitumour immunity induced by cholesterol hemisuccinate-treated syngeneic cell vaccines. *Journal of Surgical Oncology.* 1986; **33**, 145–50.
131. Rosenberg SA, Spiess P, Lafreniere R. A new approach to the adoptive immunotherapy of cancer with tumour-infiltrating lymphocytes. *Science.* 1986; **233**, 1318–21.
132. Rosenberg SA, Lotze MT, Muul LM, Chang AE, Avis FP, Leitman S, Linehan WM, Robertson CN, Lee RE, Rubin JT, Seipp CA, Simpson CG, White DE. A progress report on the treatment of 157 patients with advanced cancer using lymphokine-activated killer cells and interleukin-2 or high dose interleukin-2 alone. *New England Journal of Medicine.* 1987; **316**, 889–97.
133. Rosenstein M, Ettinghausen SE, Rosenberg SA, Extravasation of intravacular fluid mediated by the systemic administration of recombinant interleukin 2. *Journal of Immunology.* 1986; **137**, 1735–42.
134. Roszman TL. Personal communication, 1988.
135. Rutka JT, Giblin JR, Tokuda K, McCulloch JR, Aggarwal GG, Shepherd M,

Bodell WJ, Rosenblum ML. The effects of human recombinant tumour necrosis factor on glioma-derived cell lines. *Journal of Neuro-oncology.* 1987; **5**, 181.
136. Saito T, Tanaka R, Kouno M, Takai N, Yoshida S, Hara N, Washiyama K, Sekiguchi K, Kumanishi T. Immunohistological analysis of infiltrating lymphocyte subpopulations in gliomas and metastatic brain tumours. *No To Shinkei.* 1987; **39**, 339–45.
137. Salford LG, Stromblad LG, Nordstrom CH, Hornmark-Stenstam B, Brandt L, Brismar J, Brun A, Sjogren HO, Flodgran P. Intratumoural administration of interferons in malignant gliomas. *Acta Neurochirugica.* 1981; **56**, 130–1.
138. Sano K, Nagai M, Takakura K, Mogami H, Nomura K. Effects of Hu IFNβ on gliomas. Abstract, *The Third Annual International Congress for Interferon Research, Miami, Florida.* 1982.
139. Saya H, Masuko T, Hashimoto Y. Derivation of a brain tumour-selective monoclonal antibody from hybridoma between mouse myeloma and rat spleen cells immune to syngeneic glioma. *Japanese Journal of Cancer Research.* 1985; **76**, 1198–202.
140. Scuderi P, Sterling KE, Raitano AB, Grogan TM, Rippe RA. Recombinant interferon-gamma stimulates the production of human tumour necrosis fator *in vitro. Journal of Interferon Research.* 1987; **7**, 155–64.
141. Selker RG, Wolmark N, Fisher B, Moore P. Preliminary observations on the use of *Corynebacterium parvum* in patients with primary intracranial tumours. Effect of intracranial pressure. *Journal of Surgical Oncology.* 1978; **10**, 299–303.
142. Shibata S, Mori K, Moriyama T, Tanaka K, Moroki J. Randomized controlled study of the effect of adjuvant immunotherapy with Picibanil on 51 malignant gliomas. *Surgical Neurology.* 1987; **27**, 259–63.
143. Shimizu K, Okamoto Y, Miyao Y, Yamada M, Ushio Y, Hayakawa T, Ikeda H, Mogami H. Adoptive immunotherapy of human meningeal gliomatosis and carcinomatosis with LAK cells and recombinant interleukin-2. *Journal of Neurosurgery.* 1987; **66**, 519–21.
144. Shimizu K, Okamoto Y, Miyao Y, Tamura K, Yamada M, Ushio Y, Hayakawa T, Mogami H. Adoptive immunotherapy of brain tumours. *Journal of Neuro-oncology.* 1987; **5**, 182.
145. Shinitzky M, Skornick Y, Haran-Ghera N. Effective tumour immunization induced by cells of elevated membrane-lipid microviscosity. *Proceedings of the National Academy of Sciences of the USA.* 1979; **76**, 5313–6.
146. Sikora K, Alderson T, Phillips J, Watson J. Human hybridomas from malignant gliomas. *Lancet.* 1982; **i**, 11–14.
147. Sikora K, Alderson T, Ellis J, Phillips J, Watson J. Human hybridomas from patients with malignant glioma. *British Journal of Cancer.* 1983; **47**, 135–45.
148. Sikora K, Alderson T, Nethersell A, Smedley H. Tumour localization by human monoclonal antibodies. *Medical Oncology and Tumour Pharmacotherapy.* 1985; **2**, 77–86.
149. Sikora K. Human monoclonal antibodies to cancer cells. In: Strelkauskas AJ, ed, *Human Hybridomas. Diagnostic and Therapeutic Applications.* New York: Marcel Dekker, Immunology Series. 1987; **30**, 159–81.
150. Skornick Y, Danciger E, Rozin RR, Shinitzky M. Positive skin tests with autologous tumour cells of increased membrane viscosity. First Report. *Cancer Immunology and Immunotherapy.* 1981; **11**, 93–6.
151. Skornick Y, Dresdale AR, Sindelar WF. Induction of delayed hypersensitivity reactions in cancer patients by cholestero-hemisuccinate treated autologous tumour cells. *Journal of the National Cancer Institute.* 1983; **70** 465–7.
152. Skornick Y, Gorelik E, Klausner J, Shinitzky M, Sindelar WF. Inhibition of growth and metastases in mice by immunization with cholesterol hemisuccinate-enriched tumour cells. *Cancer Letters.* 1984; **25**, 153–61.
153. Skornick Y, Rong GH, Sindelar WF, Richert L, Klausner J, Rozin RR, Shinitzky M.

Active immunotherapy of human solid tumour with autologous cells treated with cholesteryl hemisuccinate. A phase I study. *Cancer.* 1986; **58**, 650-4.
154. Smith R, Anderson R, Ott K, Copeland B, Davis J, Georgiades G, Berneman L. Experimental treatment of malignant glioma with intraventricular administration of gamma interferon. *Abstracts of 2nd Annual Neuro-Oncology Update.* 1986, Tampa, Florida.
155. Smith RA, Kirstein M, Fiers W, Baglioni C. Species specificity of human and murine tumour necrosis factor. A comparative study of tumour necrosis factor receptors. *Journal of Biological Chemistry.* 1986; **261**, 14871-4.
156. Spies T, Morton CC, Nedospasov SA, Fiers W, Pious D, Strominger JL. Genes for the tumour necrosis factors alpha and beta are linked to the human major histocompatiblity compled. *Proceedings of the National Academy of Sciences of the USA* 1986; **83**, 8699-702.
157. Stavrou D, Hulten M, Anzil AP, Bilzer T. The humoral antibody response of rats immunized with chemically modified syngeneic brain cells and glioma cells. *Internationl Journal of Cancer.* 1980; **26**, 629-37.
158. Stavrou D, Hulten M, Bilzer T. Chemical modification and antigenicity of glioma cells. *Acta Neuropathologica.* 1981; (suppl) VII, 75-8.
159. Stavrou D, Suss C, Bilzer T, Kummer U, de Tribolet N. Monoclonal antibodies reactive with glioma cell lines derived from experimental brain tumours. *European Journal of Cancer and Clinical Oncology.* 1983; **19**, 1439-49.
160. Stavrou D, Glassner H, Bilzer T, Senekowitsch R, Keiditsch E, Mehraein P. Radioimaging of experimental glioma grafts using $F(ab')_2$-fragments of monoclonal antibodies. *Anticancer Research* 1986; **6**, 897-903.
161. Stavrou D, Mellert W, Mellert U, Keiditsch E, Bise K, Mehraein P. Growth inhibition of experimental glioma grafts by monoclonal antibody treatment. *Journal of Cancer Research and Clinical Oncology.* 1986; **112**, 111-18.
162. Steinbok P, Thomas JPW, Grossman L, Dolman CL. Intratumorual autologous mononuclear cells in the treatment of recurrent glioblastoma multiforme. A Phase I study. *Journal of Neuro-oncology.* 1984; **2**, 147-51.
163. Szmigielski S, Jeljaszewicz J, Pulverer G. Thermoimmunotherapy of advanced neoplasms. A concept and preliminary results. *Biomedical Pharmacotherapy.* 1987; **41**, 132-8.
164. Takakura K, Miki Y, Kubo O, Ogawa N, Matsutani M, Sano K. Adjuvant immunotherapy for malignant brain tumours. *Japanese Journal of Clinical Oncology.* 1972; **12**, 109-20.
165. Takatsu K, Kikuchi Y, Takahasi T, Honjo T, Matsumoto M, Harada N, Yamaguchi N, Tomainaga A. Interleukin 5, a T cell derived B cell differentiation factor also induces cytotoxic T lymphocytes. *Proceedings of the National Academy of Sciences of the USA.* 1987; **84**, 4234-8.
166. Takiguchi M, Ting J, Buessow S, Boyer C, Gillespie Y, Frelinger J. Response of glioma cells to interferon-gamma: increase in class II RNA, protein and mixed lymphocyte reaction-stimulating ability. *European Journal of Immunology.* 1985; **15**, 809-14.
167. Tanaka N, Nagao S, Tohgo A, Sekiguchi F, Kohno M, Ogawa H, Matsui T, Matsutani M. Effects of human fibroblast interferon on human gliomas transplanted into nude mice. *Japanese Journal of Cancer Research.* 1983; **74**, 308-16.
168. Thorpe PE, Ross WCJ. The preparation and cytotoxic properties of antibody-toxin conjugates. *Immunological Reviews.* 1982; **62**, 119-58.
169. Tilden AB, Ition K, Balch CM. Human lumphokine-activated killer (LAK) cells: Identification of two types of effector cells. *Journal of Immunology.* 1987; **138**, 1068-73.
170. Topalian SL, Muul LM, Solomon D, Rosenberg SA. Expansion of human tumour infiltrating lymphocytes for use in immunotherapy trials. *Journal of Immunological Methods.* 1987; **102**, 127-41.
171. Trouillas P, Lapras CL. Immunotherapie active des tumeurs cerebrales. A propos de 20 cas. *Neuro-Chirurgie.* 1970; **18**, 143-70.

172. Trouillas P. Carcino-fetal antigent in glial tumours. *Lancet.* 1971; **ii**, 552.
173. Trouillas P. Immunology and immunotherapy of cerebral tumours: Current status. *Revue Neurologique.* 1973; **128**, 23–38.
174. Vasquero J, Marinez, R, Barbolla L, de Haro J, de Oya S, Coca S, Ramiro J. Intrathecal injection of autologous leukocytes in glioblastoma: Circulatory dynamics within the arachnoid space and clinical results. *Acta Neurochirugica.* 1987; **89**, 37–42.
175. Vetto JT, Papa MZ, Lotze MT, Chang AE, Rosenberg SA. Reduction of toxicity of interleukin-2 and lymphokine-activated killer cells in humans by the administration of corticosteroids. *Journal of Clinical Oncology.* 1987; **5**, 496–503.
176. von Hanwehr RI, Hofman FM, Taylor CR, Apuzzo MLJ. Mononuclear lymphoid populations infiltrating the microenvironment of primary CNS tumours. *Journal of Neurosurgery.* 1984; **60**, 1138–47.
177. Wakabayashi T, Yoshida J, Kobayashi T, Kageyama N, Kanzaki M. Effect of interferon on malignant brain tumour. *Gan To Kagaku Ryoho.* 1982; **9**, 1400–6.
178. Watanabe N, Niitsu Y, Uamauchi N, Umeno H, Sone H, Neda H, Urushizaki I. Antitumour synergism between recombinant human tumour necrosis factor and recombinant human interferon-r. *Journal of Biological Response Modification.* 1988; **7**, 24–31.
179. West WH, Tauer KW, Yannelli JR, Marshall GD, Orr DW, Thurman GB, Oldham RK. Constant-infusion recombinant interleukin-2 in adoptive immunotherapy of advanced cancer. *New England Journal of Medicine.* 1987; **316**, 898–905.
180. Wikstrand CJ, Bigner SH, Bigner DD. Demonstration of complex antigenic heterogeneity in a human glioma cell line and eight derived clones by specific monoclonal antibodies. *Cancer Research.* 1983; **43**, 3327–34.
181. Wikstrand CJ, Bigner SH, Bigner DD. Characterization of three restricted specificity monoclonal antibodies raised against the human glioma cell line D-54 MG. *Journal of Neuroimmunology.* 1984; **6** 169–86.
182. Wikstrand CJ, Grahmann FC, McComb RD, Bigner DD. Antigenic heterogeneity of human anaplastic gliomas and glioma-derived cell lines defined by monoclonal antibodies. *Journal of Neuropathology and Experimental Neurology.* 1985; **44**, 229–41.
183. Wikstrand CJ, McLendon RE, Bullard DE, Fredman P, Svennerholm. L, Bigner DD. Production and characterization of two human glioma xenograft-localizing monoclonal antibodies. *Cancer Research.* 1986; **46**, 5933–40.
184. Wikstrand CJ, Bigner DD. Use of monoclonal antibodies in neurobiology and neurooncology. In: Sell S, Reisfeld RA, eds. *Monoclonal Antibodies in Cancer.* Clifton NJ: Humana Press, 1986; 365–97.
185. Wikstrand CJ, McLendon RE, Carrel S, Kemshead JT, Mach JP, Coakham HB, de Tribolet N, Bullard DE, Zalutsky MR, Bigner DD. Comparative localization of glioma-reactive monoclonal antibodies *in vivo* in an athymic mouse human glioma xenograft model. *Journal of Neuroimmunology.* 1987; **15**, 37–56.
186. Yamasaki T, Handa H, Yamashita J, Watanabe Y, Namba Y, Hanaoka M. Specific adoptive immunotherapy with tumour specific cytotoxic T lymphocyte clone for murine malignant gliomas. *Cancer Research.* 1984; **44**, 1776–83.
187. Yates AJ, Stephens RE, Elder PJ, Markowitz DL, Rice JM. Effects of interferon and gangliosides on growth of cultured human glioma and fetal brain cells. *Cancer Research.* 1985; **45**, 1033–9.
188. Yoshida J, Wakabayashi T, Kato K. Combination therapy with IFN-beta, ACNU and radiation. *Gan To Kagaku Ryoho.* 1986; **13**, 520–4.
189. Yoshida J, Kato K, Wakabayashi T, Enomoto K, Inoue I, Kageyama N. Antitumour effect of IFN-beta combined with ACNU against malignant glioma. *Journal of Interferon Research* 1986; **6**, 3.
190. Yoshida S, Tanaka R, Takai N. Local administration of autologous lymphokine activated killer cells and recombinant interleukin-2 to patients with malignant brain tumours. *Gan to Kagaku Ryoko.* 1987; **14**, 1930–2.

191. Young H, Kaplan A, Regelson W. Immunotherapy with autologous white cell infusions ("Lymphocytes") in the treatment of recurrent glioblastoma multiforme. A preliminary report. *Cancer.* 1977; **40**, 1037–44.
192. Yumitori K, Handa H, Yamashita J, Suda K, Otsuka S, Shimizu Y. Treatment of malignant glioma with mumps virus. *No Shinkei Geka.* 1982; **10**, 143–7.
193. Yung WKA, Castellanos AM, Moser RP. Intravenous recombinant beta interferon (IFNβ_{ser}) in patients with malignant gliomas. *Neurology.* 1987; **37**, 334.
194. Yung WKA, Castellanos AM, van Tassel P, Moser RP, Marcus S. Intravenous recombinant beta interferon in recurrent malignant gliomas. *Journal of Neuro-oncology.* 1987; **5**, 190.
195. Yung WKA, Castellanos AM, van Tassel P, Moser RP, Marcus S. Recombinant interferon beta (IFNβ_{ser}) given intravenously in patients with recurrent malignant gliomas. *Proceedings of the American Society for Clinical Oncology.* 1988; **7**, 84.
196. Zovickian J, Johnson VG, Youle RJ. Potent and specific killing of human malignant brain tumour cells by an anti-transferrin receptor antibody-ricin immunotoxin. *Journal of Neurosurgery.* 1987; **66**, 850–61.
197. Zovickian J, Youle RJ. Efficacy of intrathecal immunotoxin therapy in an animal model of leptomeningeal neoplasia. *Journal of Neurosurgery.* 1988; **68**, 767–74.

15 The terminal care of brain tumour patients

Margaret Wheildan and Ronald McKeran

Introduction

After the patient with a primary or secondary malignant brain tumour has been fully assessed with modern imaging techniques, received the most appropriate surgery, radiotherapy and chemotherapy, with perhaps a further attempt at treatment when the inevitable recurrence occurs, there remains the eternal problem of how best to care for the dying patient. This is an area which receives proportionally far less attention in any review of the management of brain tumours and about which very little has been specifically written. The question might then be asked whether there are any singular or novel features surrounding the terminal care of the brain tumour patient compared with any other patient dying from a malignancy. The fear and indeed the reality that the patient may not be able to communicate or understand at a relatively early stage in their terminal care can and does cause great distress both to patients and relatives. A progressive deterioration of vital functions with an intact sensorium as for example in some brain stem tumours can be very distressing when it affects breathing, swallowing and speech patterns. Given therefore the limited success in the treatment of malignant brain tumours and the present rate of progress in improving life expectancy for many of these tumours, we might serve our patients' best interests by considering in some detail the current approaches and facilities available for the care of the terminally ill patient with a brain tumour.

The place of death

Approximately 30 per cent of cancer deaths occur at home in the South East and South West Thames Regions England, whereas only 21 per cent of brain tumour patients die at home. The precise factors which lead to the decision on the part of the patient, relatives and general practitioners to choose a home or hospital death have not been closely studied. An investigation directed to this point might give useful guidance to the physicians caring for these patients. Despite the trend to specialization and a tendency to opt for hospitalization which is a characteristic of much modern medicine, for many, as the above figures suggest, the general practitioner remains the central figure in the management of terminal cancer. The recent survey conducted by Wilkes demonstrated that in 16 per cent of cases the newly bereaved relatives were highly critical of their care.[1] The criticisms directed to the practitioner included failure to inform or explain, appeared disinterested, visited only on demand, never examined the patient properly, relied too much on drugs rather than relationships, and was classed as uncaring. Far more frequently, however, the relatives were full of praise for their care, commenting on the support given, the fact that the doctor explained things well, was patient, and interested, often gave his home phone number to the next of kin, tried hard to keep the patient comfortable and arranged to make available all hospital and nursing skills when they were needed. The increase in medical costs over the last few decades has focused attention on the economic evaluation of new drug therapies and in a more general setting different forms of treatment and patterns of care. However, even in the relatively straighforward matter of the evaluation of specific drug therapies in the framework of cost-effectiveness or cost-benefit analysis, the complexity of the task is immediately apparent, particularly with respect to the benefit side of the analysis. Many of these studies either ignore treatment benefits altogether, restricting analysis to cost differentials between treatment alternatives, or have considered exclusively the impact on patients' earning capacity through reductions in morbidity or mortality. A full economic evaluation of a form of treatment (and this would apply to the different patterns of care available to the terminally ill patient with a brain tumour) requires assessment of the direct and immediate treatment benefits including the concept of life quality. Models have been devised to assess life quality with regard to the action of different drugs and similar considerations may be applicable to assessing optimal patterns of care as for example in the management of terminally ill patients.[2]

Support structures

The general practitioner is clearly a central figure in the terminal care of the patient dying from a brain tumour in the United Kingdom. The resources available to him would include:

meals on wheels
community psychiatric help
home help
night attendants
twilight nurses
care-attendant schemes
incontinence laundry services
referral to the hospice team/centre

Each patient should receive a medical, nursing and social work assessment. The benefits to the patients and relatives from this combined approach and the continued reassessment of need and care with the intelligent application of nursing models of care to the individual patient have been frequently and eloquently reported.[3] Available to many communities are a number of support networks which have grown in recent years to include the hospice movement with its domiciliary teams of workers who act in close consort with the general practitioner.

Practical and emotional support for the patient and family

This can be given by the following groups:

general practitioner
community nurses
home care teams/Macmillan nurse
Marie Curie nurses
social workers
occupational therapists
physiotherapists
day centre
community care groups
cancer support groups
bereavement support groups

The role of the specialist terminal care unit is still evolving in many parts of the country and remains flexible to local need and demand. At its best this service offers a unique core of specialist knowledge which is at the disposal of primary and secondary health care teams, offering a consistent management policy. The specialist teams available range from well-established units providing medical, nursing and social work support on a 24-hour basis, seven days a week, to those who have just started with one or two nurse advisers.

The management of specific clinical problems arising from neurological dysfunction in patients with brain tumours

The symptoms and signs arising from brain tumours derive from the effects of raised intracranial pressure, secondary focal effects on the brain resulting from displaced intracranial structures, and from the direct focal effects produced by the tumour and surrounding oedema.

Increased intracranial pressure

The headache of raised intracranial pressure demands attention in the conscious patient who can communicate distress and may be surmised in the restless, semi-comatosed patient with raised intracranial pressure. The preferred drug of choice is dexamethasone. The relatively long half-life of this drug in the range 50 h guarantees against risk from withdrawal, and indicates that it need not be given more than twice a day with meals. There is no clear evidence that is causes gastrointestinal bleeding and there is therefore little justification for recommending the routine use of cimetidine or ranitidine to protect against the risk of haemorrhage. Indeed, in the patient with a damaged blood–brain barrier around a tumour, increased brain penetration of those drugs may cause a confusional state. Doses up to 100 mg a day have been offered and it is claimed there is a linear effect with increasing dose. Maintenance doses of 4 mg three times a day are more often used, tailed off and then discontinued in the setting of terminal care when appropriate.

Seizure

Every effort is made to control seizures, partly because of the distress caused to both patients and relatives, and also because of the increased difficulties in caring for the patient freely fitting at home and in hospital. The specific pharmacokinetics of phenytoin assures its popularity, because it is possible to offer a loading dose, and to calculate from a serum drug level and the current dosage (using a nomogram) the required dosage to be within any part of the therapeutic range. Carbamazepine offers an acceptable alternative to many patients, but the same principles of monotherapy with drug level monitoring apply in this clinical context as in the more general care of the epileptic patient. Status epilepticus may be managed with intravenous diazepam or subcutaneous phenobarbitone with titration of maintenance therapy to optimal effect.

Deteriorating intellect and focal cerebral deficits

It should always be assumed that the patient with a deteriorating intellect has retained some insight into the situation and conversations with relatives should be held away from the patient where sensitive matters of prognosis are to be discussed. The patient must not be excluded from discussions but explanations must be kept simple and appropriate to the level of residual insight and intellect. Involving patient and relatives in their care provides a sound, reassuring framework for caring and being cared. This reduces anxiety. Residual cognitive ability should be stimulated and supported as much as possible. Orientation can be maintained, for example by signs, naming each room and article, and keeping a light on to reduce fears and disorientation. Admission to hospital should be accompanied by a relaxed attitude to visiting and should be actively encouraged.

The dysphasic patient can be easily frustrated and communication can be aided by speaking slowly, clearly and in an unhurried manner with appropriate gestures. The role of speech therapy is debatable unless the deficit is likely to be stable over a prolonged period, when referral should be considered. Approaching the patient with a homonymous hemianopia on the side in which the field is intact and reminding patients of this deficit when present and not apparent to them should be encouraged.

The wearing of an eye patch can remove the distress of diplopia where appropriate. Eye drops (methylcellulose) for the patient who cannot close an eye with the provision of an eye guard if the cornea is anaesthetic, may be required in the patient with a facial palsy. Dysphagia in its early stages may be reduced by thickened liquids but at the later stage a nasogastric tube may need to be passed with tube feeding. The hemiparetic patient will benefit from community physiotherapy to prevent contractures and maintain limb function for as long as possible. An arm sling may prevent subluxation and the development of a frozen shoulder or the shoulder hand syndrome in the patient with marked shoulder girdle weakness. Dependent leg oedema is usually adequately treated by elevation and recourse to elastic stockings without the need for diuretics. In the paraplegic patient the usual attention to bladder and bowel function, often with catheterization, skin care and physical therapy are the main points of emphasis in management. Constipation should be anticipated and prevented by the use of stool softeners (lactulose) and mild laxatives (bisacodyl) in the evening followed where necessary by a suppository and enema (micralax) in the morning.

The bedridden or comatosed patient

Frequent aspiration is often required but aspiration pneumonia remains a common cause of death. Frequent turning (two-hourly) whilst reducing pressure on sensitive areas also aids aspiration of secretions. Fever complicating an aspiration pneumonia indicates added infection on the initially sterile infection, and where considered appropriate and not a terminal event, penicillin G should be administered with sputum culture and adjustment of medication where necessary. Steroids are no longer considered to be indicated in this situation.

Nasogastric tube feeding or very rarely gastrostomy can maintain nutrition in the comastosed patient or in one who is unable to swallow. Dietetic advice and the involvement of the family in administering liquid food either prepared at home or commercially available with multivitamin supplements should be sought. Feeding in the upright position avoids aspiration pneumonia.

Skin care is important. Keeping the skin dry and clean, turning the patient frequently every two hours or less with careful positioning to avoid pressure on vulnerable points, protection of heels with sheepskin booties and the use of a Spenco mattress should prevent the development of pressure sores. Frequent passive movement of the limbs, and elastic stockings should prevent the occurrence of deep venous thrombosis. Careful attention to bowel and bladder function as described above applies just as much in this terminal situation, with the added complication of the need to keep the perineum clean and dry to avoid maceration. Adult diapers and incontinence pads are very useful in this situation.

Confusion

Confusion is a common symptom in terminally ill patients, especially those with primary or secondary brain tumours. It can cause distress not only to the patient, but also the relatives and friends who are caring for the patient.

Confusion may present as hallucination, memory loss, disorientation, restlessness and aggressive behaviour. The common causes of confusion include drugs, biochemical disturbances, cerebral anorexia, change of environment, sepsis, other causes of brain damage, depression or anxiety, as well as cerebral tumours.

It is therefore important to exclude any cause of the confusion that can be treated specifically. Often the confusion will have multiple causative factors and explanation and reassurance will relieve both the patient and the family.

Management of confusion should include explanation, a constant routine and the presence of close friends or family members to reassure the patient and provide company. Drugs are needed when the symptoms cause distress and are persistent. Dexamethasone 2–4 mg every six hours will reduce cerebral oedema if this is the cause of the confusion. Haloperidol 5–10 mg is useful for hallucinations and diazepam 5–10 mg will control agitation and restlessness. If more sedation is required the phenothiazine drugs should be considered (chlorpromazine 50–100 mg).

Confusion can often be treated and made more tolerable for the patient; reassurance and explanation are essential.

Symptom control

Nausea and vomiting

It is important to try and establish the cause of the nausea or vomiting before prescribing treatment. Causes in brain tumour patients will include raised intracranial pressure, disturbance of the vestibular mechanism, direct stimulation of the integrative vomiting centre by radiation therapy and by drugs acting on the chemoreceptor trigger zone in the floor of the fourth ventricle.

During the initial period of treatment it may be necessary to give antiemetic parenterally. The antiemetic of choice for patients with raised intracranial pressure is cyclizine, which is an antihistamine and acts directly on the vomiting center. Cyclizine is available in tablet, suppository and injectable form. The normal dose is 50 mg eight-hourly.

If the vomiting is thought to be caused by stimulation of the chemoreceptor trigger zone haloperidol is the antiemetic of choice. The oral recommended starting dose is 5 mg, preferably at night. It may also be given subcutaneously via an infusion pump. Another useful antiemetic is metoclopramide which acts by increasing the speed of gastric emptying. Metoclopramide 10 mg can be given orally or subcutaneously every eight hours.

The phenothiazine drugs act on the chemoreceptor trigger zone, but are more sedative than haloperidol, especially chlorpromazine, and this drug is therefore not recommended for routine use. Prochlorperazine (Stemetil) is available in suppository form and can be useful.

Pain relief

Pain is not a common sympton in patients who are terminally ill with a primary brain tumour, but 70 per cent of patients with advanced cancer will have pain as a major symptom and therefore two-thirds of patients with secondary brain tumours will experience pain which is caused by the cancer itself, treatment of the cancer or pain which is unrelated to the cancer or treatment.

It is important to remember when treating a patient with pain, that pain is not simply a physical sensation. Pain is an unpleasant sensory and emotional experience associated with actual or potential tissue damage and is always subjective.

The initial assessment of the patient is very important, because treatment will vary according to the cause of the pain. It is not uncommon for patients to have more than one site of pain, and 30 per cent of patients will have four or more pains. A body chart, as used at the first author's hospice, may be used to record the site, intensity and possible mechanisms of each individual pain (Fig. 15.1). We need to understand the physical, psychological, spiritual, interpersonal and financial components of the patient's pain.

The patient needs to understand the cause or causes of the pain and careful explanation is essential. This reduces the anxiety associated with the pain and will raise morale. It is important to set realistic targets with the patient. The initial target should be to make the patient pain-free at night so that he is able to sleep undisturbed. To achieve complete pain relief for patients with bony metastases who want to be fully mobile is possible although much more difficult.

Once treatment has been initiated it is important to reassess and review the patient regularly; the importance of this cannot be overemphasized. New pains may develop which will require assessment and explanation.

The use of analgesic drugs remains the mainstay of the treatment of pain caused by cancer. It is vital to keep the analgesic regimen simple, and when making the initial assessment to decide whether the pain is mild, moderate or severe. For mild pain a non-opioid drug such as paracetamol or aspirin should be prescribed. These drugs need to be given every four to six hours to give effective relief. There is no place for "as required" or PRN prescribing for continuous pain. Moderate pain that is not adequately relieved by regular paracetamol should respond to a weak opioid such as Co-proxamol (dextropropoxyphene and paracetamol) or codeine given regularly every four to six hours. Combining the effect of a weak opioid with a non-steroidal anti-inflammatory drug (NSAID) which acts by inhibiting prostaglandin synthesis is often effective especially for the relief of pain due to bony metastases.

For patients with severe pain, a strong opioid, morphine or diamorphine, is the drug of choice. There is nothing to be gained from changing from a weak opioid to another weak opioid if pain relief has not been achieved with the former. The decision to prescribe a strong opioid is taken in a logical step sequence along the "analgesic ladder" (non-opioid, weak opioid, strong opioid). Morphine is the strong opioid of choice for oral administration. Diamorphine is rapidly metabolized to 6-monoacetyl morphine and morphine when given orally, and has no advantages over oral morphine. The initial dose of morphine elixir will depend on the patient's age and previous analgestic requirements and is usually 5–10 mg four-hourly. Reassessment of the pain after the first dose and after 24 hours will indicate how effective the pain relief is. It there is insufficient analgesia the starting dose should be increased by 30–50 per cent. Doses should be titrated to the pain and morphine should be increased in logical steps, 5 mg/10 mg/15 mg/30 mg/45 mg/60 mg/90 mg, until pain relief is achieved. Most patients will be satisfactorily controlled on doses of between 10 and 30 mg four-hourly.

Once a patient is pain-free on morphine elixir, he may prefer to be transferred to controlled release morphine sulphate MST-Continus tablets. MST is effective over 12 hours and makes the drug regimen simpler for the patient. It is available in 10 mg, 30 mg, 60 mg and 100 mg strengths. When converting from morphine elixir to MST the total daily dose of elixir is divided by 2 to give the 12-hourly dose of MST, i.e. 180 morphine elixir (30 mg four-hourly) = 90 mg MST b.d.

For patients who are unable to tolerate oral morphine because of dysphagia, vomiting or debility, morphine is available in suppository form. The suppositories are in 10 mg, 15 mg, 30 mg and 60 mg strengths and should be given four-hourly.

Portable syringe driver

When oral administration of morphine is no longer possible, in the last few hours or days of life, or because of dysphagia or vomiting which is not controlled by antiemetics, diamorphine should be given subcutaneously. A continuous infusion subcutaneously using a syringe driver will ensure even analgesia and is acceptable to both patient and family.

A suitable syringe driver is the Graseby MS 26. This is battery driven and portable and weighs only 175 g. A butterfly cannula is inserted subcutaneously usually in the chest wall and connected to the syringe driver which slowly injects the drugs over 24 hours. This ensures continuous pain relief and eliminates the "peaks and troughs" associated with oral medication. Diamorphine is the strong opiate of choice for parenteral use and when changing from the oral to parenteral route, the parenteral dose of diamorphine will be one-third to one-half the previously satisfactory oral dose of morphine sulphate elixir. It is often advisable to combine an antiemetic with the diamorphine. Haloperiol 5–10 mg or metoclopramide 10 mg are compatible with diamorphine.

When a patient is unable to take oral anticonvulsants, these may be changed to phenobarbitone which can be given subcutaneously. Status epilepticus is rare but can be controlled with phenobarbitone given continuously via a syringe driver 100–200 mg per 24 hours.

Effective symptom control, especially of pain, remains the cornerstone of continuing or "palliative care". It will enable patients to perform to the best of their ability. Whenever possible analgesic drugs should be given orally to maintain the patient's independence and there should be satisfactory titration of the dose and side-effects should be controlled. The concept of cancer pain management using analgesic drugs 'by the clock' and 'by the ladder' should be remembered.

The role of the hospice movement

There have been considerable advances in the care of the dying patient over the last 25 years and it is well-recognized that a great deal can be done to relieve suffering and to enable the patient to die with dignity. The hospice movement owes much to Dame Cicely Saunders who in the 1960s was aware of the inadequate care provided for the dying and developed a specialist service for the dying at St Christopher's Hospice in London. Following the development of the inpatient hospice service, home care and hospital support teams have been established to improve the care of the patients nursed at home or in general hospital wards.

In-patient hospice service

The advantages of hospice-type care are many. The staff have chosen to care for dying patients and their families and form part of a specially trained multi-disciplinary team. The nurse-to-patient ratio is usually higher than in a general hospital ward and as most nurses are not in training there is continuity and security for the patient. Each hospice will normally have its own home care team to advise and support the community staff, and many hospices are developing a day-care service. Patients will be admitted to the hospice for respite care to give relatives and friends a much-needed break, for symptom control of distressing symptom and, in the terminal stages of their illness, to die.

Home-care team

This is a team of specially trained nurses with a district nursing or health-visiting background. Their role is to offer advice and support to health service staff in the community who are caring for the patient at home. Most home-care teams are based at a hospice and at the general practitioner or consultant's request will visit and assess the patient's needs at home with the hospice doctor. The home-care sister will liaise closely with the patient's district nurse and general practitioner. She will not normally be involved in the physical aspects of nursing care, but offers expert advice on symptom control and emotional support for both "the patient and the family". In the United Kingdom many home-care teams have been established with the aid of grants, for example the Macmillan nurses. To help families care for relatives at home as long as possible, many home-care teams have a "siting service" to provide people to sit with patients at home, particularly at night, so that relatives can have a good night's sleep.

Hospice day care

Many hospices now offer their home-care patients day-care facilities. Patients may wish to see the hospice doctor and medical problems can be treated as they arise and good symptom control achieved. Physical nursing care can be provided including baths, showers and dressings where appropriate. Recreational activities are usually available as well as physiotherapy, hairdressing and chiropody. Attendance at the day centre will provide the patient with an opportunity for socializing with other patients, and will allow the patient to lead a less restricted life. More importantly, it will offer respite to the relatives on a regular basis.

The hospital support team/symptom control team

This is usually a mutidisciplinary team based in a hospital. The team acts as advisers to hospital and staff who are looking after dying patients. Some teams will also work in the community caring for paitents after they have been discharged from the hospital in which they are based. They provide expertise in symptom control and offer support to the patient and the family.

The main aim of continuing care is to improve the quality of daily life for the patient, and this must include good symptom control, alleviation of loneliness and fear, and rehabilitation to enable the patient to live as normal a life as possible. It is important to remember that some people will need spiritual and pastoral care.

For patients who are terminally ill with a brain tumour, early referral to the nearest hospital and home-care team is recommended. This will ensure that the facilities and expertise that are available for these patients will be utilized to the full. The hospice movement has shown what can be achieved, not only for the patient but also for the friends and relatives of the person who is dying.

Conclusion

Death and coping with death as a process as opposed to an isolated happening are events that modern man finds increasingly difficult and his life experience prepares him poorly in many cases for this inevitable final act. The commitment of those people and organizations who have taken it upon themselves to cope with this area of care should be welcomed and developed. Ideas, current fashion and philosophy of care evolve and we should keep the planning process as flexible as possible to accomodate this inevitable change.

Index

NOTE:
Page numbers in *italics* refer to pages on which figs./tables appear. All index entries refer to brain tumours, and in particular, malignant gliomas, unless otherwise stated.

Abbreviations used in sub-entries:
- CT Computed tomography
- MRI Magnetic resonance imaging
- POGF Platelet-derived growth factor
- PET Positron emission tomography

A4 antibodies 45, *46*
A15 A5 cell line 63
Adenovirus 12, 59
Adenylate cyclase 14
Adoptive immunotherapy, *see* Immunotherapy
Aerobic glycolysis 124, 127, 128, 131
Age, as prognostic factor in astrocytomas 200, 207
Age-related incidence 137, 138
   in children *167*
Amino acid metabolism 128–129, 131
Anaerobic glycolysis 124
Analgesic(s) 289
Anaplastic change 79
   in transplanted tumour systems 63–64
Angiography, cerebral 101–102
   complications 101
   haemorrhages 105, *106*
Antibodies
   in passive immunotherapy of gliomas 258–262

   in serological analysis of gliomas 45
Antiemetics 288, 290
Antigen expression 40–50, 83
   analysis *in vitro* and *in situ* 45–48, 83, 259, 260
   FN^+ and $A4^+$ 45–*46*
   biological response modifier effect on 18
   changes induced *in vitro* 18
   established cell lines,
      gliosarcoma 5, *8*
      malignant astrocytomas 5, *6–7*, 13, *46*, 83
      medulloblastomas 9, *10, 46*
      oligodendrogliomas 9, *46*
   in glial and neuronal development 40–44, 83
   heterogeneity 13–14
   in leukaemic cells 48
   monoclonal antibodies to, *see* Monoclonal antibodies
   optic nerve cells 41–42, *43*
   see also individual antigens

293

Antioncogene 26, 30
  deletion in glioma pathogenesis 36
  in neoplastic development 27, 30
Aspiration pneumonia 287
Astroblastoma 78
Astroblasts 44
Astrocytes
  identification 47, 83
  normal, in gliomas 47
  in retina, origin 44
  type-1 41, *43*, 45
  type-2 42, 45
Astrocytic glioma, classification 198–199
  see also Astrocytoma; Glioblastoma multiforme
Astrocytoma 198, 199–204
  anaplastic (malignant) 198
    classification 82, 198
    clinical trials results 205–*206*
    established cell lines 5, *6–7*, 13
    prognostic variables and survival *199*, 207
    radiotherapy, *see* Radiotherapy
  antigenic heterogeneity 13, 45–*46*
  cell motility 4
  cerebellar 169
  cerebral hemisphere 186
  in children 169, 186
  classification 78, 81–82, 198
  computed tomography (CT) 105, *108*, *129*
  cytology 82, *86*, *87*
  gemistocytic *86*
  incidence 137, 138, *166*
  juvenile philocytic 203
  Kernohan grade IV 198
    see also Glioblastoma multiforme
  low-grade,
    CT scans *104*
    epilepsy in 146
    'good-risk' group 200
    grade influence on prognosis *202*, 203
    prognostic factors and survival 200, *201*
    radiotherapy in 199–204
  morphological vs. serological analysis 46
  pathogenesis 58
  PET images *129*
  pilocytic (piloid) 78, *86*
  prognostic factors 169, *199*, 200, *201*, 207
  radiotherapy, *see* Radiotherapy
  spontaneous transplantable murine 64, *65*
Ataxia 167
Ataxia telangiectasia 139
Attachment of glioma cells, in culture 4
Autocrine hypothesis, of glioma pathogenesis 28, 31–32

Bailey and Cushing's classification 40–*41*, 78, 198
Basal ganglia, tumours 145
B-cell growth factor-II (BCGF-II, inter-leukin-5) 255

BCG (Bacille Calmette-Guerin) immunotherapy 245
BCNU 13, 223–224
  in anaplastic astrocytoma, with radiotherapy 204–206
  bone marrow transplantation with 224
  clonogenic assays 15–16
  intra-arterial 230, *231*
    intravenous BCNU vs. 230
    radiotherapy with 232
    toxicity 230, 232
  intravenous 223–224, 230
  megadose 224, 232
  side-effects 194, 224
  supraophthalmic infusions 233
  uptake kinetics 130–131
Bedridden patients, management 287
Biochemical heterogeneity, of gliomas 14
Biological characteristics, heterogeneity 14
Biological response modifier (BRM) 18, 242–282
  classification 242–271, *243*
  examples and effects *244*
  rationale for use 242
  see also Immunotherapy
Biology of brain tumours; *in vitro* 1–25
Biopsy
  brain stem lesions 156–157
  freehand burr hole 112, 149
  mortality 149
  stereotactic, *see* Stereotactic biopsies
1, 3-Bis(2-chloroethyl)-1-nitrosourea, *see* BCNU
BK virus 59
Blindness 181
Blood flow, of cerebral tumours 125–127
Blood vessel tumours 85, 92
Blood-brain barrier
  disruption 130, 233–234
    effect on drug delivery 234
  integrity and tumour regions 112, 233
  passive immunotherapy with monoclonal antibodies 261
  formation 41
  function in tumours 129–130
  loss, imaging 112
  penetration of chemotherapeutic agents 225, 234
B lymphocytes, in glioma tissue 265
Bone metastases 174, *175*
  pain relief 289
Brachytherapy, interstitial 210, 212
Brain adjacent to tumour (BAT), tumour cells in 107, 112, 233
Brain damage, focal 141, 142–143
  management 286
Brain stem tumours
  in children 166, 176–178
  open biopsy 156
  signs and symptoms 145
  stereotactic biopsy 156–157

see also Posterior fossa tumours
Brain tumour syndromes 143-146
Bromodeoxyuridine (BUdR), cell labelling *11-12*

Calcification, imaging 108-111, *110*
Cancer Registry studies 135
Capillaries, abnormal 112
Capillary hyperplasia *87*
Carboplatin (CBDCA) 225
Carcinogenesis, after radiotherapy 173
Carcinogens, chemical 51-58
Case control studies, bias in 139
CCNU, *in vitro* chemosensitivity testing 15
Cell
 culture, *see* Culture, cell
 labelling methods *11-12*
 motility, attachment and spreading 4
 proliferation, differentiation relationship 18
Cell kinetics 9-13
 relevance to treatment 12-13
Cell-lineages
 gliomas 45-47
 neuronal and glial tumour classification *41-42*
 implications of recent studies 44
 in optic nerve 40-42, *43*
 in retina and cortex 42, 44
Cell lines, established 1, 5-9, 31
 in athymic nude mouse 68
 characteristics 5, *6-7, 8*
 chemically-induced transplantable tumours 63-64
 spontaneous transplantable murine astrocytoma 64-*65*
c-*erb* gene, amplification and expression 32-35
Cerebellum, tumours 146
Cerebral arterial oxygen extraction, regional (rOER) *125, 126*
Cerebral atrophy 196-197
Cerebral blood volume, regional (rCBV) *125, 126*
Cerebral cortex, glial and neuronal development 42, 44
Cerebral hemisphere tumours
 in children 184-189
  chemotherapy 187
  resection and radiotherapy 187
 signs and symptoms 143-144, 186-187
Cerebral oxygen utilization, regional (rCMROz) *125, 126*
Cerebrum, primitive neuroectodermal tumours (PNET) 82-83, *188*-189
c-*fos* gene *29*, 30
Chemotherapy
 in adults 222-241
  assessment of response 222-223
  blood-brain barrier disruption 225, 233-234
   limitations of 234
  cerebral hemisphere tumours in children 187
  combination 227, *228-229*, 233
  in ependymoma of fourth ventricle 176

intra-arterial 227, 230-233, *231*
 drug-characteristics 227, 230
 in medulloblastoma in children 174
 pineal region tumours 183-*184*
radiotherapy with,
 in anaplastic astrocytoma 204-206, 232
 late delayed reactions 196, 198
resistance, predicting 15-16
single-agent therapy 223-226
testing,
 in transplantable tumours 61, 62, 68
 in vitro 15-17
uptake kinetics 130-131
see also BCNU
Children, central nervous system tumours 164-192
 aetiology 164
 astrocytomas, radiotherapy in 204
 brain development 166
 cerebral hemisphere 184-189
 CT technique 95
 grading, sites and metastases 165-166
 incidence *165, 166, 167*
 late delayed reactions to radiotherapy 196, 197
 optic glioma *179*, 180-181
 pathological classification 165-166
 pineal region 182-184
 pituitary region 178-182
 posterior fossa, *see* Posterior fossa tumours in children
 spinal cord tumours 189-190
 under one year of age 189
Cholesteryl hemi succinate (CHS) 270
Chromosomal abnormalities
 gliosarcoma cell lines *8*
 malignant gliomas 4-5, 13, 35-36
  cell lines *6-7*, 36
 medulloblastomas cell lines 9, *10*
Chromosome 7 36
Chromosome 10 47
Chromosome 22 36
Cisplatin 225
 intra-arterial 232-233
Cisternography 95-96
Classification of brain tumours 77-92
 astrocytic gliomas 78, 81-82, 198-199
 in children 165-166
 cytogenetic analysis 79
 development 40, *41*, 77-82
 germ-cell tumours *91*
 grade vs. histological-based classification *199*
 Kernohan grading system 79, 198, 199
  in children 165-166
  FDG uptake correlation 127
 meningiomas 84-85, 92
 morphological analysis-based 40, *41*, 44, 78-79, 199
 nerve sheath cell tumours 83-84
 neuroepithelial tissue tumours 77-83

Bailey and Cushing classification 40, *41, 78*, 198
  revised (Russell, Rubinstein) *81*–*82*, 198
  WHO classification 79, *80*
  serological analysis 45–48, 83
  site of origin inclusion 82
  see also WHO classification of tumours
Clinical manifestations 141–147
  brain tumour syndromes 143–146
  delay before presentation 141
  focal neurological deficit 142–143
  frequency *142*
  see also Intracranial pressure, raised
Clonogenic assays 15–16
c-*myc* gene *29*, 30, 35
  amplification 35
Collagenase digestion, cell culture method 2, 3
Colloid cysts 145
Colony-stimulating factor 1 (CSF-1) 28
Comatosed patient, management 287
Computed tomography (CT) 94–96, 148
  in astrocytomas *104, 105, 108, 129*
    anaplastic, volume determination 208
  chemotherapy response, assessment 223
  degree of malignancy and growth rate 114
  dynamic 96
  early delayed reactions to radiotherapy 194
  false-negative 114
  intraoperative 157
  intrathecal contrast 95–96
  intravenous contrast 95, 111–112, 153
  optic nerve glioma *180*–181
  patient movement and sedation 95
  in posterior fossa tumours in children 169
  in postoperative patient 115–116
  scan segmentation 94–95
  stereotactic biopsy, *see* Stereotactic biopsies
  stereotactic technique, interstitial implantation 212
  tissue characterization 103
    calcification 108–109, *110*
    oedema 107, *110*
    solid components 103, *104*–105
    tumour localization 112, *113*
Computer-interactive stereotactic system 157–161
c-*onc* 27
Confusion, management 287
Constipation 286
Corpus callosum tumours 143–144
Corticosteroids, interleukin-2 therapy with 256
Corynebacterium parvum 245
Cranial nerve palsies 143, 145, 176
Craniopharyngioma 145, 178–179
Craniospinal irradiation, *see* Radiotherapy
c-*sis* gene 28, *29*
  expression in glioma cells 31–32
Culture, cell 1–14
  applications 15–19

characteristics of glioma cells 4–5
enzymatic and mechanical digestion 2–4, 14
established cell lines 1, 5–9, 31
explant, methods 3–4
from CT-directed stereotactic biopsies 153
heterogeneity of malignant gliomas 13–14
short-term 2–4, 9
Cyclizine 288
Cytogenetics, of glioma cells *in vitro* 4–5, *6–7*, 13, 35–36

Death, place of 283–284
2-Deoxy-D-glucose 115, 124
Dexamethasone 18
  cerebral blood flow, effect 127, 131
  in management of confusion 287
  raised intracranial pressure management 285
  Rb influx in tumours and 130
Diamorphine 289, 290
Dianhydrogalactitol (DAG) 225
Diaziquone (AZQ) 225
  intra-arterial 233
  for recurrent tumours *226*
Dibromodulcitol (DBD) 225
Dibutyryl cyclic AMP (dbcAMP) 14
Diethylenetriaminepentaacetic acid (DTPA) 100
Differential diagnosis, of cerebral tumours 146
Differentiation, *in vitro* induction 18
Digital subtraction angiography (DSA) 102
  intravenous/intra-arterial routes 102
Diplopia 143, 167
  management 286
DNA content, heterogeneity of gliomas 13
DNA synthesis, stimulation in tumours 47
Double minute chromosomes (DMs) 5, 35–36
Doubling times 12
  established cell lines 5, *6–7, 8, 10*
Dysphagia 286
Dysphasia 144, 286

Embryonal tumours of infancy 82–83
Embryonic chick heart fragment confrontation assay 17
Embryonic development
  optic nerve 41
  retina and cortex 42, 44
Endocrine abnormalities 181
Endothelial cells, in gliomas 47
Environmental factors, in brain tumour aetiology 137, 138–139
Enzymatic digestion, cell cultures 2–3
Ependymoblastoma 78
  murine 62
Ependymoma 78
  cerebral hemisphere, in children 186, 187–188
  fourth ventricle, in children 175–176
  infratentorial 175–176
  papillary *88*

pathogenesis 58
supratentorial 176, 186, 187-188
Epidemiology of cerebral tumours 135-140
  factors affecting interpretations 136
  incidence, prevalence rates 136
Epidermal growth factor (EGF) 28
Epidermal growth factor receptor (EGF-R) 28
  on chromosome 7 36
  gene amplification and expression 32-35
  on glioma cells 33
Epilepsy 141, 143, 144, 146
  in cerebral hemisphere tumours of children 187
  management 286, 290
Epipodophyllotoxins 225
N-Ethyl-N-nitrosourea (ENU)-induced tumours 52, 53-54
  incidence 54
  pathogenesis, theoretical scheme 57
  sites 54
  stages of induction 53-54, 55-56, 57
  transplantable 63
Etoposide (VP-16) 225
Experimental brain tumours, pathology 51-76
  in vivo heterotransplantation 67
    growth rates 68
  latency 51, 58, 59, 60
  oncogenic agents 51-60
    chemical carcinogens 51-58
    implantation sites 51-52
    oncogenic viruses 59
    pathogenesis 54-58
    radiation 59-60
  transplantable 60-69
    advantages/disadvantages 66-67
    chemically-induced 61-64
    heterotransplanted 60
    methods 60-61, 62
    spontaneous 64, 65
    syngeneic 60, 61-67
    virus-induced 64
Explant cultures 3-4, 153
Extracellular matrix material (ECM) 18

F(ab) fragments 260, 261
Family, practical and emotional care 285
Fibronectin 45, 46
  antibodies to 45, 46
  positive cells, in malignant astrocytoma cell lines 5
^{18}F-2-Fluoro-2-deoxy-D-glucose (FDG) 127
5-Fluorouracil (5-FU) 13
Focal neurological deficit 141, 142-143
  management 286
Fourth ventricle tumours 146
  ependymoma 175-176
Frontal lobe tumours 143

Gadolinium (Gd) 100

B-Galactosidase 42, 44
Gangliosides 14
Gelfoam rafts 16
Gene amplification 32-35, 36
  see also Oncogenes
General practitioner (GP), in terminal care 284
Genetic factors, in brain tumour aetiology 138-139
Germ-cell tumours, classification 91, 92
Germinoma, intracranial 183, *184*
Glial cell
  development 40-42, 44
  markers 40-50
  see also Antigen expression; *individual antigens*
Glial fibrillary acidic protein (GFAP) 4, 5, *45*, 47
  antibodies to 45
  in classification of tumours 83
  in established cell lines 5
  gliomas grown in athymic mice 69
  heterogeneity in expression 13
  in vitro modification 18
  normal astrocytes in gliomas 47, 83
Glial fibrils 86
gli gene 36
Glioblastoma 78
  classification 78, 79, 81
  cytology 87
  growth rate 114
Glioblastoma multiforme 26
  classification 78, 79, 198
  incidence 137
  mortality rate 207
  pathogenesis 26
  radiotherapy, *see* Radiotherapy
  survival and prognostic factors 222
  tumour volume 208
  see also Astrocytoma
Glioblasts 56
Glioma, malignant
  advantages of *in vitro* studies 2
  antigenic heterogeneity 13-14
  see also Antigen expression
  arising from subependymal plate, morphology 56-57
  cell characteristics in culture 4-5
  cell culture 1-3
  cell kinetics 9-13
  in children 165
  classification 40, 77-83
  see also Classification of brain tumours
  co-culture with normal brain fragments 17
  CT scans *104*
  cystic, imaging *109*
  established cell lines 5, *6-7*, 31
  experimental, *see* Experimental brain tumours
  FN^+ and $A4^+$ *45-46*
  heterogeneity 13-14
  incidence 137
  invasiveness, measurement 17

in vivo heterotransplantation 67
karyotype analysis 5, *6-7*, 13, 35-36
lineage relationships and cell-types 40, *41*
mixed 82
  cytology *88*
  pathogenesis 58
neoplasia-metaplasia feedback hypothesis 47
oncogenes in 30-36
  c-*erb* amplification and expression 32-35
  c-*myc* and N-*myc* amplification 35
  c-*sis* expression and PDGF-like factors 31-32
  karyotype analysis 35-36
pathogenesis 31-32, 34-35, 36
pathological diagnosis 149
serological analysis 45-48
see also individual gliomas, imaging techniques, therapies
Glioma RG2 63
Gliosarcoma, established cell lines 5, *8*
9L cell line 15, 16
Glucose metabolism, PET studies 127, 131
Glutamine synthetase (GS) expression 2, 13
  in vitro modification 18
Glycolysis
  aerobic 124, 127, 128, 131
  anaerobic 124
Growth factors, oncogenic potential 28, *29*, 58
  in gliomas 31-35
Growth failure, after radiotherapy 173
Growth rate of tumour
  heterogeneity 14
  imaging methods 114
Growth stimulation, autocrine, v-*sis* gene expression 28, 31
GTP-binding proteins (G-proteins) 29

Haemangioblastomas 85, 92
'Haemangiopericytoma of the meninges' 84
Haematoma, cerebral 105, *106*
Haemorrhages, imaging of 105, *106*
Halogenated pyrimidines 211
Haloperidol 287, 288
Headache 141, 142
  management 285
Helium-argon laser 159
Hemiparesis 143, 167, 286
Heterogeneity, malignant gliomas 13-14
Heterotransplanted tumours 60
Hexokinase activity 124, 127
Hexose carriers 124, 130
HNK-1 antibody 83
Home-care, of terminally ill 290-291
Hospice movement 290-291
  day care 291
  in-patient service 290
Hospital support team 291
Hydrocephalus 146, 167
  in brain stem glioma in children 176, *177*

oxygen metabolism and blood flow 126
treatment 169
Hyperdense tumours 103
Hyperosmolar agents, blood-brain barrier disruption 234
Hyperthermia 211
  with immunomodulation 271
Hypothalamus, tumours of 145, 181-182
Hypothyroidism, after radiotherapy 173
Hypovitaminosis C 256

Imaging, *see individual imaging techniques*; Neuro-radiological imaging
Immunoperoxidase histochemistry 83
Immunotherapy
  active 244, 268-271
    examples and effects 244
    methods to improve immunogenicity of cells 270
    reported trials 268-269
  adoptive 243, *244*, 263-268
    examples and effects 244
    LAK cell therapy 263-268
    reported trials *266-267*
    specific 263
    see also LAK cells
  combination and new approaches 271
  passive 244, 258-262
    antiglioma antibodies 258-262
    clinical trials *258*
    examples and effects 244
    polycloncal antisera *258*, 259
    see also Monoclonal antibodies
  restorative (non-specific) 243, *244*, 244-258
    efficacy, results *246*
    interferons, *see* Interferons
    interleukins 254-257
    microbial/synthetic agents 245-247
    rationale 245
    thymosins 257
    tumour necrosis factors 257-258
Incidence of brain tumours 136, 165
  age-related 137, 138, *167*
  in children *165, 167*
Intellectual deterioration 141
  after radiotherapy 173, 197
  management 286
Interferons 247-254
  alpha- (IFNα) 247-248, *248*, 250, 253
    clinical studies 248, 250, *251*, 253
    preclinical studies *248*
  beta- (IFNβ) 248
    clinical trials *251-252*, 253
    preclinical studies *248-249*, 253
    recombinant 253
  classification and characteristics *247*
  combination therapy 254
  gamma (immune IFNT) 248
    clinical trials *252*, 253-254

preclinical studies *250*
radiotherapy with 253–254
tumour necrosis factor receptors 258
Interleukin(s) 254–257
Interleukin-1 (IL-1) 254–255, 256
Interleukin-2 (IL-2) 243, 255
  constant infusion 256
  high-affinity receptor deficiency 245
  LAK cells with 256, 257
    preclinical studies 263–*264*
  side-effects 255–256
  as single agent 255–256
Interleukin-3 (IL-3) 255
Interleukin-4 (IL-4) 255
Interleukin-5 (IL-5) 255
Interleukin-6 (IL-6) 255
Intermediate filaments 44
Interstitial brachytherapy 210–211, 212
Intracranial pressure, raised 141, 142–143
  in cerebral hemisphere tumours of children 186
  in children 167, 168, 186
  management 285
  oxygen metabolism 126, 127
Invasiveness, measurement 17
In vitro biology 1–25
In vitro chemosensitivity testing 15–17
In vivo heterotransplantation of tumours 67–69
In vivo metabolism, *see* Metabolism, *in vivo*

JC Virus 59

Karnofsky Performance scores 207
Karyotype analysis of gliomas 5, *6–7*, 35–36
  heterogeneity 13
Kelly-Goerss computer-interactive arc-quadrant stereotactic instrument 158–*159*
Kernohan grading system, *see* Classification of brain tumours
Ki-67 labelling studies 12

Labelling index (LI) *11*, 12
  survival time correlation 12
LAK cells
  criticisms of therapy 267
  interleukin-2 with 256, 257
    preclinical studies 263–*264*
  localization, and intraturmoural injection 265, 267
  mechanism of action 265
  nature and characteristics 264
  production 265, 268
Latency, experimental tumour development 51, 58, 59, 60
Lateral ventricle tumours 145
Leukaemia, acute lymphoblastic (ALL) 196, 198
Levamisole 245–247, 269, 271
Low-density components of gliomas, imaging 105, 107

Lymphomas, cerebral and spinal 85
Lymphotoxin 257

Magnetic resonance imaging (MRI) 96–101, 148
  after radiotherapy 116
  anaplastic astrocytoma, volume of 208
  brain stem glioma in children 177
  degree of malignancy and growth rate 114
  false-negative CT 114
  intravenous contrast 100–101
  posterior fossa tumours in children 169
  principles 96–99, *98*
  radiation necrosis vs. tumour recurrence 197
  safety factors 101
  scanning protocol sequences 99–100
  sedation for 100
  spinal cord tumours *186*, 189, *190*
  stereotactic biopsies 114, 154–156
  T_1 and T_2 decay curves 97
  tissue characterization 99
    calcification 109–111, *110*
    haemorrhages 105
    low-density 105, 107
    oedema 107
Malignant phenotype expression, *see* Oncogenes; Transformation
Marker antigens, *see* Antigen expression
Medulloblastoma 78, *89*, 165
  in children 165, *170*
    chemotherapy 174
    radiotherapy 170–174, *172*
  CT scans *170*
  desmoplastic 88
  dissemination and spinal seeding 170, *171*, 174, *175*
  established cell lines 9, *10*
  short-term cultures 9, 17
Meduloepithelioma 77–78, 82
Meningioma
  classification 84–85, 92
  haemangioblastic 84
  haemangiopericytic *89*
  incidence 137
  labelling index 12
  lipomatous *89*
  ratio of gliomas to 137
  WHO classification 84, *85*
Metabolism, *in vivo* 122–134
  amino acids 128–129, 131
  blood-brain barrier function 129–130
  cerebral pH 122, 128
  in distant brain tissue, tumour effect 126
  glucose 127, 131
  oxygen 125–127, 131
  PET studies 125–127, 128, 129–131
  surface-coil NMR studies 127–128, 131
Metastases
  bone 174, 175, 289
  cerebral, imaging *110*

CNS tumours in children 166
  medulloblastoma 170, *171*, 174, *175*
  spinal 166, 170, *171*
Metastatic brain disease, incidence 138
Methionine uptake assay 15, 128
Methotrexate (MTX) 234
3-*O*-Methyl-D-glucose (MeG) 124, 130
N-Methyl-*N*-nitrosourea (MNU) 52, 53–54
  pathogenesis of tumours 57–58
Metoclopramide 288
Microtitration assays 15
Mitogen, in neoplasia-metaplasia feedback loop 47
Mitogenesis 28–*29*
Modulator genes 26
Monoclonal antibodies
  14AC1 260
  antigenic heterogeneity of gliomas 13–14, 260
  FR77 260
  Ki-67 12
  passive immunotherapy 244, *258*, 259, 260–262
    human antibodies *258*, 262
    intracarotid vs. intravenous 261–262
    localization 261–262
    murine antibodies *258*, 260–262
    specificities/cross-reactivities 260–261
  radiolabelled, in glioma therapy 259
  in serological analysis of gliomas 13, *45, 46*, 83, 259, 261
Morphine 289, 290
Mortality rates 136
Motility, cell, in culture 4
MST-Continus 289
Mucopolysaccharides, cell-surface 14
Multicellular tumour spheroids (MTS) 16–17
Mumps virus vaccination 245
myc gene family *29*, 30, 35
Myelin synthesis, inhibition 194
Myelosuppression 224

Nasogastric tube feeding 287
Natural killer (NK) cells 264
Nausea 288
Neoplasia-metaplasia feedback hypothesis 47–48
Nerve sheath cell tumours 83–84
neu gene 28, 35, 58
Neuret, definition 195
Neurilemmoma 83
Neuroblastoma, cerebral 188
Neurocutaneous, melanosis 139
Neuroepithelial tissue tumours, classification 77–83
  see also specific tumours
Neuroepithelioma 78
Neurofibroma 83
Neurofibromatosis 139, 164, 180
Neurofilament proteins 9
Neuronal development, in retina and cortex 42, 44

Neurones, antigen expression 45
Neuron-specific enolase 83
Neuroradiological imaging 94–121, 148
  techniques 94–102
  in tumour assessment 102–116, 149
    extent of tumour 114–115
    malignancy and rate of growth 114
    postoperative patient 115–116
    tissue characterization 103–114
    tumour localization 112–114, 149
    tumour size 114
  see also individual imaging techniques: Stereotactic biopsies
Neurotoxicity of chemotherapy
  after blood-brain barrier disruption 234
  of BCNU 230, 232
Neutron irradiation 211
Nitrosamide-induced tumours 52, 53–54
  incidence 54
Nitrosamines 52
Nitrosocompounds 51, 52
  actions 52–*53*
Nitrosoureas 52, 53–54
  chemotherapy with 223–224
    side-effects 224
  see also BCNU
  intra-arterial 230
  syngeneic transplantable tumours 61, 63
N-myc gene amplification 30, 35
Nuclear magnetic resonance (NMR) 123–124
  surface-coil 124, 127–128, 131
    cerebral pH 128
    tumour metabolism 127–128, 131
  see also Magnetic resonance imaging (MRI)
Nude mouse tumour system 67, 68–69
  problems 69

O-2A progenitor cells 41, 42, *43*, 44
  control of division of 44
  in cortex 44
  in optic nerve 41–42, *43*
Occipital lobe tumours 144
Ocular toxicity, of BCNU 230
Oedema, tumour
  blood flow and oxygen utilization 126
  computed tomography (CT) 107, *110*, 115
  magnetic resonance imaging (MRI) 107
Oligoblasts 44
Oligodendrocytes 41–42, 57
Oligodendrocyte-type-2 astrocyte, *see* O-2A progenitor cells
Oligodendroglioma
  antigen expression 46
  cell types in 82
  classification 78, 82
  cytology 87
  epilepsy in 146
  established cell lines 9
  pathogenesis 57–58

Oncogenes 26, *27,* 29
  activation 27-28
  functional aspects *27*-30, 58
  in glioma 30-36
  interplay with antioncogenes *27,* 30, 36
  see also Glioma, malignant; *individual oncogenes*
Oncogenic viruses, see Viruses, oncogenic
Optic chiasm tumours 145, *179,* 180-181
Optic nerve, glial cell development 40-42
Optic nerve glioma *179,* 180-181
  mortality 181
Organ culture systems 16, 17
Oxygen metabolism 122, 124-128
  arterial extraction 125, 126
  historical aspects 124
  PET studies 125-127, 131

Pain relief 288-289
  portable syringe driver 289-290
Papilloedema 142
Parietal lobe tumours 144
Partial brain external-beam irradiation 213
Pathogenesis of cerebral tumours
  earliest stages in experimental tumours *55-56*
  ENU-induced tumours 54-55, *55-57*
  oncogenes in 31-32, 34-35, 36
Pathological diagnosis, of gliomas 149
  see also Stereotactic biopsies
Pathology, see Experimental brain tumours, pathology
PCNU 224
Personality changes 143
pH, cerebral tumours 122, 128
Phenobarbitone 290
Phenotypic modification *in vitro* 18
Phosphocreatine: ATP ratio 127-128, 131
Picibanil (OK-432) 245
Picket fence localization method 151, *153*
Pinealoblastoma 183, 188
Pineal region tumours 145, 182-184
  chemotherapy 183-*184*
  in children 182-184
  germ cell and non-germ cell 182
  radiotherapy 182-183
'Pineoblastoma' 78
Pineocytoma 78
Pituitary region tumours, in children 166, 178-182
Platelet-derived growth factor (PDGF) 41
  B-subunit gene 28
  -like factors, in glioma cells 28, 31-32
  receptors in glioma cell lines 31, 32
Polyclonal antibodies
  passive immunotherapy *258,* 259
  serological analysis of gliomas *45,* 46
Polycyclic aromatic hydrocarbons 51, 52
  syngeneic transplantable tumours 61
Polyoma viruses 59

Positron emission tomography (PET) 115, 116, 122-123
  astrocytoma *129*
  blood-brain barrier function *129*-130
  cerebral pH 128
  glucose metabolism 127, 131
  oxygen metabolism and haemodynamics 125-127, 131
  radiation necrosis vs. tumour recurrence 116, 127, 129
  Rb extraction *129,* 130
  tracers 122, *123*
Posterior fossa tumours in children *166,* 167-178
  astrocytoma 169
  brain stem glioma 176-178
  clinical presentation 167-168
  ependymoma of fourth ventricle 175-176
  incidence *166, 167*
  investigations 168-169
  medulloblastoma 165, *170*
  surgical management 169-178
Postoperative patients, imaging methods 115-116
Presenting symptoms 141
Prevalence rates 136
Primitive neuroectodermal tumours (PNET) 82-83, *188*-189
Procarbazine (PCB) 15, 224
Prognosis, grade vs. histological-based classification 199
Prognostic factors 79
  age 200, 207
  glucose utilization 127
  grading (Kernohan) 79
  tumour contrast enhancement 115
  see also *individual tumours*
Prostaglandin E (PGE$_2$) 255
Protein synthesis rate (PSR), cerebral 129
Proto-oncogenes *27, 29,* 30-31
Pseudo-palisade 87
Pulmonary fibrosis 224

Radiation, experimental brain tumour induction 59-60
Radiation necrosis 115, 116, 195-198
  intra-arterial BCNU 232
  surgical resection 196
  time – dose relationship 195-196
  tumour recurrence vs. 197
  tumour recurrence vs. PET analysis 116, 127, 129
Radiofrequency heating 101
Radiography, skull 103
Radiosensitizers 211, 223
Radiotherapy
  acute reactions 193, 194
  anaplastic astrocytoma 204-210
    BCNU with 204-206
    doses 205

late delayed reactions 209
   optimal dose 209-210
   survival improvement by new approaches 212, 213
   tissue volume for irradiation 208-209
   whole brian vs. generous volume 208-209
astrocytomas 169, 193-221
   new approaches 210-213
brain stem glioma in children 177-178
cerebellar astrocytoma in children 169
cerebral hemisphere tumours in children 187
craniopharyngioma 178
early delayed reactions 193, 194-195
fractionation schemes/hyperfractionation 211-212
gamma interferon with 253-254
glioblastoma multiforme 204-210
   optimal dose 210
   volume to be irradiated 208-209
hyperfractionation plus acceleration 212
imaging after 115-116
intra-arterial BCNU with 232
late delayed reactions 193, 195-198, 209
   chemotherapy effect 196, 198
   intellectual function decrease 197
   see also Radiation necrosis
low-grade astrocytomas 199-204
   in children 204
   doses 204
medulloblastoma, in children 170-174, *172*
optic nerve glioma 181
partial brain external-beam with interstitial implant 213
pineal region tumours 182-183
resistance of hypoxic cells, reduction of 211
temporal lobe function after 127
tolerance of brain 193-198, 211
whole craniospinal axis,
   in children 170-*172*
   complications 173-174
   ependymoma of fourth ventricle 175
   pineal region tumours 183
ras genes *29*-30
Recurrence, tumour 115
   combination chemotherapy *229*
   diaziquone (AZQ) for *226*
   radiation necrosis vs. 116, 127, 129, 197
Respiration, depression in tumours 125, 127, 128, 131
Restorative immunotherapy, *see* Immunotherapy
Reticulin fibres *66*, 84
Retina, glial and neuronal development 42, 44
Retinoblastoma 30
Retroviral labelling, cell lineage studies 42, 44
Retroviruses 27, 59
   β-galactosidase expression 42, 44
   concogenes 27-28, *29*, 31
Rous sarcoma virus, Schmidt-Ruppin strain 59, 64

Rubidium (Rb) extraction *129*, 130
S100 protein 83
Sarcoma, monstrocellular 92
Schmidt-Ruppin strain of Rous sarcoma virus (SR-RSV) 59, 64
Schwannoma 83
Scout image 112, *113*
Sedation, patient
   for computed tomography 95
   for magnetic resonance imaging (MRI) 100
Seizure, management 286
Simian sarcoma virus (SSV) 28, 31
sis gene 28, *29*, 31
Size of tumour, imaging methods 114
Skin care, in comatosed and bedridden patients 287
Spinal cord tumours *186*, 189-190
   imaging *186*, 189, *190*
Spinal metastases 166
   radiotherapy 171, *172*
Spin echo (SE) sequence 97
Spongioblastoma, *see* Glioblastoma multiforme
Spontaneous animal brain tumours 64
Status epilepticus 146, 290
Stem cells 41, 42, *43*, 57
Stereotactic biopsies 149-156
   brain stem lesions 156-157
   computed-tomography (CT) 112-114, 149-153
      BRW system 149-151, *150*, 152, 156
      burr holes 152-153
      localizing frame *151*
      picket-fence localization 151, *153*
   magnetic resonance imaging (MRI) 114, 154-156
      advantages and role 154, 156
      procedure 154-156
Stereotactic techniques
   interstitial implantation of radioactive source 212
   tumour localization 112, *113*, 157
Stereotactic tumour excision, computer-interactive 157-161
   data acquisition stage 157
   digitalization of tumour edge 157, *158*
   operative procedure 158-161
   surgical planning 157-158
Steroid treatment, imaging *111*, 112
Subependymal giant cell tumours 82
Subependymal plate 55, 56, 58
Supratentorial intracerebral tumours 112, 176, 186, 187-188
Surface-coil NMR, *see* Nuclear magnetic resonance (NMR)
Surgery, advances in 148-163
   computer-interactive stereotactic excision 157-161
   objectives of treatment 148

see also Stereotactic biopsies
Survival data 138
  after computer-interactive stereotactic excision 161
  duration, as treatment response endpoint 223
  ependymoma of fourth ventricle 176
  quality of 223
  time, labelling index correlation 12
  see also individual tumours, therapies
Syngeneic transplantable tumours 60, 61–67
Syringe driver, portable 289–290

T cell growth factor (interleukin-2) 243, 255
T-cell replacing factor (TRF) 255
Temporal lobe tumours 144
Teniposide (VM-26) 225
Teratoma, intracranial 183
Terminal care 283–291
  clinical problems 285–288
  hospice movement 290–291
  support structures 284–285, 291
  symptom control 288–290, 291
Thalamus, tumours 145
Thermoimmunotherapy 271
Third ventricle region tumours 145
Thymidine, tritiated, cell labelling 11
Thymosins 257
T lymphocytes
  cytotoxic to glioma cells 263
  in glioma tissue 265, 267
  helper, deficiency 245
  helper:cytotoxic/suppressor ratio 265, 267
Todd's palsy 146
Transformation 27, 28, 58
  mitogenesis relationship 28–29, 31–32
  see also Oncogenes; Tumorigenesis
Transforming growth factor alpha (TGF-α) 28, 34
Transplantable tumours 60–69
Trypsin 3
Tuberose sclerosis 138, 186

Tumorigenesis 27–30
  gliomas 31–32, 34–35, 36
  oncogenes in 27–30
Tumour infiltrating lymphocytes (TIL) 265, 267
Tumour markers
  pineal region tumours 182
  see also Antigen expression
Tumour necrosis factor (TNF) 254, 258
  -alpha (TNFα) 257
  -beta (TNFβ) 257
Tumour suppressor genes, *see* Antioncogenes

U343MG-A glioma cell line 18

Vascular malformations 92
Vasoconstriction, dexamethasone-induced 127
Vasogenic oedema 107, *110*, 115
v-*erb* and v-*fms* 28, *29*
Vimentin 66
Vincristine (VCR) 13, 15
Viruses, oncogenic 27–28, 31, 59
  experimental tumours 59
  transplantable tumours 64
  see also Retroviruses
Visual failure 142
Visual impairment, optic nerve glioma 180
VM astocytoma model *61*, 64–*65*
Vomiting 142, 288
Von Hippel-Lindau disease 139, 164
von Recklinghausen's syndrome 139, 164, 180
v-*sis* gene 28, 31

WHO classification of tumours
  meningiomas 84, *85*
  of nerve sheath cells 83–*84*
  of nervous system, categories *90*
  of neuroepithelial tissue 79, *80*
Wilms' tumour 30

Xanthoastrocytoma, pleomorphic 82
X-ray, brain tumour incidence and 139